DIAGNOSIS
AND
TREATMENT
OF
ERECTILE
DISTURBANCES

A Guide for Clinicians

DIAGNOSIS AND TREATMENT OF ERECTILE DISTURBANCES

A Guide for Clinicians

Edited by

R. Taylor Segraves

Tulane University
New Orleans, Louisiana

(Formerly University of Chicago
Chicago, Illinois)

and

Harry W. Schoenberg

University of Chicago
Chicago, Illinois

PLENUM MEDICAL BOOK COMPANY
New York and London

Library of Congress Cataloging in Publication Data

Main entry under title:

Diagnosis and treatment of erectile disturbances.

Includes bibliographies and index.
1. Impotence—Treatment. 2. Impotence—Psychological aspects. I. Segraves, R. Taylor,
1941–   . II. Schoenberg, Harry W. III. Title: Erectile disturbances. [DNLM: 1. Impotence
—diagnosis. 2. Impotence—therapy. WJ 709 D536]
RC889.D53   1985   616.6′92   85-3714
ISBN-13: 978-1-4615-9411-6   e-ISBN-13: 978-1-4615-9409-3
DOI: 10.1007/978-1-4615-9409-3

© 1985 Plenum Publishing Corporation
Softcover reprint of the hardcover 1st edition 1985
233 Spring Street, New York, N.Y. 10013

Plenum Medical Book Company is an imprint of Plenum Publishing Corporation

Contributors

Robert J. Alonso, M.D., *Chief Resident in Neurology, Hahnemann University School of Medicine, Philadelphia, Pennsylvania 19102*

David M. Barrett, M.D., *Consultant, Department of Urology, Mayo Clinic and Mayo Foundation, and Associate Professor in Urology, The Mayo Medical School, Rochester, Minnesota 55905*

C. Sue Carter, M.D., *Professor of Psychology and Ecology, Ethology and Evolution, University of Illinois, Champaign, Illinois 61820*

John M. Davis, M.D., *Illinois State Psychiatric Institute, and Professor of Psychiatry, University of Illinois, Chicago, Illinois 60612*

William L. Furlow, M.D., *Consultant, Department of Urology, Mayo Clinic and Mayo Foundation, and Professor of Urology, The Mayo Medical School, Rochester, Minnesota 55905*

Bruce L. Gewertz, M.D., *Associate Professor of Surgery, University of Chicago, Chicago, Illinois 60637*

Larry Goldman, M.D., *Assistant Professor of Psychiatry, University of Illinois, Chicago, Illinois 60680*

Thomas M. Jones, M.D., *Associate Professor of Medicine, University of Chicago, Chicago, Illinois 60637*

Stephen B. Levine, M.D., *Associate Professor of Psychiatry, Case Western Reserve University School of Medicine, Cleveland, Ohio 44106*

Robert Madsen, M.D., *Associate, Department of Surgery, University of Iowa, Iowa City, Iowa 52240*

Elliott L. Mancall, M.D., *Professor and Chairman of Neurology, Hahnemann University School of Medicine, Philadelphia, Pennsylvania 19102*

Wendy B. Marlowe, Ph.D., *Consultant in Neuropsychology to the Department of Neurology, Hahnemann University School of Medicine, Philadelphia, Pennsylvania 19102*

Harry W. Schoenberg, M.D., *Professor of Surgery (Urology), University of Chicago, Chicago, Illinois 60637*

Kathleen A. B. Segraves, Ph.D., *Assistant Professor in Psychiatry, Tulane University Medical Center, New Orleans, Louisiana 70112*

R. Taylor Segraves, M.D., Ph.D., *Professor in Psychiatry, Tulane University Medical Center, New Orleans, Louisiana 70112*

Christopher K. Zarins, M.D., *Professor of Surgery, University of Chicago, Chicago, Illinois 60637*

Preface

This book is the result of an informal association between the editors which extends back to 1974. At the beginning, it was a tenuous alliance between physicians in quite different medical subspecialties—urology and psychiatry. As the alliance was forged, subspecialty rivalries and mistrust were replaced by a common clinical interest in the diagnosis and treatment of erectile problems. We quickly became aware of the high prevalence of such disorders, how poorly prepared we were to make accurate and responsible diagnosis and treatment plans, and how complicated an etiological diagnosis could prove to be. A variety of biological and psychological influences bear on sexual function, and in many clinical contexts, diagnosis and treatment planning involves consideration of complex interactive variables. The need for an expanded multidisciplinary team became obvious. The requisite knowledge base extended across too many subspecialty boundaries, and the necessary information was not available in a convenient source. As we began accumulating the information base, we became aware that this information might be of value to other physicians. The authors enjoy the luxury of an academic setting in which special expertise can be readily assembled. Such resources are often unavailable to the physician in practice. Thus, it is our hope that this text can serve as a multispecialty team for the physician in solo practice.

R. TAYLOR SEGRAVES

New Orleans, Louisiana

HARRY W. SCHOENBERG

Chicago, Illinois

Acknowledgments

The editors would like to express their appreciation to Donald King, Dean of the Pritzker School of Medicine, and James Hamlin, Dean of the Tulane University School of Medicine, for providing academic climates in which interdisciplinary efforts of this sort are encouraged and fostered. The editors would also like to acknowledge their appreciation to Eberhard Uhlenhuth, Professor and Acting Chairman of the Department of Psychiatry at the Pritzker School of Medicine; Joseph Green, Chairman of the Department of Psychiatry and Neurology at Tulane University School of Medicine; and David Skinner, Chairman of the Department of Surgery at the Pritzker School of Medicine, for their encouragement and patience during the preparation of this text.

Last but not least, we would like to express our appreciation to Ms. Runae Hartfield and Ms. Amelia Spenser for their laborious and patient persistence during the preparation of this manuscript.

Contents

1. Diagnosis and Treatment of Erectile Problems: Current Status..   1
   R. Taylor Segraves and Harry W. Schoenberg

2. Erectile Dysfunction Associated with Pharmacological Agents..   23
   R. Taylor Segraves, Robert Madsen, C. Sue Carter, and John M. Davis

3. Sexual Dysfunction in Neurological Disease......................   65
   Elliott L. Mancall, Robert J. Alonso, and Wendy B. Marlowe

4. The Psychological Evaluation and Therapy of Psychogenic
   Impotence   87
   Stephen B. Levine

5. Vasculogenic Impotence...   105
   Bruce L. Gewertz and Christopher K. Zarins

6. Hormonal Considerations in the Evaluation and Treatment of
   Erectile Dysfunction..   115
   Thomas M. Jones

7. Other Causes of Erectile Impotence   159
   Harry W. Schoenberg

8. Evaluation of the Etiology of Erectile Failure...................   165
   R. Taylor Segraves, Harry W. Schoenberg, and Kathleen A. B. Segraves

9. Psychiatric Evaluation of Penile Prosthesis Candidates   197
   Larry Goldman and R. Taylor Segraves

10. Penile Prosthesis Implantation 219
   David M. Barrett and William L. Furlow

11. Erectile Impotence: Training and Research Needs 241
   R. Taylor Segraves, Harry W. Schoenberg, and Kathleen A. B. Segraves

Index 247

DIAGNOSIS AND TREATMENT OF ERECTILE DISTURBANCES

A Guide for Clinicians

1

Diagnosis and Treatment
of Erectile Problems

Current Status

R. TAYLOR SEGRAVES and HARRY W. SCHOENBERG

In the last decade, there have been tremendous gains in knowledge concerning the diagnosis and treatment of male erectile dysfunction. Many problems previously felt to be beyond help have responded to current therapeutic approaches. Unfortunately, this new information is not readily available to most clinicians, and most professionals treating erectile problems are poorly prepared to evaluate these complaints. Nonmedical professionals are understandably ill prepared to evaluate and appreciate biological influences on sexual behavior. Many physicians are minimally trained in the evaluation and treatment of patients with complaints of impotence. It is comparatively recently that medical schools have included instruction in the evaluation and treatment of sexual problems.[1] With the recent advances in knowledge concerning human sexuality, it is nearly impossible for any subspecialist's knowledge and clinical experience to encompass all the relevant information concerning the diagnosis and treatment of erectile problems. An additional problem is that the necessary knowledge base cuts across traditional medical subspeciality boundaries. For example, a thorough evaluation of a complaint of impotence might require nocturnal

R. TAYLOR SEGRAVES • Department of Psychiatry, Tulane University Medical Center, New Orleans, Louisiana 70112.   HARRY W. SCHOENBERG • Department of Surgery, Section of Urology, University of Chicago, Chicago, Illinois 60637.

penile tumescence testing in a neurophysiology laboratory, penile blood flow studies in a vascular laboratory, full evaluation of endocrine status, a careful review of the patient's medical and pharmacological history, a thorough physical examination, as well as a specialized psychiatric interview focusing on sexual behavior and marital interaction. Within each of these medical subspecialty areas, technical subtleties and controversial procedures and techniques abound. For example, standard accepted criteria for the use of nocturnal tumescence testing to differentiate organic from psychogenic impotence are lacking, and considerable controversy exists over whether the absence of nocturnal penile tumescence is definitive of an organic etiology.[2-4] Although exogenous testosterone is frequently used in the management of erectile problems,[5] it is still unclear whether testosterone levels have any direct influence on erectile function.[6] Many physicians use psychological testing to help identify candidates for penile prosthesis surgery,[7] although current evidence indicates that such information may be useless in differentiating psychogenic from organogenic impotence.[8] A further complication in the evaluation of erectile problems is that many subspecialists are relatively inexperienced in the area of human sexuality. Referral of an impotent patient to a psychiatrist unskilled in the area of human sexuality might well prove to be a waste of time. Similarly, an endocrinologist with an interest in male infertility will provide a different perspective on male impotence than a general internist.

It is clear that complaints of erectile problems are encountered in most medical practices as well as in the practices of clinical psychologists and psychiatric social workers.[9] It is also clear that, because of shame and anxiety, many patients do not volunteer information regarding their sexual lives.[10] If the physician does not specifically question his patients regarding their sexual activities, he probably will grossly underestimate the prevalence of impotence in his clinical practice. This assertion of the authors is partially corroborated by a recent study of 1180 outpatients at the Minneapolis Veterans Administration Medical Center.[11] In this sample of men with an average age of 59 years, 401 (approximately one third) were found to be impotent. These problems are often highly difficult to evaluate because of the diversity of ways in which the disorder may present as well as the diversity of psychological and physical disorders which may account for the symptom.[12]

Erectile function is the end product of complicated, interactive biological and psychological influences. Thus, erectile failure can have its etiology in a myriad of biological and psychological systems. Many impotent patients have multisystem disease,[13] and thus one has to entertain the possibility of a variety of organic as well as psychogenic etiologies. The relative contribution of each component may be difficult to evaluate, yet essential to treatment planning. Diagnosis of organogenic impotence is often only the beginning of a diagnostic evaluation. Identification of the precise etiology might result in a range of possible interventions including judicious modification of pharmacological agents, vascular reconstructive surgery, penile prosthesis implantation, administration of exogenous testosterone, bromocriptine therapy, or surgical adenomectomy.

An increasing proportion of the United States population is elderly. Many elderly men continue to have active sexual interest and active sexual lives.[14] With the change in sexual mores and the increasing attention in the press to human sexuality, one can expect increasing numbers of elderly men requesting help for sexual concerns. Many of these men will present with complicated medical histories, making precise diagnosis of the etiological factor more complicated.

Most patients with problems of erectile impotence present to the physician with considerable embarrassment and urgency for a solution. For many men, loss of erectile potency means much more than the simple loss of the ability to perform sexually. It also symbolizes the loss of manhood.[15] Understandably, these men are often desparate for a solution. The recent reports in the popular press concerning organic causes for impotence may exert considerable pressure on the physician to find the etiological factor. Although a variety of conditions are known to be associated with impotence, it is often difficult to determine the disease process responsible for the complaint in the individual patient. A hasty and erroneous clinical decision regarding etiology can be a disservice to the patient. It is obviously a disservice to refer a man who is impotent secondary to an autonomic neuropathy for psychotherapy. The complaint will not be reversed, and the patient may develop a sense of demoralization and hopelessness as he searches unproductively for the illusive psychological cause of his problem. Similarly, one would not wish to refer a patient for penile prosthesis surgery if simpler procedures, such as change of medication or couple psychotherapy, might reverse the problem.

The scope of the problem in differential diagnosis and treatment planning becomes obvious when one begins to catalog the diseases and conditions known to affect potency. A variety of surgical procedures, medical conditions, commonly prescribed drugs, psychological syndromes, and situations are known to adversely influence potency. Potency disturbances are frequently encountered in most medical practices.

PREVALENCE OF ERECTILE DIFFICULTIES

Although various authors have commented on the frequency of occurrence of sexual disorders in the general population, very little empirical evidence is available to estimate the prevalence of erectile problems. Kinsey and his colleagues[16] were among the first to address this question. Using cross-sectional survey data, they reported that the frequency of marital coitus declines and the frequency of impotence increases with advancing age. Their data are difficult to evaluate for several reasons. First, it is unclear whether this decline represents a decrement in biological capacity in males or boredom with repetition of sex with the same partner.[17] More important, Kinsey's samples were not random samples; thus, his estimate cannot be used to estimate population parameters.[18]

Frank and her co-workers[19] recently reported the results of a questionnaire study of 100 couples in Pittsburgh. Their population had an average age of 36.2 years, was predominately white and middle class, and was not randomly selected. Couples at various gatherings who felt that "their marriages were working" were asked to complete a 15-page self-report questionnaire. Although 36% of the men reported difficulty with rapid ejaculation, only 7% complained of difficulty obtaining an erection and 9% reported difficulty maintaining an erection. The use of a self-report questionnaire and the absence of a random sample limit the generalizations one can make from this study. A properly constructed study by Nettelbladt and Uddenberg[20] reported similar findings. A representative sample of 58 married Swedish men were studied by means of a semi-structured interview. Premature ejaculation was reported by 36% of the sample whereas only 7% reported impotence. The average age of the men was 31 years. It is also of interest that sexual problems occurred more frequently in men reporting poor contact with their fathers and a domineering mother. Eysenck[18] administered a sexual questionnaire to 423 male and 379 female university students in Great Britain. This 158-item questionnaire inquired about the frequency of impotence, among other things. Of those students reporting sexual intercourse, 120 (42%) answered yes to the question whether they had suffered from impotence one or more times. College students reporting erectile problems also had higher scores on the neuroticism scales. Various other surveys[21-23] have reported on the frequency of sexual problems in various specialized clinics.

One would expect surveys of older patients to indicate a higher incidence of erectile dysfunction. With increased age, there is, of course, an increased liklihood of chronic disease and concomitant pharmacological intervention.[24] In the absence of physical disease, sexual activity persists into old age.[25] For example, Pfeiffer[26,27] at the Duke University Center for the Study of Aging and Human Development has reported that approximately 80% of men aged 68 years are still regularly sexually active. By age 78, only 25% remain sexually active.

In medical subpopulations, the prevalence of erectile dysfunction clearly exceeds that of the general population. Impotence appears to occur most frequently in patients with diabetes mellitus, multiple sclerosis, hypertensive arterial disease, or renal failure. It has long been recognized by the medical profession that impotence frequently accompanies diabetes mellitus.[28,29] Recent surveys by various investigators suggest that the prevalence of impotence approaches 50% in diabetic males.[30-34] In a recent survey, Kolodny and associates[35] closely interviewed 175 male diabetic outpatients. Eighty-five (49%) were found to be impotent. The average age of the sample was 53.2 years. The incidence of impotence was not correlated with the duration of diabetes, the mode of treatment, or the incidence of retinopathy, nephropathy, or hypertension. The incidence of peripheral neuropathy was significantly higher in impotent diabetics than in nonimpotent diabetics. It is also of note that impotence was the first symptom of diabetes in 14 men and preceded the diagnosis of diabetes. Rubin and Babott[30] also reported that impotence in diabetics is unassociated with either the severity or the duration of the disease. The frequency of impotence does, however, increase with the age of the patient. Whereas only 25% of diabetic males between the ages of 30 and 34 were impotent, 74% of men between the ages of 60 and 64 were impotent. Although diabetics can suffer from psychogenic impotence[35] and some have recovered potency after psychiatric counseling,[36-38] current evidence suggests that organic factors explain the predominance of sexual problems in diabetic men.[39,40] Various etiologies have been hypothesized for the frequent association of diabetes with erectile dysfunction. Both vascular[4] and endocrine[33,42] etiologies have been proposed. Current evidence suggests that a peripheral autonomic neuropathy is the most common etiological factor.[43-47]

Chronic renal failure has also been documented to be associated with a high frequency of erectile problems. The disease state is associated with a variety of metabolic and endocrine abnormalities. Infertility, gynecomastia, azoospermia, and testicular atrophy have been reported in end-stage renal disease.[48] Various degrees of impaired libido and erectile dysfunction have been reported, and a variety of mechanisms, including retention of unidentified uremic toxins,[49] excess circulating parathyroid horomone,[50] abnormalities in zinc metabolism,[51] abnormalities in the pituitary testicular hormonal axis,[52-54] uremic neuropathy,[55] and psychosocial factors,[56-60] have been proposed as causative. A number of case reports and surveys of patients in various degrees of renal failure have been reported. In general, it appears that impotence occurs frequently in renal failure, both before and during dialysis, and may remit in some men after renal transplant surgery. These studies have used varying methodologies, including interviews and self-administered questionnaires.

Various studies have indicated that approximately 50–100% of male patients experience sexual difficulties after the onset of renal insufficiency but before renal dialysis is began.[61-63] These studies predominantly relied on the retrospective memory of patients currently on dialysis. Surveys of patients on renal dialysis have reported that from 28 to 88% of patients complain of impotence.[62,64-70] It is unclear whether patients with end-stage renal disease have an improvement in sexual function after dialysis has begun.[71] Studies of patients with renal failure who receive renal transplants suggest that sexual function usually improves[72,73] although some patients remain sexually impaired.[69,70,74,75] Karacan and co-workers[71] reported an investigation of nocturnal tumescence recordings in a small sample of men with end-stage renal disease. Nocturnal tumescence was definitely suppressed in men with end-stage renal disease, before and after renal dialysis, suggesting an organic component to the erectile problem. Nocturnal penile tumescence improved after renal transplantation, suggesting that the improvement in sexual function after transplant surgery is due to organic rather than psychogenic factors.

Sexual symptoms are common early symptoms of multiple sclerosis, and capacity for erection is frequently diminished.[76,77] The degree of erectile impairment appears to be a function of the duration of the disease process. Ivers and Goldstein[78] reported that impotence occurred in 26% of male patients with multiple sclerosis at the Mayo Clinic. It is of note that impotence was the presenting symptom in 3% of the cases. Vas[79] reported on the incidence of impotence in a series of 37 patients with multiple sclerosis. Forty-three percent of his series of male patients complained of partial or total impotence. The degree of erectile incapacity appeared related to the duration of the disease process. His totally impotent men had suffered from multiple sclerosis for 12 years, whereas his partically impotent patients had been diagnosed as having multiple sclerosis for 9 years. His potent group had suffered from multiple sclerosis for only 5 years. Vas emphasized that sexual symptoms can remit and relapse similar to the other symptoms of multiple sclerosis. He also emphasized that the frequency of impotence might be expected to be much higher in a series of chronically impaired patients. This may explain the higher incidence of erectile failure (80%) reported by Lilius and co-workers.[76]

Sexual problems occur frequently in patients with cardiovascular disease, and especially in the post-myocardial-infarction group. Statistics indicate that there are approximately 650,000 survivors of myocardial infarction annually.[80] Various studies[81-83] have demonstrated a decrease in coital frequency after myocardial infarction. The mechanism for this is unknown, although psychosexual factors and especially the fear of a "coital coronary" have been implicated.[84-94] The claim that postcoronary sexual problems are psychologically based has to be viewed with a degree of skepticism as few authors considered the possibility of impotence as a drug side effect in these patients. In a fascinating report, Wabrek and Burchell[95] interviewed 131 male patients admitted to the hospital with a diagnosis of acute myocardial infarction. Each patient was interviewed closely regarding his sexual function prior to the myocardial infarction. Surprisingly, 57 (44%) of the patients reported impotence prior to the myocardial infarction. The report by Wabrek and Burchell, if replicated would suggest that erectile problems are common in men with cardiovascular disease even before the first myocardial infarction and that stress associated with myocardial infarction may not be the explanation for postcoronary impotence. Similarly, few authors considered the possibility that vascular disease might be present in the pelvis as well as the coronary arteries. As well as suffering a general decline in frequency of sexual activities, some patients develop impotence after myocardial infarction. Some authors report that after myocardial infarction 60% of patients experience erectile difficulties in at least 50% of coital attempts. Tuttle and colleagues[94] interviewed men attending a cardiac evaluation unit about their sexual activity and reported that 10% of the patients had become permanently impotent after myocardial infarction. It is also of note that two thirds of the men reported that they had received no advice regarding the prevalence of sexual problems in men after myocardial infarction.

Erectile problems are also quite common in men with arterial hypertensive disease. The incidence of impotence has ranged from 33% to 55% depending on the pharmacological agent used.[96,97]

OTHER MEDICAL CONDITIONS ASSOCIATED WITH ERECTION PROBLEMS

A large number of other diseases have been reported to be associated with erectile problems. In most cases, there is insufficient evidence to indicate the frequency with which such cases appear in medical populations or even the frequency with which men suffering from the condition also suffer from impotence. These conditions will be briefly reviewed to remind the clinician of the magnitude of the problem of differential diagnosis.

Leriche in 1923[98] described a syndrome involving ischemia to the lower extremities and erectile impotence due to occlusion of the abdominal aortic bifurcation. It is now well known that men with occlusive aortoiliac disease have some impairment of erectile function.[99] The degree of impairment appears related to the degree of occlusion.[100] Although most men with vasculogenic impotence will have other signs of peripheral vascular disease, impotence may be the first sign of vascular disease in men who are otherwise asymptomatic.[101] Another vascular disorder producing erectile impotence is the so-called "pelvic steal syndrome."[102] This occurs in patients with unilateral occlusion of the external iliac artery and contralateral stenosis of the internal iliac artery. The ipsilateral internal iliac artery may thus act as the main supply to the lower extremity. During active coital thrusting, blood may be shunted from the pelvic region to the lower extremity, producing a loss of erection. Several authors have reported that venous abnormalities may contribute to the failure to maintain an erect state,[103,104] but this claim remains controversial.[99]

A variety of syndromes other than diabetes may be associated with autonomic neuropathies and thus are capable of producing erectile problems. These include hepatic neuropathies, thyroid disease, alcoholic neuropathy, inflammatory neuropathies (e.g., Guillain-Barré syndrome), carcinomatous neuropathy,[105] peripheral nerve trauma, tabes dorsalis, and nutritional neuropathies.[106] Impotence in alcoholics may also be dependent on hormonal factors.[107] Spinal-cord-injured patients are widely recognized to have erectile difficulties.[108–110] The degree and type of remaining erectile function appear dependent on the level of the cord lesion.[111]

Impotence associated with brain lesions has been minimally studied to date. A small number of male patients develop impotence after cerebral vascular accidents.[112–114] The small number of cases and lack of precise information concerning the site of the lesion make these reports difficult to evaluate. However, considerable evidence suggests that temporal lobe lesions are frequently associated with decreased libido and erectile problems.[115–118]

As is well known, impotence has been frequently reported to be associated with abnormalities in the pituitary–gonadal axis.[119,120] More recently, pituitary microadenomas have been discovered to present with impotence as the primary symptom.[121,122] Anecdotal evidence suggests that abnormalities in thyroid[123] function may be associated with impotence.

Impotence and diminished libido have been reported in men with adrenoleukodystrophy. Adrenoleukodystrophy is a rare, fatal sex-linked disease which primarily affects the central nervous system and adrenal cortex. This syndrome would be suspected if the clinician noted any signs of ataxia, spasticity, visual defects, or hyperpigmentation. Impotence has also been reported to be the initial symptom in progressive systemic sclerosis. The erectile diminution occurs in the presence of normal libido and is not associated with abnormal urological or neurological findings.

A list of disease processes reported to be associated with erectile disturbances is contained in Table 1. Any number of chronic debilitating diseases interfere with sexual function although they may not impair the

Table 1. Diseases Associated with Erectile Problems

Diabetes mellitus	Spinal cord injury or compression
Renal failure	Temporal lobe lesions
Multiple sclerosis	Myocardial infarction
Aortoiliac disease	Hypertensive arterial disease
Hepatic failure	Pituitary adenomas
Thyroid disease	Hypogonadism
Alcoholic neuropathy	Adrenoleukodystrophy
Inflammatory neuropathy	Progressive systemic sclerosis
Peripheral nerve trauma (pelvic	Priapism
fracture)	Peyronie's disease
Tabes dorsalis	Adrenal disease (Cushing's, Addison's)
Nutritional neuropathies	Adrenocortical tumor

erectile mechanism per se. For example, sexual activity is generally decreased in men with chronic heart failure and emphysema. Similarly, urological problems such as Peynonie's disease and priapism may interfere with erectile function.

SURGICAL PROCEDURES ASSOCIATED WITH ERECTILE DISTURBANCE

The clinician's attempt to make a differential diagnosis as to the etiology of an erectile complaint is complicated by the number of medical conditions associated with erectile problems. A variety of surgical procedures have also been reported to result in erectile problems. These include cystectomy,[123] proctectomy,[124,125] abdominal–perineal colon resection,[126] aortoiliac vascular reconstruction, abdominal aneurysmectomy,[127] radical perineal or retropubic prostatectomy,[123] retroperitoneal lymphadenectomy,[123] and sympathectomy.[128] Pelvic radiation has also been reported to be associated with erectile impairment.[129] This information is summarized in Table 2.

Table 2. Surgical Procedures Associated with Impotence

Cystectomy	Radical perineal prostatectomy
Proctectomy	Radical retropubic prostatectomy
Abdominoperineal colon resection	Retroperitoneal lymphadenectomy
Aortoiliac vascular reconstruction	Sympathectomy
Abdominal aneurysmectomy	Pelvic radiation

DRUGS AND ERECTILE DISTURBANCE

The effects of commonly prescribed drugs on human sexuality have been extensively reviewed elsewhere.[96,130–135] Impotence has been reported to be a side effect of many of the commonly prescribed psychotropic medications and hypotensive agents. Among psychotropic agents, antipsychotic drugs, tricyclic antidepressants, monoamine oxidase inhibitors, and lithium carbonate have been associated with erectile problems. Hypotensive agents such as methyldopa, guanethidine, clonidine, reserpine, spironolactone, ganglionic blocking agents[96] and diuretics[11] have been reported to cause impotence. Other drugs associated with impotence include

Table 3. Drugs and Impotence

Psychotropic agents	
Fluphenazine (Prolixin)	
Thioridazine (Mellaril)	
Lithium carbonate (Eskalith)	
Imipramine (Tofranil)	
Protriptyline (Vivactil)	
Tranylcypromine (Perofran)	
Desmethylimipramine (Pertofran)	
Mebanazine (Actomol)	
Clomipramine (Anafranil)	
Phenelizine (Nardil)	
Amitriptyline (Elavil)	
Chlorpromazine (Thorazine)	
Thiothixene (Navane)	
Haloperidol (Haldol)	
Hypotensive agents	
Methyldopa (Aldomet)	Hexamethonium chloride (Methium Cl)
Guanethidine (Esmelin)	Mecamylamine HCl (Inversine)
Clonidine (Catapres)	Trimethaphan camsylate (Artonad)
Reserpine (Serpasil)	
Spironolactone (Aldactone)	
Diuretics (eg., Diuril)	
Chlorthalidone (Hygroten)	
Prazosin (Minipres)	
Other drugs	
Clofibrate (Atromid-S)	Trihexyphenidyl (Artane)
Methantheline (Banthine)	Benztropine (Cogentin)
Cimetidine (Tagamet)	Propantheline bromide (Pro-Banehise)
Propranolol (Inderal)	Disulfiran
Heroin	Digoxin (Lanoxin)
Methadone (Dolophine)	Cancer chemotherapy agents
Baclofen (Lioresal)	
Ethionamide (Trecator)	
Perhexilene (Pexid)	

clofibrate,[136] methantheline,[137] cimetidine,[138-140] and propranolol.[141,142] Heroin and methadone usage are also frequency associated with erectile difficulties.[96] Drugs causing erectile problems are listed in Table 3. It is also of note that phenothiazines such as thioridazine, mesoridazine, and chlorpromazine have been reported to cause priapism.[143] Repeated bouts of priapism can, of course, lead to permanent impotence.[144,145]

PSYCHIATRIC CONDITIONS AND ERECTILE PROBLEMS

A variety of psychiatric conditions and psychosocial problems can result in erectile impotence. Many times, the differential diagnosis of the etiology of psychogenic impotence will prove even more frustrating than the search for the etiology of organic impotence. Segraves and co-workers[8] discussed psychogenic etiologies in a series of 51 impotent men:

> ...cases of chronic psychogenic impotence constitute an extremely heterogenous group. Within this sample, the appearance of psychologic erectile dysfunction appeared related to a myriad of causes ranging from individual psychopathology to chronic marital dysfunction in otherwise healthy individuals. In other cases, the onset of impotence appeared clearly related to a significant psychosocial stress such as widowhood, becoming divorced, or the death of a child or parent [p. 236].

Maurice and Guze[146] assessed 20 consecutive admissions at a sex therapy clinic and found evidence of concurrent psychiatric disorder in only a minority of the patients. Of course, the small sample size in this study seriously limits any generalizations. Sexual and erectile problems have been reported in patients with schizophrenia[147,148] and affective disorders.[149] Meyer and collaborators[150] and O'Connor and Stern[151] reported a high overall presence of neurotic and character pathology in patients with sexual problems. The frequent presence of relationship problems in cases of erectile problems has also been noted.[152, 153]

In the typical case of psychogenic impotence, the clinician usually looks for origins in the patients' interpersonal world. Thus one suspects such things as unexpressed anger with a spouse or guilt over a transgression. In divorced men, erectile problems may be a reflection of ambivalence about reinvolvement with the opposite sex. In widowers, erectile problems may reflect guilt about fogetting the deceased or even evoke a delayed grief reaction. The sexual intimacy of a new partner evokes similar memories of the deceased. In cases of impotence of long duration, it may be impossible to pinpoint an etiology. In these cases, one may simply observe a vicious cycle of fear of erectile failure contributing to continual erectile failure.[154] Psychiatric factors associated with impotence are listed in Table 4.

Table 4. Psychiatric Conditions and Erectile Problems

Schizophrenia	Unexpressed anger
Bipolar disorder, depressed	Guilt
Major depression	Ambivalence regarding attachment
Character pathology	Delayed grief reactions
Marital discord	Situational anxiety

RELATIVE PREVALENCE OF PSYCHOGENIC AND ORGANOGENIC IMPOTENCE

For many years, it was assumed that the majority of cases of impotence were psychogenically based.[155–160] In the past few years, it has become recognized by many clinicians that cases of organic impotence are more common that previously recognized.[161–163] Psychiatrists as a group tend to emphasize the frequency of psychogenic impotence, whereas nonpsychiatric physicians tend to stress the frequency of organogenic impotence. For example, Spark and colleagues[164] recently reported that 35% of a series of 105 impotent men were found to have abnormalities in the hypothalamic–pituitary axis. This report was also disturbing in that many of these men had previously been in psychotherapy on the assumption that the problem was psychogenic. Slag and co-workers[11] recently reported a survey of sexual function in 1180 men in the medical outpatient clinic at the Minneapolis Veterans Administration Medical Center. Only 14% of these men were considered to have psychogenic impotence. The most common causes of impotence in this population were medication effects, 25%; neurological problems, 7%; urological problems, 6%; primary hypogonadism, 10%; secondary hypogonadism, 9%; diabetes mellitus, 9%; hypothyroidism, 5%; hyperthyoidism, 1%; and hyperprolactinemia, 4%. The average age of this sample was 59.4 years.

One clearly needs to exercise caution in generalizing about population characteristics of impotent men from clinical series. Clearly, the etiologies of impotence will vary among the medical subspeciality clinics as a certain degree of patient self-selection can be expected to occur. The prevalence of organogenic impotence would, of course, be expected to be much lower in younger patient populations. Segraves and co-workers[165] have reported one of the few studies of differences in patient characteristics of impotent men as a function of the specialist originally consulted. All patients were assessed by the same multidisciplinary team, and criteria for diagnosis of organogenic or psychogenic impotent were clearly specified. In the urology clinic, 31% of impotent men were found to have organic etiologies. In the psychiatry clinic, only 5% were found to have organic etiologies. This difference was highly significant statistically. The authors concluded:

> It is of note that the relative frequencies of organic etiologies in the two series roughly parallel reports from other investigations; psychiatric series have usually reported a much lower incidence of organic causes of impotence than clinical series reported by nonpsychiatric physicians. The results of this investigation suggest that such differences may be the result more of sampling different populations than the result of subspecialty bias in diagnosis [p. 232].

RECENT ADVANCES IN THE DIAGNOSIS AND TREATMENT OF ERECTILE PROBLEMS

During the last decade, there has been a renewed interest in understanding the basic physiology of the human sexual response. Contemporary investigators are questioning widely held assumptions about neural mediation[166-172] and vascular mechanisms[173-176] of the erectile response. With this increase in knowledge, a variety of new diagnostic procedures have become available permitting a much more sophisticated evaluation of erectile complaints. At this point, most medical centers utilize some form of nocturnal penile testing[3] to aid in the differential diagnosis of erectile problems. Doppler studies of penile blood flow and direct tests of pudendal nerve conduction are becoming more widely available.[177] At the same time, endocrinological evaluation of erectile complaints has become more sophisticated,[178] and the psychiatric evaluation of these men has evolved toward a more exact science.[179] This rapid advance in knowledge mandates a multidisciplinary approach to treatment planning in many cases, for few clinicians' expertise includes all the necessary information.

Treatment approaches have also undergone tremendous change. The possibility of correction of vasculogenic impotence by vascular surgery exists;[180] technical problems with the inflatable implantable prosthesis have decreased to the point where this is a highly successful treatment for many men with organogenic impotence.[181,182] There has been an explosion of literature concerning the treatment of psychogenic impotence, and a variety of techniques exist including systematic desensitization,[183] biofeedback training, hyponotherapy,[184] focal dynamic psychotherapy, [185] conjoint behavioral sex therapy,[186] combined behavior and psychodynamic therapy,[187] and group psychotherapy.[188] Slowly, a knowledge base is building regarding which patients will benefit from different types of psychiatric approaches,[152,165,189] how long treatment gains will be sustained,[190] and which men will be likely to experience a spontaneous remission without formal treatment.[191]

OVERVIEW

Clearly, knowledge of the recent advances in the diagnosis and treatment of erectile complaints is of importance to most physicians and allied health professionals. The purpose of this text is to assemble a multidisciplinary team of experts in differing subspecialty areas. Each expert will describe the state of the art and science in his respective area concerning diagnosis and treatment of erectile problems. Thus, chapters will be devoted to the diagnosis and treatment of neurogenic, vasculogenic, pharmacologically induced, endocrinological, and psychogenic impotence. Additional chapters will be devoted to the differential diagnosis of impotence, penile prosthesis surgery, and the screening of candidates for such surgery. To the authors' knowledge, this information has never before been brought together in one text. It is our hope that this information will be of help to practicing clinicians and their patients.

REFERENCES

1. Rosenzwig N, Pearsall FP: Introduction, in Rosenzweig N, Pearsall FP (eds): *Sex Education for the Health Professional: A Curriculum Guide.* New York, Grune and Stratton, 1978
2. Wasserman MD, Pollak CP, Speilman AJ, et al: The differential diagnosis of impotence. *JAMA* 243:2038–2042, 1980
3. Wasserman MD, Pollak CP, Speilman AJ, et al: Theoretical and technical problems in the measurement of nocturnal penile tumescence for the differential diagnosis of impotence. *Psychosom Med* 42:575–585, 1980
4. Allen RP: Erectile impotence: Objective diagnosis from sleep related erections (nocturnal penile tumescence). *J Urol* 126:353, 1981
5. Shrom SH, Lief HI, Wein AJ: Clinical profile of experience with 130 consecutive cases of impotent men. *Urology* 13:511–515, 1979
6. Bancroft J, Wu FCW: Changes in erectile responsiveness during androgen replacement therapy. *Arch Sex Behav* 12:59–66, 1983
7. Melman A, Redfield J: Evaluation of the DSFI as a test of organic impotence. *Sexual Disabil* 4: 108–114, 1981
8. Segraves RT, Schoenberg HW, Zarins CK, et al: Discrimination of organic verses psychological impotence with the DSFI: A failure to replicate. *J Sex Marital Ther* 7: 230–238, 1981
9. Burnap DW, Golden JS: Sexual problems in medical practice. *J Med Educ* 42:673–680, 1967
10. Lief HI: Why sex education for health practitioners? in Green R (ed): *Human Sexuality: A Health Practitioner's Text.* Baltimore, Williams and Wilkins, 1979

11. Slag MF, Morlem JE, Elson MK, et al: Impotence in medical clinic outpatients. 249:1736–1740, 1983
12. Norell JS: Psychosexual problems seen in general practice, in Crown S (ed): *Psychosexual Problems: Psychotherapy, Counseling and Behavioral Modification.* New York, Academic Press, 1976
13. Schumaker S, Lloyd CW: Physiological and psychological factors in impotence. *J Sex Res* 17:40–53, 1981
14. Pfeiffer E: Sexuality and the aging patient, in Green R (ed): *Human Sexuality: A health practitioner's Text.* Baltimore, Williams and Wilkins, 1979
15. Segraves RT, Schoenberg HW, Zarins CK: Psychosexual adjustment after penile prosthesis surgery. *Sexual Disabil,* 5:222–229, 1982
16. Kinsey AC, Pomeroy WB, Martin CE: *Sexual behavior in the human male.* Philadelphia, WB Saunders, 1948
17. Udry JR: Changes in the frequency of marital intercourse from panel data. *Arch Sex Behav* 9:319–325, 1980
18. Eysenck HJ: *Sex and Personality.* Austin, University of Texas Press, 1976
19. Frank E, Anderson C, Rubinstein D: Frequency of sexual dysfunction in normal couples. *N Engl J Med* 299:111–115, 1978
20. Nettelbladt P, Uddenberg N: Sexual dysfunction and sexual satisfaction in 58 married Swedish men. *J Psychosom Res* 23:141–147, 1979
21. Catalan J, Bradley M, Gallwey J, et al: Sexual dysfunction and psychiatric morbidity in patients attending a clinic for sexually transmitted diseases. *Br J Psychiatry* 138:292–296, 1981
22. Swan M, Wilson LJ: Sexual and marital problems in a psychiatric outpatient population. *Br J Psychiatry* 135:310–314, 1979
23. Kawano T: Sexual problems seen in medical practice at a psychosomatic clinic. *Shinshin-Igaku* 20:7–14, 1980
24. Wise TN: Sexuality in the aging and incapacitated. *Psychiatr Clin North Am* 3:173–188, 1980
25. Masters WH, Johnson VE: Sex after sixty-five. *Reflections* 12:31–43, 1977
26. Pfeiffer E, Verwoerdt A, Wang HS: The natural history of sexual behavior in a biologically advantaged group of aged individuals. *J Gerontolo* 24:193–197, 1969
27. Pfeiffer E: Sexuality in the aging individual. *J Am Geriatr Soc* 12:481–484, 1974
28. Rollo J: *An Account of Two Cases of Diabetes Mellitus: With Remarks as They Arose During the Progress of the Cure.* London, C Dilly, 1979
29. Naunyn B: *Der Diabetes Mellitus.* Vienna, Alfred S Holder, 1906
30. Rubin A, Babott D: Impotence and diabetes mellitus. *JAMA* 168:498–500, 1958
31. Ellenberg M: Impotence in diabetes: The neurologic factor. *Ann Intern Med* 75:213–219, 1971
32. Montenero P, Donatone E: Diabete et activite' sexuelle chez l'homme. *Diabete* 8:327–332, 1982
33. Schoffling K, Federlin K, Ditschuneit H, et al: Disorder of sexual function in male diabetes. *Diabetes* 12:519–527, 1963
34. Rundles RW: Diabetic neuropathy. *Medicine* 24:111–116, 1945
35. Kolodny RC, Kahn CB, Goldstein H, et al: Sexual dysfunction in diabetic men. *Diabetes* 23:306–309, 1974
36. Renshaw DC: Sexual function and diabetes. *Psychosomatics* 20:54–60, 1979
37. Renshaw DC: Diabetic impotence: A need for further evaluation. *Med Aspects Hum Sexuality* 12:19–25, 1978

38. Schiavi RC: Psychological treatment of erectile disorders in diabetic patients. *Ann Intern Med* 92:337–339, 1980
39. Melman A: The diagnosis and therapy of impotence associated with diabetes. *Sexual Disabil* 1:52–56, 1978
40. Karacan I, Salis PJ, Ware JC, et al: Nocturnal penile tumescence and diagnosis in diabetic impotence. *Am J Psychiatry* 135:191–197, 1978
41. Abelson D: Diagnostic value of the penile pulse and blood pressure: A Doppler study of impotence in diabetics. *J Urol* 113:636–639, 1975
42. Wright AD, Holden G, Williams JW, et al: Luteinizing release hormone tests in impotent diabetic males. *Diabetes* 25, 975–977, 1976
43. de Groat WC, Booth AM: Physiology of male sexual function. *Ann Intern Med* 92:329–331, 1980
44. Masteri AR: Neuropathology of diabetic neurogenic bladder. *Ann Intern Med* 92:316–318, 1980
45. Waxman SG: Pathophysiology of nerve conduction: Relation to diabetic neuropathy. *Ann Intern Med* 92:297–301, 1980
46. Duchen LW, Anjorin A, Watkins PJ, et al: Pathology of autonomic neuropathy in diabetes mellitus. *Ann Intern Med* 92:301–308, 1980
47. Bradley WE: Autonomic neuropathy and the genitourinary system. *J Urol* 119:299–302, 1978
48. Soffer 0: Sexual dysfunction in chronic renal failure. *Southern Med J* 73:1599–1600, 1980
49. Levy NB: Symposium on sexual problems of chronic renal failure patients. *Dialysis and Transplant* 7:870–871, 1978
50. Massry SG, Procci WR, Kletzky OA: Impotence in patients with uremia. *Dialysis Transplant* 7:916–923, 1978
51. Antoniou LD: Zinc in the treatment of impotence in chronic renal failure. *Dialysis Transplant* 7:912–915, 1978
52. Horton R, Chopp R: Testicular function in uremia. *Dialysis Transplant* 7:909–910, 1978
53. Holdsworth S, Atkins RC, de Kretser DM: The pituitary-testicular axis in men with chronic renal failure. *N Engl J Med* 296:1245–1249, 1977
54. Lim VS, Avletta F, Kathpalia S: Gonadal dysfunction in chronic renal failure. *Dialysis Transplant* 7:896–906, 1978
55. Golden JS, Milne JF: Somatopsychic sexual problems of renal failure. *Dialysis Transplant* 9:879–889, 1979
56. Finkelstein FO: Sexual dysfunction and chronic renal failure. *Dialysis Transplant* 9:921–923, 1979
57. Berkman AH: Sexuality counseling with hemodialysis patients. *Dialysis Transplant* 7:924–942, 1978
58. McKevitt PM: Role of the nephrology social worker in treating sexual dysfunction. *Dialysis Transplant* 7:928–937, 1978
59. Finkelstein FO, Finkelstein SH, Steele TE: Assessment of marital relationship of hemodialysis patients. *Am J Med Sci* 271:21–28, 1976
60. De Nour, AK: Hemodialysis: Sexual functioning. *Psychosomatics* 19:229–235, 1978
61. Rager K, Bundschu H, Gupta D: The effect of HCG on testicular androgen production in adult men with chronic renal failure. *J Reprod Fertil* 42:113–120, 1975
62. Levy NB, Sexual adjustment to maintenance hemodialysis and renal transplantation. National survey by questionnaire. Preliminary report. *Trans Am Soc Artifi Intern Organs* 19:138–143, 1973
63. Chen JC, Vidt DG, Zorn EM: Pituitary–Leydig cell function in uremic males. *J Clin Endocrinol Metab* 31:14–17, 1970

64. Schmitt GW, Shehadeh L, Sawin CT: Transient gynecomastia in chronic renal failure during chronic intermittent hemodialysis. *Ann Intern Med* 69:73–79, 1968
65. Sherman FP: Impotence in patients with chronic renal failure on dialysis. *Fertil Steril* 26:221–223, 1975
66. Hagen C, Olgaard K, McNelly AS: Prolactin and the pituitary–gonadal axis in male uremic patients on regular dialysis. *Acta Endocrinol* 82:29–38, 1976
67. O'Brien KM, Rawl J, Binkley L: Sexual dysfunction in uremia. *Proc Clin Dial Transplant Forum* 5:98–101, 1975
68. Bommer J, Ritz E, Tschope W: Life on hemodialysis. *Lancet* 2:511, 1975
69. Pradke AG, MacKinnon KJ, Dosse Tor JB: Male fertility in uremia. Restoration by renal allographs. *Can Med Assoc J* 102:607–608, 1970
70. Salvatierra 0, Fortmann JL, Belzer FO: Sexual function in males before and after renal transplantation. *Urology* 5:64—66, 1975
71. Karacan I, Dervent A, Cunningham G, et al: Assessment of nocturnal penile tumescence as an objective method for evaluating sexual functioning in ESRD patients. *Dialysis Transplant* 7:872–876, 1978
72. Abram HS, Hester LR, Epstein GM: Sexual activity and renal failure, *Proceedings of the Fifth International Congress of Nephrology*. in Villareal H (ed): Basel, Skargen, 1974.
73. Abram HS, Hester LR, Sheridan WF: Sexual functioning in patients with chronic renal failure. *J Nerv Ment Dis* 160:220–226, 1975
74. Proccl WR, Hoffman KI, Chatterjee SN: Persistent sexual dysfunction following renal transplantation. *Dialysis Transplant* 7:891–894, 1978
75. Proccl WR, Hoffman KI, Chatterjee SN: Sexual functioning of renal transplant recipient. *J Nerv Ment Dis* 166:402–407, 1978
76. Lilius H, Valtonen E, Wilkstrom J: Sexual problems in patients suffering from multiple sclerosis. *J Chron Dis* 29:643–647, 1976
77. Smith BH: Multiple sclerosis and sexual dysfunction. *Med Aspects Hum Sexuality* 34:34–35, 1976
78. Ivers R, Goldstein N: Multiple sclerosis: A current appraisal of signs and symptoms. *Proc Mayo Clin* 38:457–466, 1963
79. Vas C: Sexual impotence and some autonomic disturbances in men with multiple sclerosis. *Acta Neurol Scand* 45:166–182, 1969
80. Sanders JD, Sprenkle DH: Sexual therapy for the post coronary patient. *J Sex Marital Ther* 6:174–186, 1980
81. Masur FT: Resumption of sexual activity following myocardial infarction. *Sexual Disabil* 2:98–114, 1979
82. Rahe RH, Ward HW, Hayes V: Brief group therapy in myocardinal infarction rehabilitation: Three to four-year follow-up of a controlled trial. *Psychosom Med* 41:229–242, 1979
83. Hellerstein HK, Friedman EH: Sexual activity and the post-coronary patient. *Arch Intern Med* 125:987–998, 1970
84. Kushnir B, Fox KM, Tomlinson IW, et al: Primary ventricular fibrillation and resumption of work, sexual activity, and driving after the first acute myocardinal infarction. *Br Med J* 4:609–611, 1975
85. Stern MJ, Pascale L: Psychosocial adaptation post-myocardial infarction: The spouse's dilemma. *J Psychosom Res* 23:83–87, 1979
86. Cole CM: A treatment strategy for postmyocardial sexual dysfunction. *Sexual Disabil* 2:122–129, 1979
87. Cole CM, Levin EM, Whitley JO, et al: Brief sexual counseling during cardiac rehabilitation. *Heart Lung* 8:124–129, 1979

88. Waxberg JD: Sexual counseling techniques for coronary bypass patients. *Behav Med* 6:30–33, 1979
89. Mayou R: The course and determinants of reactions to myocardinal infarction. *Br J Psychiatry* 134:588–594, 1979
90. Weinstein SA, Como J: The relationship between knowledge and anxiety about postcoronary sexual activity among wives of postcoronary males. *J Sex Res* 16:316–324, 1980
91. Krop H, Hall D, Mehta J: Sexual concerns about myocardinal infarction. *Sexual Disabil* 2:91–97, 1979
92. Mehta J, Krop HD: The effect of myocardial infarction on sexual functioning. *Sexual Disabil* 2:115–120, 1979
93. McClaine M, Krop H, Mehta J: Psychosexual adjustment and counseling after myocardial infarction. *Ann Intern Med* 92:514–519, 1980
94. Tuttle WB, Cook WL, Fitch E: Sexual behavior in postmyocardial infarction patients, *Am J Cardiol* 13:140, 1964
95. Wabrek AJ, Burchell RC: Male sexual dysfunction associated with coronary artery disease. *Arch Sex Behav* 9:69–75, 1980
96. Segraves RT: Pharmacological agents causing sexual dysfunction. *J Sex Marital Ther* 3:157–176, 1977
97. Bulpitt CJ, Dollery CT: Side effects of hypotensive agents evaluated by a self-administered questionnaire. *Br Med J* 3:485–490, 1973
98. Leriche R, Morel A: The syndrome of thrombotic obliteration of the aortic bifurcation. *Ann Surg* 127:193, 1948
99. Kedia KR: Vascular disorders and male erectile dysfunction. *Urol Clin North Am* 8:153–168, 1981
100. May AG, De Weese JA, Rob CE: Changes in sexual function following operation on the abdominal aorta. *Surgery* 65:41–45, 1969
101. Scheer A: Impotence as a symptom of arterial vascular disorder in the pelvic region. *Munich Med Wochenschur* 102:1713–1715, 1960
102. Michal V, Krammar R, Pospichal J: External iliac steal syndrome. *J Cardiovasc Surg* 19:355–357, 1978
103. Fitzpatrick TJ: Venography of the deep dorsal venous and valvular system. *J Urol* 111:518–520, 1974
104. Fitzpatrick T: The corpus cavernosum intercommunicating venous drainage system. *J Urol* 113:494–496, 1975
105. Brady WE: Autonomic neuropathy and the genitourinary system. *J Urol* 119:299–302, 1978
106. McDowell FH: Sexual manifestations of neurologic disease. *Med Aspects Hum Sexuality* 20:13–21, 1968
107. Wagner G, Jensen SB: Alcohol and erectile failure, in Wagner G, Green R., (eds): *Impotence: Physiological, Psychological, Surgical Diagnosis and Treatment.* New York, Plenum Press, 1981
108. Bors E, Comarr AE: Neurological disturbances of sexual function with special references to 529 patients with spinal cord injury. *Urol Rev* 10:191–222, 1960
109. Bord E, Turner RD: Neurologic urology, in Kaufman JJ (ed): *Advances in Diagnostic Urology.* Boston, Little, Brown, 1964
110. Munro D, Horne HW, Paull DP: The effect of injury to the spinal cord and cauda equina on the sexual potency of men. *N Engl J Med* 239:903–911, 1948
111. Chapelle PA, Durand J, Lacert P: Penile erection following complete cord injury in man. *Br J Urol* 52:216–219, 1980

112. Allsup-Jackson, G: Sexual dysfunction in stroke patients. *Sexual Disabil* 4:161–168, 1981
113. Bray GP, De Frank RS, Wolfe TL: Sexual functioning in stroke survivors. *Arch Phys Med Rehabil* 62:286–288, 1981
114. Kalliomarki JL, Markkanen TK, Mustonen VA: Sexual behavior after cerebral vascular accident. *Fertil Steril* 12:156–158, 1961
115. Saunders M, Rawson M: Sexuality in male epileptics. *J Neuro Log Sci* 10:577–583, 1970
116. Niedermeyer E, Walker AE, Blumer D: EEG and behavioral findings in temporal lobe epileptics (before and after temporal lobectomy). *Electroenceph Clin Neurophys* 23:493, 1967
117. Hierons R, Saunders M: Impotence in patients with temporal-lobe lesions. *Lancet* 1:761–763, 1966
118. Blumer D, Walker EA: Sexual behavior in temporal lobe epilepsy. *Arch Neurol* 16:38–43, 1967
119. Rose RM: The psychological effects of androgens and estrogens—a review, in Shader RI (ed): *Psychiatric Complications of Medical Drugs.* New York, Raven Press, 1972
120. Weideman CL, Northcutt RC: Endocrine aspects of impotence. *Urol Clin North Am* 8:143–151, 1981
121. Franks S, Jacobs HS, Martin N, et al: Hyperprolactinaemia and impotence. *Clin Endocrinol* 8:277–287, 1978
122. Carter JN, Tyson JE, Tolis G, et al: Prolactin-secreting tumors and hypogonadism in 22 men. *N Engl J Med* 299:847–852, 1978
123. Gonick P: Urologic problems and sexual dysfunction, in Oaks WW, Melchiode GA, Ficher I (eds): *Sex and the Life Cycle.* New York, Grune & Stratton, 1976
124. Goligher JC: Sexual function after excision of rectum. *Proc Roy Soc Med* 44:824–825, 1951
125. Corman ML, Veidenheimer MC, Coller JA: Impotence after protectomy for inflammatory disease of the bowel. *Dis Colon Rectum* 21:418–419, 1978
126. Yeager ES, Van Heerden JA: Sexual dysfunction following proctocolectomy and abdominoperineal resection. *Ann Surg* 188:169–170, 1980
127. May A, DeWeese J, Rob C: Changes in sexual function following operation or the abdominal aorta. *Surgery* 65:41–47, 1969
128. Whitelaw GP, Smithwick RH: Some secondary effects of sympathectomy. *N Engl J Med* 245:121–130, 1951
129. Ray GR: Potency after radiation therapy of prostatic carcinoma. *Med Aspects Hum Sexuality* 9:132–137, 1975
130. Munjack DJ: Sex and drugs. *Clin Toxicol* 15:75–89, 1979
131. Carver JR, Oaks WW: Sex and hypertension, in Oaks WW, Melchiode GA, Ficher I (eds): *Sex and the Life Cycle.* New York, Grune & Stratton, 1976
132. Hollister LE: Drugs and sexual behavior in man. *Life Sci* 17:661–668, 1977
133. Bancroft JHT: Evaluation of the effects of drugs on sexual behavior. *Br J Clin Pharmacol* (suppl):83–90, 1960
134. Stony NL: Sexual dysfunction resulting from drug side effects. *J Sex Res* 10:132–149, 1974
135. Carter CS, Davis JM: Effects of drugs on sexual arousal and performance, in Meyer J (ed): *Clinical Management of Sexual Disorders.* Baltimore, Williams & Wilkins Co, 1976
136. Schneider J, Kaffarnik H: Impotence in patients treated with clofibrate. *Atherosclerosis* 12:455–457, 1975
137. Schwartz NH, Robinson BD: Impotence due to methantheline bromide. *NY State J Med* 52:1530, 1952
138. Peden NR, Cargill JM, Browning MCK, et al: Male sexual dysfunction during treatment with cimetidine. *Br Med J* 10:659, 1979

139. Adaikan PG, Karim SMM: Male sexual dysfunction during treatment with cimetidine. *Br Med J* 1:1282–1283, 1979

140. Wolfe MM: Impotence of cimetidine treatment. *N Engl J Med* 300:94, 1979

141. Bathen J: Propranolol erectile dysfunction relieved. *Ann Intern Med* 88:716–717, 1978

142. Miller RA: Propranolol and Impotence. *Ann Intern Med* 85:682–683, 1976

143. Gottlieb JI, Lustberg T: Phenothiazine-induced priapism: A case report. *Am J Psychiatry* 134:1445–1446, 1977

144. Dorman BW, Schmidt JD: Association of priapism in phenothiazine therapy. *J Urol* 116:51–53, 1976

145. Bastecky J, Gregova L: Priapism as a possible complication of the chlorpromazine treatment. *Activ Nerv Suppl* (suppl. 16):175, 1974

146. Maurice WL, Guze SB: Sexual dysfunction and associated psychiatric disorders. *Compr Psychiatry* 11:539–543, 1970

147. Akhtar S, Thompson JA: Schozphrenia and sexuality: A review and a report of twelve unusual cases—Part I. *J Clin Psychiatry* 41:134–142, 1980

148. Akhtar S, Thompson JA: Schizophrenia and sexuality: A review and a report of twelve unusual cases—Part II. *J Clin Psychiatry* 41:166–174, 1980

149. Tamburello A, Seppecher MF: The effects of depression on sexual behavior: Preliminary results of research, in Geine R, Wheeler CC (eds): *Progress in Sexology.* New York, Plenum Press, 1977

150. Meyer JK, Schmidt CW, Lucas MJ, et al: Short-term treatment of sexual diabetes. Interim report. *Am J Psychiatry* 132:172–176, 1975

151. O'Connor JF, Stern LO: Developmental factors in functional sexual disorders. *NY State J Med* 42:1838–1842, 1972

152. Ansari J: Impotence prognosis (a controlled study). *Br J Psychiatry* 128:194–198, 1976

153. Lobitz CW, Lobitz GK: Clinical assessment in the treatment of sexual dysfunctions, in LoPiccolo J, LoPiccolo L (eds): *Handbook of Sex Therapy,* New York, Plenum Press, 1978

154. Segraves RT; Treatment of sexual dysfunction. *Compr Ther* 4:38–43, 1978

155. Tyler EA: Sexual-incapacity therapy, in Freedman DX, Dyrud JE (eds): *American Handbook of Psychiatry, Vol V, Treatment.* New York, Basic Books, 1975

156. Kaplan HS: *The New Sex Therapy.* New York, Brunner/Mazel, 1974

157. Strauss EB: Impotence from a psychiatric standpoint. *Br Med J* 1:697–699, 1950

158. Thorn GW: Disturbances of sexual function, in Thorn GW, Adams RD, Braundald E (eds): *Harrison's Principles of Internal Medicine,* 8th ed. New York, McGraw-Hill, 1977

159. Wershub LP: *Sexual Impotence in the Male.* Springfield, Illinois, Charles C Thomas, 1959

160. Burger H, Rose N: Sexual impotence. *Med J Aust* 2:24–26, 1979

161. Ellenberg M: Sexual function diabetic patients. *Ann Intern Med* 92:331–333, 1980

162. Montague DK, James RE, DeWolfe VG: Diagnostic evaluation, classification and treatment of men with sexual dysfunction. *Urology* 14:545–548, 1979

163. Legrass JJ, Mormont C, Servais J: A psychoneuroendocrinological study of erectile psychogenic impotence: A comparison between normal patients and patients with abnormal reactions to glucose tolerance test, in Carenza L, Pancheri P, Zichella L (eds): *Clinical Psychoneuroendocrinology in Reproduction.* New York, Academic Press, 1978

164. Spark RF, White RA, & Connolly PB: Impotence is not always psychogenic. *J Amer Med Assoc* 243:750–755, 1980

165. Segraves RT, Schoenberg HW, Zarins CK, et al: Characteristics of erectile dysfunction as a function of medical care system entry point. *Psychosom Med* 43:227–234, 1981

166. Domer FR, Wessler G, Brown RL, et al: Involvement of the sympathetic nervous system in the urinary bladder internal sphincter and in penile erection in the anesthetized cat. *Invest Urol* 15:404–407, 1978

167. Penttila 0: Acetycholine, biogenic amines and enzymes involved in their metabolism in penile erectile tissue. *Ann Medicinal Exp Biol Fenniae* 44 (suppl 9):7–42, 1966
168. Dail WG, Evan AP: Experimental evidence indicating that the penis of the rat is innervated by short adrenergic neurons. *Am J Anat* 141:203–217, 1974
169. Gilmore DP, McGrath JC: Effects of castration on the mechanical response to motor nerve stinulation of the rat vas deferens. *Br J Pharmacol* 61:473–474, 1977
170. Krane RJ, Siroky MB: Neurophysiology of erection. *Urol Clin North Am* 8:91–102, 1981
171. McConnell J, Benson GS, Wood J: Autonomic innervation of the mammalian penis: A histochemical and physiological study. *J Neural Transmission* 45:227–238, 1979
172. Holmquist B, Olin T: Angiography of the internal pudental artery at electrical stimulation of the pelvis nerves and at injection of posterior pituitary hormones. *Scand J Urol Nephrol* 3:291–296, 1969
173. Dorr LD, Brody MJ: Hemodynamic mechanisms of erection in the canine penis. *Am J Physiol* 213:1526–1531, 1967
174. Newman HF, Northup JD, Devlin J: Mechanism of human penile erection. *Invest Urol* 1:350–353, 1963
175. Benson GS, McConnell J, Lipschultz HI, et al: Neuromorphology and Neuropharmacology of the human penis. *J Clin Invest* 65:506–513, 1980
176. Benson GS, McConnell J, Schmidt WA: Penile polsters: Functional structures or atherosclerotic changes? *J Urol* 125:800–803, 1981
177. Vliet LW, Meyre JK: Erectile dysfunction: Progress in evaluation and treatment. *Johns Hopkins Med J* 151:246–258, 1983
178. Cooper AJ: Diagnosis and management of endocrine impotence. *Br Med J* 1:34–36, 1972

179. Abel GG, Beck JV, Cunningham-Rather J, et al: Differential diagnosis of impotence in diabetes. The validity of sexual symptoms. *Neurol Urodynamics,* 1:157–169, 1982
180. Michal V, Kramar R, Pospichal J, et al: Arterial epigastrico cavernnosus anastomosis for the treatment of sexual impotence. *World J Surg* 1:515–520, 1977
181. Melman A: Development of contemporary surgical management for erectile impotence. *Sexual Disabil* 4:272–281, 1978
182. Furlow WL: Surgical treatment of erectile impotence using the inflatable penile prosthesis. *Sexual Disabil* 1:299–306, 1978
183. Friedman D: The treatment of impotence by brietal relaxation therapy. *Behav Res Ther* 6:257–261, 1968
184. Reynolds BS: Psychological treatment models and outcome results for erectile dysfunction: A critical review. *Psychol Bull* 84:1218–1238, 1977
185. Courtenay M: *Sexual Discord in Marriage.* London, Taristock, 1968
186. Masters WH, Johnson VE: *Human Sexual Inadequacy.* Boston, Little Brown, 1970
187. Kaplan HS: *The New Sex Therapy.* New York, Quadrangle Books, 1974
188. Zilbergold B: Alternatives to couple counseling for sex problems: Group and individual therapy. *J Sex Marital Ther* 6:3–18, 1980
189. Cooper AJ: Disorder of sexual potency in the lame: A clinical and statistical study of some factors related to short-term prognosis. *Br J Psychiatry* 115:709–719, 1969
190. Levine SB, Agle D: The effectiveness of sex therapy for chronic secondary psychological impotence. *J Sex Marital Ther* 4:235–258, 1978
191. Segraves RT, Knopf J, Camic P: Spontaneous remission in erectile impotence. *Behav Res Ther* 20:89–91, 1982

2

Erectile Dysfunction Associated with Pharmacological Agents

R. TAYLOR SEGRAVES, ROBERT MADSEN,
C. SUE CARTER, and JOHN M. DAVIS

INTRODUCTION

The purpose of this chapter is to review pharmacological effects on male erectile dysfunction. As will be documented in this chapter, a wide variety of pharmacological agents have been reported to have sexual side effects. Drugs may influence male sexual function at various levels including (1) sexual interest or desire (also termed libido), (2) the capacity to achieve and maintain an erection sufficient for coitus, (3) ejaculation, and (4) fertility. Although the issue of fertility is beyond the scope of this review, drugs that inhibit fertility often suppress hormonal secretions and may thus influence sexual behavior. This text is concerned primarily with erectile function. However, libido and ejaculation problems often coexist and interact with erectile problems. The effects of drugs on these sexual activities will also be reviewed.

A more complete knowledge of the interactive effects of hormones and other biochemical processes in normal sexual behavior would obviously enhance our understanding of the actions of pharmacological agents

R. TAYLOR SEGRAVES • Department of Psychiatry, Tulane University Medical Center, New Orleans, Louisiana 70112.   ROBERT MADSEN • Department of Surgery, University of Iowa, Iowa City, Iowa 52240.   C. SUE CARTER • Departments of Psychology and Ecology, Ethology and Evolution, University of Illinois, Champaign, Illinois 61820.   JOHN M. DAVIS • Illinois State Psychiatric Institute, and Department of Psychiatry, University of Illinois, Chicago, Illinois 60612.

on human sexuality. In the absence of this knowledge, the current review will depend largely on empirical observations of drugs that reportedly affect human behavior.

Available sources of information concerning drug effects on sexual capacity are typically limited to case reports or questionnaires. Case reports are, of course, limited by the small number of individuals investigated, their retrospective nature, and the possiblity of contamination of the drug effect by numerous extraneous variables including physician and patient expectations. However, case reports can provide important information concerning suspected relationships. Physician surveys and questionnaire studies may draw on a broader sample but are again retrospective and subject to physician and patient bias. Survey studies have the additional problem of combining data from individuals with diverse medical histories and therapies which may invalidate attempts to properly characterize the effects of the drug in question.

For sexual function, as for any other aspect of human behavior, individual differences can influence the evaluation of pharmacological effects. Personal history, marital situation and life-style, moral systems, diet, drinking and smoking habits, age, general health, and numerous other factors influence sexual behavior. Any drug effect acts within this complex milieu. Furthermore, because of the personal nature of sexual activity, it is likely that many sexual side effects of drugs are unreported unless the physician or investigator specifically probes this issue.

APHRODISIACS

Folk medicine has long attributed to various chemicals the power to influence sexual behavior. Both modern and historical attempts to alter sexual activity have typically focused on methods for enhancing either sexual pleasure or potency. Among food substances that have been proposed as aphrodisiacs are ginseng, olives, oysters, truffles, and potatoes. Aside from their nutritional value, there is little evidence for any direct sexual benefits from these. It is generally assumed that these foods were selected as aphrodisiacs based on their "doctrine of signatures."[1] In other words, the food substances were derived from bulbous plants or parts of plants that physically resembled the reproductive organs. Benedek[1] compiled a list of substances recommended as aphrodisiacs in at least two medical texts between 1890 and 1920. There is little evidence that any drugs in this extensive list actually have any beneficial pharmacological effect on sexual function. Many of these agents may be highly effective placebos.

The reproductive organs or glands of animals have been assumed to contain substances with aphrodisiac powers, and preparations derived from animal testes have commonly been used to treat sexual dysfunction. In the late nineteenth century, the aged physician Brown-Sequard[2] self-administered an aqueous extract of testicular tissue and reported a marked increase in energy and sexual interest. Although Brown-Sequard's aqueous testicular solution was later shown to be biologically inactive, his claims generated great interest (both medical and commercial) in the sexual effects of testicular secretions. "Monkey gland" preparations were marketed well into the twentieth century. The scientific community subsequently documented the fact that testicular hormones (which are not readily water-soluble) are behaviorally active. Research on the physiological effects of these hormones continues to the present.

It has been repeatedly reported that declines in sexual activity follow castration and that sexual behavior can be maintained or restored with androgen replacement therapy.[3] However, the sites and mechanisms of the behavioral effects of androgen are not well defined. Other investigators have reported that penile erection and sexual activity persist for many years after castration.[4,5] Bancroft[6] found that androgen replacement therapy in hypogonadal men had no effect on erections to erotic slides but appeared to enhance erectile responsiveness to sexual fantasy. He hypothesized that the primary role of androgen in the human is via hormonal effects on cognitive aspects of sexual arousal. Davidson and his associates[3] also found that hypogonadal males were essentially identical to normal controls in their ability to show penile erection in the presence of erotic stimuli. On the basis of such data and an extensive animal literature, Davidson and colleagues extended Bancroft's hypothesis and suggested that androgens influence sensory functions including the genital sensory receptors or the pathways connecting these receptors to the brain. It was specifically proposed that androgens modulate the sensory input and hedonistic interpretation of sexual stimuli. In the absence of adequate androgen levels, erection might require very powerful visual, tactile, or cognitive stimuli. A more complete knowledge of the interactive effects of hormones and other biochemical processes in normal sexual behavior would obviously enhance our understanding of the actions of pharmacological agents on human sexuality.

It was recently proposed that central serotonin pathways have an inhibiting effect on sexual behavior and that central dopamine pathways play an activating role.[7] This hypothesis is based mainly on animal experiments in which serotonin inhibitors such as parachlorophenylalanine (which inhibits tryptophan hydroxylase) have been observed to lead to compulsive sexual activity in rabbits, cats, and rats. This "hypersexual" behavior is reversed by the administration of 5-hydroxytryptophan. Increased sexual activity is also observed after administration of 5-6-di-hydroxytryptamine (an inhibitor of serotonin neurons) and a tryptophan-free diet. Agents increasing central serotonin levels, such as 5-hydroxy-tryptophan, pargyline, phenelzine, and proniazid, have been observed to decrease sexual activity in laboratory animals. By contrast, L-dihydroxy-phenylalanine (L-dopa) and apomorphine have been observed to increase sexual activity; this increase in this activity was blocked by the administration of haloperidol.[8] Unfortunately, the aphrodiasiac effects of serotonin antagonists and dopamine agonists in humans are less clear. Various clinicians have reported an increase in sexual interest in a small percentage of patients on L-dopa.[9,10] Other investigators have suggested that this effect of sexual activation is associated with other symptoms of hypomania[11] or have questioned its existence.[12] It is also of note that L-dopa has been reported to inhibit ejaculation.[13] It is well known that bromocriptine (a dopaminergic agonist) restores sexual function in impotent men with hyperprolactinemia.[14,15] Pierini and Nusimovich[16] administered two dopaminergic agents (3-4-dihydroxyphenylalanine and bromcriptine) to impotent male diabetics and reported that both agents improved sexual function. However, the criteria for evaluating sexual performance were not specified, and Ambrosi and colleagues[17] in a double-blind study found that bromocriptine was no more effective than placebo in treating men with impotence and normal prolactin levels.

The evidence regarding the effect of antiserotoninergic agents on sexual performance in human males with sexual problems is similarly inconclusive. Parachlorophenylalanine (PCPA) has been sporadically reported by migraine sufferers to cause sexual excitement.[18] However, in a controlled clinical trial in men complaining of reduced libido, PCPA alone was not more effective than placebo in modifying the number of daily erections.[19] Similarly, methysergide and metergoline (antiserotoninergic agents) have been found to be ineffective in the treatment of men with sexual impotence.[20]

Although alcohol is often used as a sexual disinhibitor, there is considerable evidence that alcohol may produce sexual dysfunction. Both acute and chronic use of alcohol may lead to erectile problems.[21,22] In studies of the effect of alcohol on direct measures of sexual responsiveness (penile strain gauge), penile tumescence has been observed to decrease as alcohol consumption increases.[23,24] Studies in animals have similarly reported inhibitory effects of large doses of alcohol on penile tumescence.[25]

Sexual studies have documented that chronic alcoholism may result in permanent impotence. The prevalence of impotence in populations of chronic alcoholics has ranged from 8%[26] to 54%[27] in different studies. It is also of note that one investigator reported[28] that 18% of alcoholics suffer from ejaculatory incompetence and that acute alcohol ingestion has been documented to prolong ejaculatory latency.[29] In alcoholic males, potency does not necessarily return after alcohol consumption has ceased.[26] Similarly, androgen therapy did not reverse the potency problem.

The mechanism by which alcohol inhibits the erectile process is unclear. Both animal[30] and human[31] studies indicate that alcohol may have a direct effect on the spinal reflex mediating erections. In chronic alcoholism, polyneuropathy is not an uncommon occurrence,[32] and a peripheral autonomic neuropathy may explain the occurrence of impotence in chronic alcoholics. Chronic alcohol abuse also results in Leydig cell damage and inhibition of the hypothalamic–pituitary gonadal axis. It similarly can result in hepatic dysfunction, leading to increased accumulation of estrogens in the body.[25]

There have been reports that marijuana in high doses[33] or after chronic use[34] may reduce sexual function and fertility. These findings remain controversial.[35] Although cannabis is often used as a sexual stimulant and may act to alter sensory perceptions, there is little evidence for an aphrodisiac effect of this drug.

DRUGS INHIBITING SEXUAL FUNCTION

ANTIHYPERTENSIVE AGENTS

Sexual disturbances have been associated with the use of virtually all the antihypertensive agents. The exact incidence of such side effects is difficult to determine for several reasons. Much of the evidence concerning the relationships of antihypertensive pharmacotherapy to erectile impairment comes from clinical series. In a small number of series, the physicians directly inquired about sexual problems. In other series, the problem was indexed only if the patient made an unsolicited complaint or questionnaires were used. It is reasonable to assume that because of embarrassment many men do not volunteer information about sexual difficulties. Very few of the clinical series even approach a minimally adequate research design. Another problem in the evaluation of these data is the necessity for an estimate of the frequency of impotence occurring in untreated hypertensives. Oaks and Moyer[36] reported that 8–10% of untreated hypertensive patients have potency problems and that once on pharmacotherapy, many of these patients erroneously blame the hypotensive drugs for their difficulty. Unfortunately, Oaks and Moyer did not include the average age of their untreated group. The incidence of impotence is known to increase with age in the general population,[37] and hypertensive disease is more common in older individuals. Clinical series are difficult to interpret in that patients in the series may also have coexisting physical disease (e.g., diabetes mellitus, renal disease) which may cause erectile problems independent of the pharmacotherapy regime. Drugs reported to be associated with male sexual problems are listed in Table 1.

Diuretics

Diuretic agents are generally the first drugs used in the treatment of essential hypertension. Other drugs are added if diuretics provide insufficient control of blood pressure.[38] With the exception of spironolactone, diuretics alone apparently rarely cause sexual disturbances,[39-43] although there are case reports of impotence and decreased libido with these agents. Hogan and co-workers[44] at the Naval Medical Center in Oakland, Cali-

Table 1. Sexual Side Effects of Hypotensive Agents[a]

Drug and reference(s)	Dose (mg/day)	Decreased libido	Impaired ejaculation	Erectile failure
Diuretics				
Hydrochlorothiazide[44-47]	100	3%	0	9%
Chlorthalidone[48,49]	100	0	0	+
Bendrofluazide[50]	10	0	0	36%
Spironolactone	50–400	+	0	4–30%
Alpha-methyldopa[44,49,51,60-70]	500–4000	11%	11%	20%
Reserpine[46,51,68,71-73]	0.5–1	2%	+	46%
Guanethidine[51,65,66,70,73,74,77-85]	33–95	28%	40%	24%
Clonidine[44,64,68,89-92]	0.5–1.8	0	0	4–41%
Propranolol[93-102]	320	+	0	13.8
Oxprenolol[95]	160	+	0	0
Atenolol[97,105,106]	50–100	0	0	+
Pindolol[105-107]	30	0	0	+
Hydralazine[44,110-112]	50–100	0	0	+
Phenoxybenzamine[113-117]	30–50	0	+	0
Guanoxan[65,77,117]	30–31	0	35–92%	20–35%
Guanoclor[65,120]	?	0	15%	15%
Bethanidine[51,66]	31–52	0	41–92%	20–67%
Debrisoquine[68]	40	0	+	0
Prazosin[123-125]	3–20	0	0	+
Indoramin[127-129]	60	0	+	0

[a] 0, No reported effect; +, reported effect. In clinical series of more than 20 patients, actual percentages with the side effect(s) are used. Where several reports are available for the same drug, figures from the largest series are utilized or the data are pooled.

fornia, gave an impotence questionnaire to 861 male patients receiving antihypertensive medication. A positive history of impotence was found in 9% of patients taking hydrochlorothiazide alone. There have also been several case reports of impotence associated with this drug,[45,46] and Yendt and associates[47] reported that 3% of men taking this agent complain of loss of libido. It is important to note that many authors do not clearly specify how they discriminated between libido and erection disturbances and the two terms are often used interchangeably. Thus, the reader has to be wary of concluding a specific effect on libido by a certain drug. Chlorthalidone, a thiazidelike diuretic, has also been reported to cause erectile problems. In two separate case reports,[48,49] administration of this drug was associated with impotence, and potency returned with its discontinuation. In one of these case reports,[48] the patients were part of a double-blind study of another hypotensive agent, and the code was broken because of the complaint of impotence. The Medical Research Council of Great Britain[50] examined the effect of bendrofluazide on potency in a single-blind study. After 3 months of bendrofluazide therapy, 36% of the patients reported impotence. Two other studies are of relevance to the association of erectile dysfunction with thiazide treatment. Bulpitt and Dollery[51] administered a questionnaire to 477 patients in a hypertension clinic. Thirty-one percent of the men on diuretics alone complained of impotence. Neither the diuretic nor its dose was specified. Slag and coworkers[52] assessed the prevalence of impotence in medical clinic outpatients at the Minneapolis Veterans Administration Medical Center. Medication side effect was the most frequent diagnosis, and impotent men were frequently on diuretics.

It is well known that spironolactone has numerous sexual side effects including irregular menses, amenorrhea, postmenopausal bleeding, and hirsutism in women as well as decreased libido, impotence, gynecomastia, and mastodynia in men.[53,54] Spark and Melby[55] reported that almost all patients noted a decrease in libido and that 30% had "relative impotence" in a series of 42 patients receiving 400 mg/day of spironolactone. A smaller clinical series[56] reported by a different clinical investigation team reported that only 1 male of 26 (4%) on spironolactone complained of impotence. The dose in this series ranged from 50 to 400 mg. Several other case reports associate decreased libido[57] and impotence[57,58] with doses in the 50 to 100 mg/day range.

Alpha-Methyldopa

Methyldopa is a synthetic phenylalanine derivative related to naturally occurring dopa. Methyldopa has an action intermediate between the more potent adrenergic blockers and the milder diuretics. Various mechanisms of action have been proposed to explain the action of methyldopa including inhibition of dopa decarboxylase, false neurotransmission (conversion to alpha-methylnorepinephrine), inhibition of renin release, and stimulation of central alpha receptors. Its precise mechanism of action remains unclear.[59]

Numerous clinical series have reported erectile problems,[44,49,51,60-67] decreased libido,[49,63,68] and ejaculatory inhibition[44,57,63,66,67,69,70] associated with methyldopa treatment of arterial hypertensive disease. The information contained in these clinical series does not allow the reviewer to ascertain if the frequency of sexual side effects is dose-dependent. The frequency of impotence during methyldopa treatment ranges from 2%[62] to 80%[49] in different series. The total number of cases in 11 clinical series specifically inquiring about impotence totals 808 male hypertensives. Twenty percent (163) of these men complained of impotence. Three clinical series specifically inquired about decreased libido. Eleven percent (9 of 80 men studied) complained of decreased libido. Seven reports concern ejaculatory inhibition. Eleven percent (29 of 264 men) reported ejaculatory inhibition. Bauer and his associates[67] compared the frequency of sexual complaints before and after starting methyldopa therapy and concluded that methyldopa therapy definitely increased the frequency of complaints of both erectile and ejaculatory impairment. Two authors[44,51] reported the frequency of sexual side effects in patients on methyldopa plus diuretics as compared to diuretics alone. Chi-square statistics computed by the authors of this chapter revealed nonsignificant differences in the frequency of sexual complaints on the two therapeutic regimes.

Reserpine

Rauwolfia alkaloids were used in primitive medicine for the treatment of hypertension and insanity. The most commonly used of the alkaloids is reserpine, which is given for mild hypertension by itself or as adjunctive therapy with other drugs for moderate to severe hypertension. Reserpine depletes stores of catecholamines and 5-hydroxytryptamine in the brain, myocardium, blood vessels, and adrenergic nerve endings. It is unclear whether depletion of biogenic amines in the brain or in the peripheral nervous system is mainly responsible for the hypotensive effect of reserpine. Case reports have linked reserpine administration with complaints of impotence,[46,51,68,71,72] decreased libido, and inability to ejaculate.[51,68,72,73] The largest series was reported by Laver,[68] who found that 46% of patients on 0.5 mg of reserpine reported reduced or absent sexual activity which they attributed to drug therapy. Bulpitt and Dollery[51] reported that 33% of patients on an average dose of 0.34 mg of reserpine per day complained of erectile problems and that 14% complained of ejaculatory failure. These figures are not significantly higher than the frequency of those complaints in patients taking diuretics alone. However, patients on reserpine report an average of only six coital episodes per year. The average for patients on diuretics is 42.1%. It is unclear whether the decreased coital frequency in reserpine patients is due to decreased libido or other factors.

Guanethidine

Guanethidine, a guanidine derivative, is an adrenergic blocking agent with a selective action on peripheral sympathetic neurons. It is used primarily for moderate to severe hypertension and interferes with neuro-transmission in adrenergic postganglionic nerve terminals by depleting nor-epinephrine. It is well known that guanethidine interferes with male sexual function,[73,74] and some authors have investigated whether the sexual side effects of this drug are reversible.[67,75,76] Several studies employing a within-subjects design have demonstrated that the administration of guanethidine significantly increases the incidence of complaints of impotence, retarded ejaculation, and decreased libido over the drug-free state.[67,77] At least nine separate studies including a total of 222 patients have studied the complaint of impotence in patients on guanethidine.[51,65–67,77–81] Fifty-four patients (24%) of this total experienced erectile failure. In 12 separate studies of the effect of guanethidine on ejaculation, 40% of the 307 hypertensive patients reported retarded ejaculation.[65–67,77–79,81–85] Bauer and his associates[67] specifically inquired about loss of libido as well as other sexual side effects and reported that 28% of men on an average dose of 50 mg/day of quanethidine reported loss of sexual desire. Not all these clinical series reported the doses utilized. However, in those reporting the average dosage,[51,65–76,77–79,81–83] there was no clear relationship between the dosage employed and the incidence of sexual problems.

Clonidine

Clonidine is frequently utilized when other hypotensive agents fail as it appears to work by a different mechanism than most other drugs. The exact mechanism of action is unclear, although current evidence suggests that clonidine probably works by central alpha-receptor stimulation in the medulla which results in decreased sympathetic activation. Various investigators have reported that clonidine does not have sexual side effects.[86–88] Raftos and associates[86] reported that some patients who were impotent while on methyldopa recovered their potency upon being switched to clonidine. Numerous other authors have reported that impotence occurs in a small number of patients on clonidine.[44,64,68,89-92] The highest frequency of impotence on clonidine was reported by Onesti and colleagues.[92] They reported that 24 of 59 patients (41%) complained of impotence while on an average dose of 0.6 mg/day. The increase in impotence while on clonidine as compared to the baseline off drugs was highly statistically significant. Retarded ejaculation does not appear to be associated with clonidine.

Beta Blockers

Beta blockers are used primarily for the control of hypertension, angina, and cardiac arphythmias. They appear to act peripherally by blocking beta-adrenergic receptors although they may have additional central effects. They were initially felt to have few sexual side effects;[71] however, numerous case reports have associated impotence and decreased libido with propranolol, the most widely prescribed of the beta blockers.[93-102] The largest study of sexual side effects associated with propranolol was reported by the Medical Research Council[50] of Great Britain; 13.8% of 1130 men on propranolol doses up to 320 mg/day complained of impotence. The incidence of impotence while on propranolol was statistically significant (p < 0.001) far more commonly than while on placebo. Hollifield and co-workers[103] at Vanderbilt University reported that sexual problems were nonexistent on propranolol doses of 160 mg/day. However, seven male patients received doses ranging from 480 to 960 mg/day, and two complained of impotence and three of decreased libido. This suggests that sexual side effects with propranolol may be dose-dependent. Other investigators have also reported dose-dependent sexual side effects.[99] Other beta blockers have received less study. Gavras and associates[95] reported that impotence was not associated with oxprenolol, and Bathen[97] reported that impotence while on propranolol disappeared when a patient was switched to atenolol. Greminger and co-workers[104] similarly reported that sexual disturbances were more common on pindolol than atenolol. However, there have been case reports of impotence associated with both atenolol and pindolol.[105,106] It is also of note that Peyronie's disease has been associated with propranolol[107,108] and that priapism has been related to the administration of Lebetalol.[109]

Hydralazine

Hydralazine, a peripheral vasodilator, was given alone or with ganglionic blocking agents when it was first introduced. Currently hydralazine is used as part of "triple combination therapy" along with beta-blocking agents and a diuretic. Hydralazine may diminish total peripheral vascular resistance by as much as 60%. Its primary mechanism of action appears to be a direct relaxation of smooth muscle in the peripheral vascular bed, although it may also cause central inhibition of sympathetic discharge as well. Hydralazine has a far greater effect on the relaxation of arterioles and small arteries than it does on venules and small veins. Several case reports[44,110-112] have suggested that hydralazine therapy may induce impotence in a small number of male hypertensives. In these reports, hydralazine was combined with other hypotensive agents, and thus it is difficult to be certain that hydralazine caused the sexual symptoms. However, Keidan[110] reported that a 33-year-old sexually active schoolteacher on 50 mg hydrochlorothiazide became impotent when 100 mg hydralazine was added to his therapeutic regime. His symptoms disappeared when hydralazine was discontinued. Similarly, Ahmad[111] reported a case of a sexually active patient who became impotent when hydralazine was added to a regime of propranolol and furosemide. When hydralazine was discontinued, his erectile function returned.

Phenoxybenzamine

Phenoxybenzamine and phentolamine are alpha-adrenergic blocking agents which have limited utility in the management of arterial hypertensive disease. They reduce blood pressure by inhibiting vasoconstriction. Their limited ability is related to the other serious side effects produced by alpha-adrenergic blockade. Several reports[113-117] have associated inhibited ejaculation with this drug. Although it has been assumed that these drugs produce retrograde ejaculation, an examination of postorgasm urine samples suggested that retrograde ejaculation did not occur.[117] Presumably, these drugs inhibit ejaculation by blocking alpha-adrenergic receptors that enervate the vas deferens, seminal vesicles, epididymis, prostate, and internal urethral sphincter.[118] The inhibition of ejaculation produced by phenoxybenzamine may be dose-dependent. Vlachakis and Mendlowitz[113] reported that ejaculatory function tended to return when the dosage was reduced.

Other Hypotensive Agents

A variety of drugs resembling guanethidine in structure and/or mechanism of action have been reported to have sexual side effects. Some of these agents are not approved for use in the United States. Guanoxan, 2-guanidenomethylbenzo-1,4-dioxan, is a guanethidine ring with a benzodioxane side chain. It depletes catecholamines both peripherally and in the

the hypothalamus. Several authors[64,65,119] have reported guanoxan administration to be associated with both erectile failure and impaired ejaculation. Reudy and Davies,[77] in a study of 25 patients on guanoxan, reported that 20% complained of impotence and that 92% complained of retarded ejaculation. The average dose was 31.3 mg/day. Another study[65] utilizing a similar dosage reported a 45% incidence of impotence and a 35% incidence of impaired ejaculation. Guanoclor, 2-(2,6-dichlorphenoxy) ethylamino-guanidine, also depletes catecholamines both centrally and peripherally and has also been reported to be associated with both erectile and ejaculatory impairment.[120]

Bethanidine is believed to exert its antihypertensive effect by inhibiting the release of norepinephrine at sympathetic postganglionic junctions. It has been reported to be associated with both retarded ejaculation and erectile impotence.[51,66] Bulpitt and Dollery[51] reported that 66.7% of men on bethanidine complained of erectile problems and that 41.2% complained of ejaculatory failure. Complaint rates of patients on diuretics alone were 31.8% for impotence and 13.6% for ejaculatory problems. Chi squares computed by the authors of this chapter reveal that the incidence of both complaints on bethanidine is significantly higher ($p < 0.05$) than the frequency of these complaints in men on diuretics alone. Debrisoquine, another agent interfering with norepinephrine release at postganglionic sympathetic nerves, has been reported to cause ejaculatory inhibition.[68] Prazosin, a guinazoline derivative, has been proposed as a replacement for hydralazine in combination drug therapy for hypertensive disease. It appears to have both a direct smooth-muscle-relaxant effect as well as postsynaptic alpha-blocking activity.[121] Although some authors report[122] that sexual side effects are notably infrequent on this agent,[123-125] others have reported a low incidence of erectile failure with this drug.

Sexual side effects were associated with the ganglionic-blocking agents,[126] such as trimethaphan camsylate, but these drugs have been totally replaced by newer agents for the treatment of hypertensive arterial disease. Indoramin[127-129] (3-2-4-benzamidopiperid-1-yl-ethylindole), an alpha-adrenergic blocking agent under investigation in Great Britain, has been associated with ejaculatory failure.

PSYCHIATRIC DRUGS

Like the drugs used in the treatment of arterial hypertension, most of the pharmacological agents used in modern psychiatry have been reported to have sexual side effects. (Table 2). It is especially important that the physician be aware of the side effects so that sexual complaints of pharmacological etiology are not erroneously attributed to the psychological condition being treated by the drug in question.

Table 2. Side Effects of Psychiatric Drugs[a]

Drug and reference(s)	Dose (mg/day)	Decreased libido	Impaired ejaculation	Erectile failure
Thioridazine[130-156]	30–2400	+	49%	44%
Chlorpromazine[161-163]	400–100	0	+	0
Chlorprothixine[170]	300	0	+	0
Mesoridazine[171]	60	0	+	0
Fluphenazine[173,174]	25/2 weeks	+	0	+
Thiothixine[175,176]	20	0	0	+
Perphenazine[177]		0	+	0
Trifluoperazine[177]		0	+	0
Butaperazine[177]		0	+	0
Butyrophenones[177]		0	+	0
Phenelzine[180-184]	60–75	0	+	+
Pargyline[187,188]	50	0	+	0
Mebanazine[188]	20	0	+	0
Iproniazid[189]	50–100	0	+	0
Isocarboxazid[189]	20–40	0	+	0
Imipramine[184,189,190-193]	75–150	0	+	+
Chlomipramine[191,200-205]	50–300	+	+	+
Amoxapine[195,206,207]	75–150	?	+	?
Amitriptyline[191,194-196]	75–150	?	+	+
Protriptyline[188]	20	0	0	+
Desmethylimipramine	150–225	0	+	+
Lithium	0.5–0.9 meq/liter	0	0	+
Clorazepate[212,213]	15 mg	?	0	0
Diazepam[212,213]	15 mg	?	0	0
Chlordiazepoxide[214,215]	30 mg	0	+	?

[a] 0, No reported effect; +, reported effect.

Major Tranquilizers (Antipsychotic Drugs)

Most classes of major tranquilizers have been reported to have sexual side effects. This is especially true of the drugs that have been in use for long periods of time such as the piperazine phenothiazines, the piperidine phenothiazines, the dimethylaminoprapyl phenothiazides, the thioxanthenes, and the butyrophenones. To varying degrees, these agents are antidopaminergic, anticholinergic, and alpha-adrenergic blockers. Antipsychotic agents have been reported to cause changes in libido, impotence, retarded ejaculation (or retrograde ejaculation), and aspermia.

Thioridazine. It is well known that thioridazine can cause sexual dysfunction.[130-136] This agent has been reported to cause retarded ejaculation,[137-156] disturbances in libido,[137] and erectile impairment.[139,145,155] The most common complaint of patients on thioridazine is the absence of ejaculation. This was first reported by Singh[143] approximately 2 years after thioridazine was introduced by Sandoz. He reported that a 35-year-old man complained of the complete inhibition of ejcaulation while on 300 mg/day of thioridazine for 1 week. Libido, erectile function, and the subjective sense of orgasm were unaffected. When thioridazine was discontinued, normal ejaculatory function returned. Numerous other clinicians have reported similar findings. Some clinicians have utilized lower doses of thioridazine to treat premature ejaculation.[144,147] Thioridazine has also been reported to decrease the frequency of nocturnal emission.[141,146] Ejaculatory inhibition has been reported to occur at doses as low as 30 mg/day.[152] Although some authors[140] have suggested that thoridazine may cause retrograde ejaculation, Kedia and Markland[118] found no evidence for this in their study of postmasturbatory urine samples of men on thioridazine. The largest clinical series was reported by Kotin and associates.[155] They interviewed 57 patients on thioridazine and found that 28 (49%) reported either decreased amounts of ejaculate or no ejaculate at orgasm. Forty-four percent of these patients complained of erectile problems. It is also of note that priapism has been reported to be associated with thioridazine therapy.[157-159] There has also been one case report of nocturnal enuresis caused by thioridazine.[160]

Chlorpromazine. There have been two case reports[161,162] of chlorpromazine causing ejaculatory inhibition. A controlled study[163] of the erectile response to erotic stimuli found no effect of chlorpromazine administration on erections. However, this study utilized only 125 mg chlorpromazine, a dose much smaller than usually employed in clinical practice. There have also been reports of priapism occurring in patients on this drug.[164-169].

Chlorprothixine. Ditman[170] reported one case of absence ejaculation in the presence of normal erectile capacity in a patient on 300 mg of chlorprothixine. The ejaculatory reflex was restored when this drug was stopped. It is of note that this same patient had previously experienced similar difficulties on 200 mg of thioridazine.

Mesoridazine. Shader[171] reported one case of failure to ejaculate in a man on 60 mg of mesoridazine. This drug has also been reported to be associated with priapism.[172]

Fluphenazine. Bartholomew[173] studied the sexual side effects of 25 mg (1 ml) fluphenazine enanthate every 2 weeks in two groups of psychiatric outpatients. Psychiatric outpatients with a history of sexual deviancy experienced a reduction in libido at this dose level. Patients without a history of sexual deviacy experienced both erectile problems and decreased libido. Dillon and Bates[174] also reported one case of impotence at this dose level.

Thiothixine. There have been two case reports[175,176] of impotence being associated with thiothixine therapy. This side effect was reported to occur at a dose level of only 20 mg/day.

Other Major Tranquilizers

Blair and Simpson[117] reported that ejaculatory disturbances occur with perphenazine, trifluoperazine, butaperazine, and butyrophenones. However, Kotin and associates[155] reported the absence of sexual side effects on both perphenazine and trifluoperazine. Tennett and co-workers[163] reported that haloperidol did not influence erectile capacity. Berger[178] also reported that pain on ejaculation occurred in patients receiving 5 mg/day of haloperidol or 10 mg/day of trifluoperazine. This complaint is noteworthy in that Bors and Comarr,[179] in their review of sexual difficulties in patients with spinal cord injuries, reported that pain on ejaculation occurred exclusively in patients with an incomplete upper motor neuron lesion. Thus, one might speculate that this symptom is related to an incomplete central dopamine blockade induced by neuroleptis.[37] Painful ejaculation has also been reported with thioridazine.[155]

MONOAMINE OXIDASE INHIBITORS

Monoamine oxidase inhibitors (MAOI) act by blocking oxidative deamination of endogenous norepinephrine, epinephrine, dopamine, and serotonin. The catecholamine hypothesis of depression assumes that MAOI work by increasing the neuronal levels of monoamines; however, the exact mechanism by which these drugs alleviate depression and lower blood pressure is unknown. MAOI are less commonly used than tricyclic antidepressants because of their potentially dangerous interactions with other drugs. However, these drugs are used in the treatment of depression refractory to other antidepressants, of certain subtypes of depression, and of certain phobias. The first MAOI, isoniazid, was withdrawn from the market because of hepatotoxicity. Two groups of MAOIs currently exist— the hydrazines including phenelzine, nialamide, and isocarboxazid—and the nonhydrazines, tranylcypromine.

Phenelzine

Both erectile failure[180] and ejaculatory impairment[181-184] have been reported with phenelzine. This effect appears to be dose-dependent and may occur as late as 3–4 weeks after therapy is begun. Sexual side effects have usually been reported at the 60 to 75-mg/day dose range. It is also of note that several authors have reported that phenelzine may increase sperm counts.[185–186]

Other MAOIs

There have also been case reports of pargyline[187,188] and mebanazine[188] causing ejaculation inhibition. Bennett[189] reported successfully using both iproniazid and isocarboxazid to treat premature ejaculation.

TRICYCLIC ANTIDEPRESSANTS

The major tricyclic antidepressants—imipramine, desipramine, amitriptyline, nortriptyline, and protriptyline—are structurally similar to the phenothiazines. Imipramine and amitriptyline are partially metabolized to their desmethyl derivatives, desipramine and nortriptyline. These drugs may exert their affect on affective disease through influences on biogenic amines.

Imipramine

There have been case reports of both impotence[188,190–193] and impaired ejaculation[184,188,191] in patients taking imipramine. Impotence was reported at doses as low as 75 mg/day,[192] and inhibited ejaculation has been reported at a 125-mg dose level. These effects may be dose-related, as two investigators reported that the difficulty remitted when the dosage was lowered.[184,191] Painful ejaculation has also been reported with imipramine.[188] The sexual side effects of tricyclic antidepressants have been postulated to be the result of peripheral anticholinergic activity associated with these drugs. In this regard, it is of note that Everett[190] reported that bethanechol, a cholinergic drug, did not relieve sexual problems in two male patients taking imipramine. It is of note that bethanechol is unable to cross the blood–brain barrier and thus would not influence the central toxicity of anticholinergic drugs.

Amitriptyline

There have also been case reports of impotence[191,194–195] and ejaculatory inhibition[191,196] associated with amitriptyline. These side effects have occurred at doses as low as 75 mg/day. It is reassuring that at least one author[196] reported that sexual function may return as early as 1 day after drug discontinuation.

Clomipramine

Clomipramine, a tricyclic antidepressant with extensive usage in Great Britain, has been frequently reported to have sexual side effects.[197-199] This agent has been reported to be associated with impotence,[200-203] retarded ejaculation,[191,200,203,204] and decreased libido.[191,200,202,203] One investigator[205] reported that the incidence of sexual side effects on this agent did not increase over baseline levels off medication. However, this investigation involved only ten male patients. One investigator,[204] noting that retarded ejaculation is a frequent side effect in the use of this drug, employed lower doses (40–75 mg/day) to successfully treat premature ejaculation in 12 of 13 patients. It is of note that from 2 weeks to 2 months of drug administration was required to cure premature ejaculation. There has been one report of spontaneous orgasm associated with yawning in patients on clomipramine.[206] The significance of this unusual report is unclear. The senior author (RTS) has been unsuccessful in using this drug to treat inhibited male orgasm.

Amoxapine

Amoxapine is a relatively new antidepressant in the United States. Three separate investigators[195,207,208] have reported sexual side effects with this agent. Hekimian and co-workers[195] reported that 8 of 19 male patients on an average daily dose of 176 mg experienced loss of libido or impotence on this agent. Schwarcz[207] reported a case of dry, painful orgasm in a 33-year-old man on 150 mg of amoxapine. Kulik and Wilbur[208] reported that a 29-year-old male experienced "an abnormally protracted spasmotic ejaculation that he characterized as painful and burning" on 75 mg of this agent. This problem disappeared when the drug was stopped. Amoxapine has also been reported to interfere with orgasm in female patients.[209]

Other Tricyclic Antidepressants

Simpson and co-workers[188] have reported sexual side effects occurring with both protriptyline and desmethylimipramine. One male patient became impotent on 20 mg of protriptyline and resumed normal sexual function when the drug was discontinued. Two patients experienced urinary hesitancy and urgency on desmethylimipramine. One of these patients also experienced impotence at 150 mg/day, which was relieved when the dose was lowered to 75 mg. The other patient reported painful orgasm on 225 mg/day, which ceased when the drug was discontinued. There has been one case report[210] of norpramin causing a decrease in sperm motility. The significance of this isolated report is difficult to assess. It is of note that priapism has been associated with trazodone.[212]

LITHIUM

Two separate investigators have reported erectile impotence to be associated with the use of lithium carbonate in affective disorders. In both reports, the effect was substantiated under double-blind conditions in therapeutic serum lithium levels. Vinarova and associates[211] first noted the problem of impotence in an open clinical trial of lithium therapy in bipolar affective illness. A double-blind study comfirmed this effect in two male patients of ten studied. Blay and co-workers[213] also reported two cases of impotence associated with lithium. In one man, the problem remitted gradually after 2 months of therapy. In the other case, double-blind substitution of placebo repeatedly restored erectile function which was impaired during lithium therapy.

MINOR TRANQUILIZERS

Although minor tranquilizers are frequently assumed to interfere with sexual function, the actual evidence supporting this assumption is meager. Magnus and co-workers[214] compared clorazepate and diazepam in a double-blind crossover study of the treatment of anxiety. Complaints of decreased libido for both agents were not significantly different from the frequency of such complaints on placebo. The dosage of each agent was 15 mg/day. The General Practitioner Research Group of Great Britain[215] also reported that similar dosages of both agents had nonsignificant effects on libido. There has been one case report of impotence occurring on chloridazepoxide,[216] but the problem spontaneously resolved without discontinuance of the drug. Hughes[217] reported one case of a male receiving 30 mg of chlordiazepoxide daily who experienced ejaculatory failure. Discontinuance of the drug led to restoration of sexual function.

OTHER PHARMACOLOGICAL AGENTS

Cimetidine, a histamine antagonist at H_2-receptor sites, has dramatically changed the medical treatment of duodenal ulcer (Table 3). This drug crosses the blood-brain barrier and has been linked with numerous side effects including mental confusion. Several authors have reported both diminished libido[218,219] and impotence[219-221] with this drug. This side effect may be dose-dependent, as Biron[218] reported a case in which libido was diminished at 600 mg/day but restored to normal when the dose was reduced to 300 mg/day. Other clinicians have reported that sexual function is promptly restored when cimetidine therapy is discontinued.[220,221] The usual dosage associated with impotence is 1 g/day[221] The evidence of sexual

Table 3. Other Pharmacological Agents[a]

Drug and reference(s)	Dose	Decreased libido	Impaired ejaculation	Erectile failure
Cimetidine[216–219]	600–1200	+	0	+
Digoxin[223]	1–2 ng/ml per day	?	0	+
Heparin[227]	75–150 mg/day	0	0	Secondary to priapism
Clofibrate[228,229]	1.8 g/day	+	0	+
Disopyramide[230,231]	300 mg/day	0	0	+
Acetazolamide[238,239]	500–1000 mg/day	+	0	0
Methazolamide[238,239]	100–200 mg/day	+	0	?
Ethoxzolamide[238]	500 mg/day	+	0	0
Dichlorphenamide[238]	100–200 mg/day	+	0	?
Methantheline bromide[233]	?	0	0	+
Baclofen[240]	30 ng/day	0	0	+
Epsilon-aminocaproic acid[241]	24 g/day	0	+	0
Diethylpropion HCl	?	0	0	?
Disulfiram[243]	250 mg/day	0	0	+
Cyclic combination cancer chemotherapy[246]	—	+	0	+
Ketamine[b][244,245]	0.5–0.1 mg/kg per day	0	0	+
Naproxen[251]	750 mg/day	0	+	0
Thiabendazole[251]	50 ng/kg per day	0	0	+
Cyproterone acetate[261–267]	50–200 ng per day	+	0	?
Medroxyprogesterone[268]	200–600 mg/wk	+	0	?
Medrogesterone[269]	15–30 mg	+	0	?
Gesterorone[270]	200 ng/1–2 wk	0	0	+
Hydroxyprogesterone[271]	?	0	0	+
Ethinyl estradiol[266]	0.02 mg/day	+	0	0
Fenfluramine[252]	?	+	0	+
Perhexiline[253,254]	100–600 mg/day	0	0	+

[a] 0, No reported effect; +, reported effect.
[b] See text.

side effects with this agent is unclear. Gifford and colleagues[219] pooled case report forms from 1232 physicians concerning 9907 patients and reported only three cases of sexual dysfunction. However, the case report form did not specifically inquire about sexual problems. The mechanism by which cimetidine interferes with sexual function is unclear. Several authors[219,222] have reported gynecomastia in patients on this drug. Elevated prolactin levels have been suggested as a mechanism.[222,223] Adaikan and Karim[224] pointed out that the evidence that the sacral parasympathetics are cholinergic is equivocal and that histamine could be the neurotransmitter. In vitro studies indicate that histamine both contracts and relaxes smooth muscle of the corpus cavernosa. The contraction effect is abolished by mepyramine (a histamine H_1-receptor antagonist), and the relaxant effect is abolished by burimamide, a drug similar to cimetidine. Thus, these authors suggest that cimetidine may interfere with erections by blocking peripheral H_2 receptors.

Several drugs commonly used in cardiovascular medicine have been reported to cause sexual dysfunction. These drugs include digoxin, heparin, clofibrate (a hypolipidemic drug), and disopyramide (an antiarrhythmic). Neri and associates[225] from Tel Aviv studied the effects of long-term (> 2 years) digoxin therapy on sexual behavior and endocrine function. A control group of patients not on dignoxin but with a similar cardiac functional capacity was utilized. The ratings of sexual function were performed by a blind interviewer. The patients on digoxin had a statistically significant increased frequency of impotence and a decreased frequency of sexual relations as compared to the control group. The patients on digoxin had significantly elevated estrogen levels and depressed testosterone and lu-teinizing-hormone levels. The authors speculated that the sexual inhibition might be due to changes in endocrine function. Other investigators have noted endocrine changes in patients on digoxin therapy.[226–228] Duggan and Morgan[229] reported four cases of priapism in patients on heparin therapy. Two of these men subsequently became permanently impotent. Schneider and Kaffarnik[230] reported three cases of impotence in men with hyperli-poproteinemia taking clofibrate. With discontinuance of the drug, sexual function was restored. The largest series of patients on clofibrate was reported by the Coronary Drug Project Research Group.[231] The clofibrate group contained 1065 patients receiving 1.8 g/day of this drug. The incidence of impotence or decreased libido in the clofibrate group was 14.1%. Only 10% of the placebo group had this complaint. This difference was statistically significant. Their mechanism of classifying sexual side effects does not allow the reader to clearly differentiate the incidence of impotence as opposed to decreased libido. There have been two separate reports[232,233] of impotence associated with disopyramide therapy for ectopic ventricular contractions. In one case,[232] lowering of the dose restored sexual function without compromising the drug's antiarrhythmic effect. In the other case, both sexual function and a life-threatening arrhythmia returned upon discontinuance of the drug. One of the authors of this chapter (RTS) has observed impotence associated with disopyramide therapy. In one case, discontinuance of the drug restored sexual function. In the other case, the drug could not be permanently discontinued because of the recurrence of a serious arrhythmia. The effect of this drug on erectile function has been attributed to its strong anticholinergic action.

Numerous anticholinergic agents are utilized in medicine for a variety of purposes including preanesthetic medication, and in combination with other agents to treat a variety of gastrointestinal disorders.[234] In view of their wide usuage, it is interesting that surprisingly few sexual side effects have been reported with these agents. Schwartz and Robinson[235] reported that methantheline bromide frequently causes impotence. However, they failed to report dosages utilized or the actual incidence of this side effect. Although it has long been assumed that penile erection and vaginal vasocongestion are governed by cholinergic nerves, the evidence for this is equivocal. Wagner and co-workers[236,237] reported that atropine infusion (0.035 mg/kg) had no effect on erectile latency or turgidity. Similarly, atropine failed to block erections produced in baboons by electrical stimulation of sacral roots. A separate report[238] also indicated that atropine (0.35 mg/kg) and methylatropine (1 mg) have no effect on vaginal blood flow and orgasm in healthy female volunteers.

Carbonic anhydrase inhibitors are often used in opthalmological practice in the long-term management of glaucoma. The agents most commonly used are acetazolamide, ethoxzolamide, dichlorphenamide, and methazolamide.[239] All of these agents have been reported to have sexual side effects.[240,241] The most commonly reported sexual problem is decreased libido, which can be relieved by supplemental sodium bicarbonate therapy or by discontinuing the drug. This side effect may be secondary to the general malaise produced by this agent rather than a specific effect on libido.

A variety of other pharmacological agents in medical practice have been reported to have sexual side effects. Baclofen [β(4-chlorophenyl) γ-aminobutyric acid], a muscle relaxant and a gamma-aminobutyric acid derivative, was reported to be associated with impotence in 1 of 23 male patients with multiple sclerosis.[242] The dosage employed was 30 mg. Epsilon-aminocaproic acid, a drug utilized in the treatment of hemophilic patients because of its inhibition of the fibrinolytic system, was reported to cause inhibited ejaculation in 4 of 25 patients receiving 24 g/day.[243] Diethylpropion hydrochloride, an appetite suppressant, was reported to cause impotence in one male patient,[244] however, one patient on placebo reported the same complaint. The dosage utilized was unclear. Snyder and colleagues[245] investigated the effects of 250 mg of disulfiram (Antabuse) on nocturnal penile tumescence in a random double-blind study. Disulfiram was found to impair nocturnal erections, and they speculated that the central norepinephrine-depleting action of the drug might be responsible. Ketamine, a dissociative anesthetic, has been reported to successfully inhibit reflex erections during urological surgery such as cystoscopy and hypospadias repair.[246,247] Decreased libido, impotence,[248] infertility,[249-251] and gynecomastia[252] have been reported during cancer chemotherapy. Cyclical combination therapy (nitrogen mustard, vinblastine, procarbazine, and prednisolone) has specifically been associated with erectile problems although other agents may also produce this side effect. Naproxen, an antiinflammatory agent used in the treatment of arthritis, has been reported to cause ejaculatory inhibition, and thiabendazole, an anthelmintic, has been associated with erectile failure.[253] Fenfluramine, an appetite suppressant, has been reported to be associated with both decreased libido and impotence.[254] Similarly, two authors[255,256] have reported that perhexiline maleate use may be associated with erectile failure. Perhexiline is utilized to decrease symptoms of angina pectoris.

OCCUPATIONAL POLLUTANTS

Impotence has been reported in farm workers exposed to a heterogenous group of insecticides,[257,258] and in workers exposed to the industrial solvent carbon disulfide.[253] Layzer[259] reported 15 patients with myeloneuropathy after prolonged exposure to nitrous oxide. Seven of these patients were impotent. It is of note that 14 of the patients were dentists.

HORMONES

The role of androgens in maintaining sexual arousal in males was discussed briefly earlier in this chapter and is dealt with more extensively in Chapter 6 in this text by Thomas M. Jones. This subject has also been excellently reviewed elsewhere.[260-262] Thus, this section will focus on endocrinologically active agents that have been reported to decrease sexual performance in the human male. Cyproterone acetate (progestin) is employed as an antiandrogen in the treatment of sexual offenders and has been reported to markedly decrease libido and sexual activity.[263-268] It may also influence erectile capacity,[269] although this is less clear. Medroxyprogesterone acetate has also been employed to reduce libido in habitual sex offenders.[270] Progestins are used in males to treat benign prostatic hyperplasia causing urinary-outlet obstruction. Several of these agents, including medrogesterone,[271] gestonorone,[272] and hydroxyprogesterone,[273] have been reported to cause decreased libido and possibility erectile dysfunction as well. Estrogens used to treat prostate carcinoma in the male may cause decreased libido as a side effect. Bancroft and co-workers[268] reported that ethinyl estradiol was as effective as cyproterone acetate in lowering sexual activity and interest in sexual deviants.

SUBSTANCE ABUSE

Various pharmacological agents have been used to enhance sexual pleasure by members of the substance-abuse population. As Hollister[274] emphasizes, many of these claims are probably more illusory than real. Although certain agents may have disinhibiting effects and strong placebo effects, most drugs when abused lead to a decline in actual sexual performance (Table 4). There are numerous difficulties in evaluating data concerning the effects of substance abuse. Potential confounding variables include drug purity, drug dose, duration of administration, the setting for drug use, user expectation, and deviant sexual patterns prior to drug use.

AMPHETAMINES

Among the actions of amphetamines are the release of and prevention of the reuptake of catecholamines. Amphetamines are general stimulants and commonly increase sexual interest and activity in animals.[275] However, dose-dependent effects of amphetamines on sexual activity in laboratory animals have been noted, with higher doses inhibiting sexual activity.[276] The effect of amphetamines on human sexual behavior is not clear. Although several investigators have reported an intensification of sexual interest and erotic sensations in amphetamine abusers,[277-282] this has not been consistently reported, and some amphetamine abusers experience decreased libido.[283-287] It is of note that delayed ejaculation has been reported with chronic amphetamine abuse.[282,285,287,289] Spontaneous erections have been reported to be associated with amphetamine injection.[290] Several authors have stressed that the premorbid personality patterns of this population seriously contaminate efforts to isolate drug effects on sexual performance.[283-291]

Table 4. Substance Abuse[a]

Drug and reference(s)	Decreased libido	Impaired ejaculation	Erectile failure
Amphetamines[275-288]	?	+	?
Marijuana[290-292]	?	0	0
Cocaine[273,283,285,295]	?	0	+
Heroin[298-300,310-313]	61–100%	52–57%	28–43%
Methadone[301-307,310,311,314,315]	22–96.5%	14–22%	40–50%
Methadyl acetate[316]	+	0	0

[a] 0, No reported effect; +, reported effect.

CANNABIS

Delta-9-tetrahyocannabinol is the active ingredient in marijuana. In moderate doses, this drug has been reported to enhance the sensory experience of coital activity.[253] However, there have been reports that high doses or chronic use may reduce sexual function and fertility.[292] Gynecomastia[293] and depressed serum testosterone levels[295] have been reported in marijuana users. The effect of marijuana on testosterone levels was not replicable by another investigator.[295] In animal studies, tetrahydrocannabinol has been reported to decrease sexual interest and performance.[296]

COCAINE

Cocaine is both a local anesthetic and a central nervous system depressant. It is regarded as an aphrodisiac among cocaine users, and has been reported to cause spontaneous erections.[275,285] However, erectile failure has been reported with cocaine use.[287,297]

AMYLNITRITE

Amylnitrite is used in the treatment of angina pectoris. However, it is purported to prolong orgasm if it is inhaled prior to orgasm.[298] The vasodilator action of amylnitrite might have an effect on the perception of orgasm, although this remains unproven. It is of note that volatile nitrites have been used to produce penile detumescence in urological surgical procedures.[299]

PSYCHEDELICS

Although psychedelic drugs (e.g., lysergic acid diethylamide, psilocybin, mescaline) may produce intense sexual–emotional experiences, there is no evidence of a direct action of these drugs on sexual performance or libido.[253]

OPIATES

It is well known that both heroin addicts[300–302] and patients on methadone maintenance[303–309] experience a decline in sexual functioning. Delayed or absent ejaculation, erectile problems, and diminished libido are common complaints. It is unclear whether these complaints are more frequent with heroin or with methadone. There is some evidence that the frequency of sexual complaints with methadone is dose-related.[310] These complaints tend to diminish when detoxification is complete and abstinence status is achieved.[311] Several studies have documented that the frequency of sexual complaints is significantly elevated during heroin or methadone use as compared to the drug-free state.[312-314] It is also of note that premature ejaculation may be one of the symptoms associated with opiate withdrawal.[311] The usual frequency of such complaints in heroin addicts is difficult to ascertain because of differences in dosages, frequency of administration, duration and strength of addiction, associated health problems, and unknown purity of substance utilized. Diminished libido has been reported to occur in 61-100% of heroin addicts.[313,315] The frequency of erectile problems has been estimated at 28–43%,[312,315] and the incidence of ejaculatory impairment has been estimated to be from 52 to 57%.[312-315] In methadone patients, the reported incidences for diminished libido, erectile problems, and ejaculatory disturbance are as follows: libido, 22–96.5%;[312,316,317] impotence, 40–50%;[312,317] and retarded ejaculation, 14–22%.[316,317] It is of note that Senay and colleagues[318] at the University of Chicago reported that methadyl acetate may have more severe sexual side effects than methadone. The mechanism by which opiates interfere with sexual function is unclear. It has been speculated that opiates may suppress luteinizing-hormone release and thus secondarily depress circulating testosterone levels,[319] although this remains controversial.[253,320] The role of endogenous opiate systems in the control of sexual behavior is also unclear.[321]

MECHANISM OF SEXUAL SIDE EFFECTS OF DRUGS

A coherent theory concerning the mechanisms by which pharmacological agents interfere with sexual function is difficult to evolve because of significant gaps in our knowledge of the physiology of the normal erectile response. Studies in spinal-cord-injured patients suggest the presence of two different erectile pathways—the so-called psychogenic and reflexogenic pathways.[179-322] Psychogenic stimuli (imaginary, visual, auditory, olfactory, nongenital tactile) are purported to arouse erotic centers in the brain and are mediated by a sympathetic nervous system thoracolumbar outflow from the T12–L1 region of the cord. Although part of the sympathetic nervous system, these fibers are vasodilator in action. Reflexogenic erections can be produced by exteroceptive stimuli (stroking the penis) or interoceptive stimuli (full bladder or rectum). The afferent branches of the reflexogenic reflex arc are the pudendal and pelvic nerves. The efferent pathway is a parasympathetic outflow (nervi erigentes) from the sacral cord, S_2–S_4. Most researchers have concluded that erections are mediated psychogenically by the sympathetic nervous system and reflexogenically by the parasympathetic system and that both pathways involve cholinergic transmission.[39,323] However, the evidence for this is far from conclusive. Atropine does not block human erections,[236] and acetylcholine does not produce erections in laboratory animals.[324,325] Choline acetyltransferase has not been found in penile erectile tissue, whereas norepinephrine has been found in such tissue.[326] Similarly, only a small number of acetylcholinesterase-positive fibers have been found in human penile tissue.[327] The hemodynamics of erection are also unclear. Blood from the internal pudendal arteries fills the erectile tissue of the two corpora cavernosa and the corpus spongiosum to produce tumescence. Detumescence occurs when blood is shunted into the veins. This shunting process is under control of the autonomic nervous system. Erection has been hypothesized to result when smooth-muscle valvelike structures (polsters) located at the anastomoses between the arterioles and vascular spaces in the erectile tissue of the penis relax;[323] however, the existence of these structures has been questionned.[328] The role of venous constriction in the erectile process is similarly unclear. There is minimal evidence concerning central mechanisms regulating sexual arousal and performance. Experiments in laboratory animals suggest that there is reciprocal control of sexual behavior, with brain serotonin pathways inhibiting and brain dopamine pathways facilitating sexual behavior.[78,329] However, the evidence for this mechanism in the human is less clear.

Ejaculation can be conceptualized as consisting of three stages: emission, bladder neck closure, and true ejaculation. Emission consists of release of the ejaculate into the pelvic urethra and is caused by contraction of the vas deferens, seminal vesicles, and smooth muscle of the prostate. The efferent outflow mediating emission is from the sympathetic nervous system thoracolumbar outflow. These fibers travel with the hypogastric nerve and synapse in ganglia close to the innervated organs. Thus, these fibers belong to a specific group of adrenergic fibers known as the short adrenergic neurons. They also appear to belong to the alpha-adrenergic system. Bladder neck closure, preventing retrograde ejaculation, is transmitted over similar pathways.[39, p 159] Ejaculation proper occurs when rhythmic contractions of the bulbocavernosus, ischiocavernosus, and urethral muscles are stimulated by impulses from the perineal branch of the pudendal nerve.

Current knowledge suggests various mechanisms by which pharmacological agents might interfere with sexual function. Some drugs cross the blood–brain barrier and thus might influence central mechanisms controlling both libido and sexual performance. Agents with central dopamine-blocking activity (e.g., neuroleptics), agents that modify brain serotonin levels (e.g., antidepressants), and agents with central sympathetic inhibition (e.g., clonidine) might interfere with sexual function by this mechanism. The role of central cholinergic pathways in sexual function is unknown at present. Pharmacological agents often have central as well as peripheral anticholinergic effects. Sexual libido might be influenced by the direct central actions mentioned previously. However, there are other mechanisms by which libido might be affected. Many pharmacological agents (e.g., carbonic anhydrase inhibitors) cause dysphoria and general malaise, which may have an indirect effect on libido. Certain agents (e.g., cimetidine, spironolactone, digoxin, methadone) have been suspected to interfere with androgen and estrogen production metabolism and thus could exert an antilibido effect via this mechanism. Other agents (e.g., neuroleptics, cimetidine) influence prolactin secretion, and it is well established that decreased libido is associated with elevated serum prolactin levels. In this regard, it is of note that it has been reported that sexual dysfunction associated with antipsychotic medication is associated with elevated prolactin levels.[330]

Although erectile function is mediated by the autonomic nervous system, the specific neurotransmitters involved remain unclear. Numerous pharmacological agents associated with erectile dysfunction have significant anticholinergic side effects. Gross[331] reported that impotence associated with MAOI was relieved by the addition of bethanechol, a cholinergic drug. However, Shen and Mallya[332] reported that impotence associated with neuroleptics was relieved by benztropine, an anticholinergic agent. Nurnberg and Ambrosini[333] noted that urinary incontinence and impotence are associated with neuroleptic drugs and have been attributed to anticholinergic activity of these drugs. They reported that drug-induced urinary incontinence is not relieved by anticholinergic agents. As previously reviewed, the evidence for acetylcholine as the major peripheral neurotransmitter involved in penile erection is far from conclusive. Histamine and noradrenaline[326] have been proposed as the effective neurotransmitter. The role of beta receptors in erectile function is also unclear.

Drug-induced ejaculatory impairment has been routinely attributed to the peripheral alpha-adrenergic blocking activity of numerous pharmacological agents (e.g., thioridazine, phenoxybenzamine). Shenoy[334] noted the frequent lack of association between the symptoms of enuresis and inhibited ejaculation in patients on neuroleptics. Both these problems have been attributed to drug-induced alpha-adrenergic blockade. The frequent independence of these complaints suggested that more than alpha-adrenergic blockade might be needed to explain these effects. Nakanishi and Kaneko[335] reported that thioridazine and chlorpromazine were equally effective in depressing the contractile response of rabbit vas deferens. Noting

that thioridazine interferes with ejaculation far more frequently than chlorpromazine, they speculated that thioridazine-induced ejaculatory failure
may be due to more than just its peripheral adrenergic inhibition.

CONCLUSION

Clearly, a wide variety of pharmacological agents have been reported
to be associated with sexual disturbances in the male. Unfortunately, the
paucity of adequately designed studies in this area makes definitive statements about these associations impossible. The number of such reports
suggests that male sexual function is highly susceptible to interference
from commonly prescribed drugs. This is an area that clearly merits further
study utilizing sound methodology.

REFERENCES

1. Benedek TG: Aphrodisiacs: Facts and fable. *Med Aspects Hum Sexuality* 5:42–45, 1971
2. Brown-Sequard CE: Des effets produits chez l'homme par des injections sauscutanees d'un liquide retine des testicules frais de cubaze et de chien. *Seane Soci Biol* 1:420–430, 1889
3. Davidson JM, Kwan M, Greenleaf WF: Hormonal replacement and sexuality in men. *Clin Endocrinol Metab* 11:599, 1982
4. Bremer J: Asexualization: A follow-up study of 244 cases. New York, Macmillan, 1959
5. Segraves RT, Schoenberg HW, Ivanoff J: Serum testosterone and prolactin levels in erectile dysfunction. *J Sex Marital Ther* 9:19–26, 1973
6. Bancroft J: Endocrinology of sexual function. *Clin Obstet Gynecol* 7:253, 1980
7. Gessa GL, Tagliamonte A: Role of brain monoamines in male sexual behavior. *Life Sci* 14:425–436, 1974
8. Gessa GL, Tagliamonte A: Role of brain serotonin and dopamine in male sexual behavior, in Sandler M, Gessa GL (eds): *Sexual Behavior: Pharmacology and Biochemistry.* New York, Raven Press, 1975
9. Goodwin FK: Behavioral effects of L-dopa in man, in Shader R (ed): *Psychiatric Complications of Medical Drugs.* New York, Raven Press, 1972
10. O'Brien CP, DiGiacomo JN, Fahn S, et al: Mental effects of high-dosage levodopa. *Arch Gen Psychiatry* 24:61–72, 1971
11. Angrist B, Gershon S: Clinical effects of amphetamine and L-dopa on sexuality and aggression. *Compr Psychiatry* 17:715–722, 1976
12. Brogden RN, Speight TM, Avery GS: Levodopa—Review of its pharmacological properties and therapeutic uses with particular reference to parkinsonism. *Drugs* 2:257–409, 1971
13. Hallstrom T, Persson T: L-dopa and non-emission of semen. *Lancet* 1:1231–1232, 1970
14. Thorner MO, Besser GM: Hyperprolactinaemia and gonadal function: Results of brom-ocriptine treatment, in Crosignani PG, Robyn C (eds): *Prolactin and Human Reproduction.* London, Academic Press, 1977
15. Carter JN, Tyson JE, Tolis G, et al: Prolactin-secreting tumors and hypogonadism in 22 men. *N Engl J Med* 229:847–851, 1978

16. Pierini AA, Nusimovich B: Male diabetic sexual impotence: Effects of dopaminergic agents. *Arch Androl* 6:347–350, 1981
17. Ambrosi B, Bara R, Travaglini P, et al: Study of the effects of bromocriptine on sexual impotence. *Clin Endocrinol* 7:417–421, 1977
18. Sicuteri F: Serotonin and sex in man. *Pharmacol Res Communi* 4:403–411, 1974
19. Sicuteri F, Bene ED, Anselmi B: Aphrodisiac effects of testosterone in parachloro-phenylalnine-treated sexually deficient men, in Sandler M, Gessa GL (eds): *Sexual Behavior: Pharmacology and Biochemistry.* New York, Raven Press, 1985
20. Ambrosi B, Travaglini P, Gaggini M, et al: Effects of serotonin antagonists in sexually impotent men. *Andrologia* 6;475–477, 1979
21. Masters WH, Johnson VE: *Human Sexual Response.* Boston, Little Brown, 1966
22. Kaplan HS: *The New Sex Therapy.* New York, Brunner/Mazel, 1974
23. Farkas GM, Rosen RC: Effects of alcohol on elicited male sexual response. *J Stud Alcohol* 37:265, 1976
24. Bridell DW, Wilson JT: Effect of alcohol and expectancy set on male sexual arousal. *J Abnorm Psychol* 85:225–234, 1976
25. Abel EL: A review of alcohol's effects on sex and reporduction. *Drug Alcohol Dependence* 5:321–332, 1980
26. Lemere F, Smith JW: Alcohol-induced sexual impotence. *Am J Psychiatry* 130:212–213, 1973
27. Whalley LJ: Sexual adjustment of male alcoholics. *Acta Psychiatr Scand* 58:281–288, 1978
28. Akhtar MJ: Sexual disorders in male alcoholics, in Madden JS, Walker R, Kenyon WH (eds): *Alcoholism and Drug Dependence. A Multidisciplinary Approach.* New York, Plenum Press, 1977
29. Malatesta VJ, Pollack RH, Wilbanks WA, et al: Alcohol effects on the orgasmic-ejac-ulatory response in human males. *J Sex Res* 2:101–107, 1979
30. Hart BL: Effects of alcohol on sexual reflexes and mating behavior in the male rat. *Psychopharmacologia* 14:377–382, 1969
31. Sheldon CH, Bors E: Subarachnoid alcohol block in paraplegia: Its beneficial effect on mass reflexes and bladder dysfunction. *J Neuro Surg* 5:385–391, 1948
32. Novak DJ, Victor M: The vagus and sympathetic nerves in alcoholic polyneuropathy. *Arch Neurol* 30:273–284, 1974
33. Hollister LE: Drugs and sexual behavior in man. *Life Sci* 17:661–666, 1975
34. Kolodny RC, Masters WH, Kolodner RM, et al: Depression of plasma testosterone levels after chronic intensive marijuana use. *N Engl J Med* 290:872, 1974
35. Mendelson JH, Kuehnle L, Ellinbgo J: Plasma testosterone levels before during and after chronic marijuana smoking. *N Engl J Med* 291:1051, 1974
36. Oaks WW, Moyer JH: Sex and hypertension. *Med Aspects Hum Sexuality* 61:128–137, 1972
37. Berman EM, Lief HI: Sex and the aging process, in Paks WW, Melchiode GA, Ficher I (eds): *Sex and the Life Cycle.* New York, Grune & Stratton, 1976
38. McMahon FG: *Management of Essential Hypertension.* Mount Kisco, New York, Futura, 1978
39. Segraves RT: Pharmacological agents causing sexual dysfunction. *J Sex Marital Ther* 3:157–176, 1977
40. Munjack DJ: Sex and drugs. *Clin Toxicol* 15:75–89, 1979
41. Mills LC: Drug-induced impotence. *Am Fam Physician* 12:104–106, 1975
42. Horowitz JD, Goble AJ: Drugs and impaired male sexual function. *Drugs* 18:206–217, 1979
43. Story NL: Sexual dysfunction resulting from drug sale effects. *J Sex Res* 10:132–149, 1974
44. Hogan MJ, Wallin JD, Baer RM: Antihypertensive therapy and male sexual dysfunction. *Psychosomatics* 12:234–237, 1980

45. Keidan H: Impotence during antihypertensive treatment. *Can Med Assoc J* 114:874, 1976
46. Boyden TW, Nugent CA, Ogihara T, et al: Reserpine hydrochlorothiazide and pituitary-gonadal hormones in hypertensive patients. *Eur J Clin Pharmacol* 17:329–332, 1980
47. Yendt ER, Gray GF, Garcia DA: The use of thiazides in the prevention of renal calculi. *Can Med Assoc J* 102:614–620, 1970
48. Stressman J, Ben-Ishay D: Chlorthalidone-induced impotence. *Br Med J* 281:714, 1980
49. Pillay VKG: Some side-effects of alpha-methyldopa. *S Afr Med J* 50:625–626, 1976
50. Medical Research Council working party on mild to moderate hypertension. *Lancet* 2:539–542, 1981
51. Bulpitt CJ, Dollery CT: Side-effects of hypotensive agents evaluated by a self-administered questionnaire. *Br Med J* 3:485–490, 1973
52. Slag MF, Morley JE, Elson MK, et al: Impotence in medical clinical outpatients. *JAMA* 249:1736–1740, 1983
53. Papadopoulos C: Cardiovascular drugs and sexuality. *Arch Intern Med* 140:1341–1345, 1980
54. Loriaux DL, Menard R, Taylor A, et al: Spironolactone and endocrine dysfunction. *Ann Intern Med* 85:630–636, 1976
55. Spark RF, Melby JC: Aldosteronism in hypertension. *Ann Intern Med* 69:685–691, 1968
56. Zarren HS, Black PM: Unilateral gynecomastia and impotence during low-dose sporonolactone administration in men. *Mili Med* 140:417–419, 1975
57. Brown J, Davies DL, Ferriss JB, et al: Comparison of surgery and prolonged spironolactone therapy in patients with hypertension, aldosterone excess, and low plasma renin. *Br Med J* 1:729–734, 1972
58. Greenblatt DJ, Koch-Weser J: Gynecomastia and impotence complications of spironlactone therapy. *JAMA* 233:82, 1973
59. Frohlich ED: Adrenergic inhibiting drugs, Hunt JC, Cooper T, Frohlich ED (eds): in *Hypertension Update: Mechanisms, Epidemiology, Evaluation, Management.* Bloomfield, New Jersey, Health Learning Systems, 1980
60. Johnson P, Kitchin AH, Lowther CP, et al: Treatment of hypertension with methyldopa. *Br Med J* 1:133–137, 1966
61. Newman RJ, Salerno HR: Sexual dysfunction due to methyldopa. *Br Med J* 4:106, 1974
62. Dollery CT, Harington M: Methyldopa in hypertension. *Lancet* 1:759–763, 1962
63. Horwitz D, Pettinger WA, Oruis H, et al: Effects of methyldopa in fifty hypertensive patients. *Clin Pharmacol Thera* 8:224–234, 1967
64. Mroczer WJ, Leibel BA, Finnerty FA: Comparison of clonidine and methyldopa in hypertensive patients receiving a diuretic. *Am J Cardiol* 29:712–717, 1972
65. Vejlsgaard V, Christensen M, Clasen E: Double-blind trial of four hypotensive drugs (methyldopa and three sympatholytic agents). *Br Med J* 2:598–600, 1967
66. Prichard BNC, Johnston AW, Hill Id, et al: Bethanidine guanethidine, and methyldopa in treatment of hypertension: A within-patient comparison. *Br Med J* 1:135–144, 1968
67. Bauer GE, Hull RD, Stokes GS, et al: The reversibility of side-effects of guanethidine therapy. *Med J Aust* 1:930–933, 1973
68. Laver MC: Sexual behavior patterns in male hypertensives. *Aust NZ J Med* 4:29–31, 1974
69. Lauwers P, Verstraete M, Joossen JV: Methyldopa in the treatment of hypertension. *Br Med J* 1:295–300, 1963
70. Bulpitt CJ, Dollery CT: Side effects of hypotensive agents evaluated by a self-administered questionnaire. *Br Med J* 1:485–490, 1973
71. VA Cooperative Study Group on Antihypertensive Agents: Propranolol in the treatment of essential hypertension. *JAMA* 237:2303–2310, 1977
72. Tuchman H, Crumptom CW: A comparison of Rauvolfia serpentia compounds cruderoot, alseroxylon derrivative and single alkoloid in the treatment of hypertension. *Am Heart J* 49:742–750, 1955

73. Girgis SM, Etriby A, El-Hefnawy H, et al: Aspermia: A survey of 49 cases. *Fertil Steril* 19:580–588, 1968
74. Sah HJ, Sah PPT, Peoples SA: The new antihypertensive agent, guanethidine—a review. *Arzneimittelforsch* 16:199–202, 1966
75. Evans B, Iwayama T, Burnstock G: Long-lasting hypersensitivity of the rat vas defers to norepinephrine after chronic guanethidine administration. *J Pharmacol Exp Ther* 185:60–69, 1973
76. Evans B, Gannon BJ, Heatin JW, et al: Long-lasting damage to the internal male genital organs and their adrenergic inervation in rats following chronic treatment with the antihypertensive drug guanethidine. *Fertil Steril* 23:657–667, 1972
77. Reudy J, Davies RO: A comparative clinical trial of guanoxan and guanethidine in essential hypertension. *Clin Pharmacol Ther* 8:38–47, 1967
78. Schinger A, Gifford RW: Guanethidine, a new antihypertensive agent: Experience in the treatment of patients with severe hypertension. *Mayo Clin Proc* 37:100–108, 1962
79. Seedat YK, Pillay VKG: Further experiences with guanethidine—a clinical assessment of 103 patients. *S Afr Med J* 40:140–143, 1966
80. Eagen JT, Orgain ES: A study of 38 patients and their response to guanethidine. *JAMA* 1975:550–553, 1961
81. Brown WJ, FIK: The use of guanethidine and hydrochlorothiazide in the long-term treatment of essential hypertension. *Curr Ther Res* 17:544–554, 1975
82. Lowther CP, Turner RW: Guanethidine in the treatment of hypertension. *Br Med J* 2:776–781, 1963
83. Bauer GE, Croll FJT, Goldrick RB, et al: Guanethidine in treatment of hypertension. *Br Med J* 2:410–415, 1961
84. Oats JA, Seligmann AW, Clark MA, et al: The relative efficacy of guanethidine, methydopa, and pargyline as antihypertensive agents. *N Engl J Med* 273:729–734, 1965
85. Page IH, Hurley RE, Dustan HP: The prolonged treatment of hypertension with guanethidine. *JAMA* 175:543–549, 1961
86. Raftos J, Bauer GE, Lewis RG, et al: Clonidine in the treatment of severe hypertension. *Med J Aust* 30:786–793, 1973
87. Saunders E, Kong B: Sexual activity in male hypertensive patients while taking clonidine. *Urban Health* 9:22–26, 1980
88. Amery A, Verstraete M, Bossaert H, et al: Hypotensive action and side effects of clonidine–chlorthalidone and methyldopa–chlorthalidone in treatment of hypertension. *Br Med J* 4:392–395, 1970
89. MacDougall AI, Addis GJ, MacKay N, et al: Treatment of hypertension with clonidine. *Br Med J* 3:440–443, 1970
90. Ebringer A, Doyle AE, Dawborn JK, et al: The use of clonidine (catapres) in the treatment of hypertension. *Med J Aust* 1:524–526, 1970
91. Khan A, Camel G, Perry HM: Clonidine (catapres): A new antihypertensive agent. *Curr Ther Res* 12:10–18, 1970
92. Onesti G, Bock KD, Heimsoth V, et al: Clonidine: A new antihypertensive agent. *Am J Cardiol* 28:74–83, 1971
93. Miller RA: Propranolol and impotence. *Ann Intern Med* 85,683:683, 1976
94. Knarr JW: Impotence from propranolol. *Ann Intern Med* 85:295, 1976
95. Gavras I, Gavras H, Sullivan PC, et al: A comparative study of the effects of oxpernolol versus propranolol in essential hypertension. *J Clin Pharmacol* 19:8–14, 1979
96. Husserl FE, Messerli FH: Adverse effects of antihypertensive drugs. *Drugs* 22:188–210, 1981
97. Bathen J: Propranolol erectile dysfunction relieved. *Ann Intern Med* 88:716–717, 1978
98. Forsberg L, Gustauvil B, Hojerbach T, et al: Impotence, smoking, and B-blocking drugs. *Fertil Steril* 31:589–591, 1979

99. Burnett W, Chaline R: Sexual dysfunction as a complaint of propanolol therapy in men. *Cardiovasc Med* 4:811–815, 1979

100. Serlin MS, Orme M, Baber N, et al: Propranolol in the control of blood pressure. *Clin Pharmacol Ther* 27:586–592, 1980

101. Warren SG, Brewer DL, Orgain ES: Long-term propranolol therapy for angina pectoris. *Am J Cardiol* 37:420–426, 1976

102. Warren SC, Warren SG: Propranolol and sexual impotence. *Ann Intern Med* 86:112, 1977

103. Hollifield JW, Sherman K, Zwagg RU, et al: Proposed mechanisms of propranolol's antihypertensive effect in essential hypertension. *N Engl J Med* 295:68–73, 1976

104. Greminger P, Vetter HH, Boerlin HJ, et al: A comparative study between 100 mg atenolol and 20 mg pindolol slow-release in essential hypertension. *Drugs* 25(supp 12):36–41, 1983

105. Ambrosioni E, Costa FV, Montebugnoli L, et al: Comparison of antihypertensive efficacy of atenolol, oxprenolol and pindolol at rest and during exercise. *Drugs* 25(suppl 2):30–36, 1983

106. Heel RC, Brodgen RN, Speight TM, et al: Atenolol: A review of its pharmacological properties and therapeutic efficacy in angina pectoris and hypertension. *Drugs* 17:425–460, 1979

107. Osborne DR: Propranolol and Peyronie's disease. *Lancet* 1:1111, 1977

108. Wallis AA, Bell R. Sutherland PW: Propranolol and Peyronie's disease. *Lancet* 1:980, 1977

109. Law MR, Copeland RFP, Armistad JG, et al: Lebetalol and priapism. *Br Med J* 1:115, 1980

110. Keidan H: Impotence during antihypertensive treatment. *J Can Med Assoc* 114:874, 1976

111. Ahmad S: Hydralazine and male impotence. *Chest* 78:358, 1980

112. Jandhyala BS, Clarke DE, Buckely JP: The effects of prolonged administration of certain antihypertensive agents. *J Pharmacol Sci* 63:1497–1513, 1974

113. Vlachakis ND, Mendlowitz M: Alpha and beta-adrenergic receptor blocking agents combined with a diuretic in the treatment of essential hypertension. *J Clin Pharmacol* 111:352–360, 1976

114. Lowew S, Puttuck SL: Anti-ejaculatory effect of sympatholytic gangliolytic and spasmolytic drugs. *J Pharmacol Exp Ther* 107:379–384, 1953

115. Green M, Berman S: Failure of ejaculation produced by dibenzyline. *Conn State Med J* 18:30–34, 1954

116. Caine M, Perlberg S, Shapiro A: Phenoxybenzamine for benign prostatic obstruction. *Urology* 17:542–546, 1981

117. Kedia KR, Persky L: Effect of phenoxybenzamine (Dibenzyline) on sexual function in man. *Urology* 18:620–622, 1981

118. Kedia K, Markland C: Effect of sympathectomy and drugs on ejaculation, in Sciarra JJ, Markland C, Speidel JJ (eds): *Control of Male Fertility.* Hagerstown, Maryland, Harper & Row, 1975

119. Peart WS, MacMahan MT: Clinical trial of 2-guanidinomethylc (1,4) benzodioxan (compound 1003) *Br Med J* 1:398–402, 1964

120. Lawrie TDV, Lorimer AR, McAlpine DSG, et al: Clinical trial and pharmacological study of compound 1029 ("vatensol"). *Br Med J* 1:402–406, 1964

121. Brogen RN, Heel RC, Speight TM, et al: Prazosin: A review of its pharmacological properties and therapeutic efficacy in hypertension. *Drugs* 14:163–197

122. Stokes GS, Oates HF: Prazosin: New alpha-adrenergic blocking agent in treatment of hypertension. *Cardiovasc Med* 3:41–57, 1978

123. Amery A, Verhiest W, Croonenberghs J, et al: Double-blind crossover study with a

new vasodilator-prazosin-in the treatment of mild hypertension. *Exerpta Med Int Congress Series* 331:100–110, 1974

124. Kochar M, Zeller J, Itskovitz H: Prazosin in hypertension with and without methyldopa. *Clin Pharmacol Ther* 25:143–148, 1979

125. Pitts NE: A clinical evaluation of prazosin, a new antihypertensive agent. *Postgrad Med* 58:117–127, 1975

126. Moser M, Prandoni AG, Orbison JA, et al: Clinical experience with sympathetic blocking agents in peripheral vascular disease. *Ann Intern Med* 38:1245–1246, 1953

127. Pentland B, Anderson DA, Critchley JAJ: Failure of ejaculation with indoramin. *Br Med J* 282:1433–1434, 1981

128. Lewis PJ, George CJ, Dollery CT: Clinical evaluation of indoramin, a new antihypertensive agent. *Eur J Clin Pharmacol* 6:211–216, 1973

129. Faerchtein I, Roque AF, Kastansky I, et al: A placebo controlled trial of the alpha-blocker, indoramin, in the treatment of arterial hypertension. *Curr Med Res Opinion* 3:675–684, 1976

130. Hollister LE: Drugs and sexual behavior in man. *Life Sci* 17:661–667, 1977

131. Mitchell JE, Popkin MK: Antipsychotic drug therapy and sexual dysfunction in men. *Am J Psychiatry* 139, 633–637, 1982

132. Zaratzian VL: Psychotropic drugs-neurotoxicity. *Clin Toxicol* 17:231–270, 1980

133. Barnes TRE, Bamber RWK, Watson JP: Psychotropic drugs and sexual behavior. *Br J Hosp Med* 12:594–599, 1979

134. Nestoros JN, Lehmann HE: Neuroleptics and male sexual dysfunction. *Int Drug Ther Newsletter* 14:21–23, 1979

135. Laughren T, Brown W, Petrucci J: Effects of thioridazine on serum testosterone. *Am J Psychiatry* 135:982–984, 1978

136. Amdur M: Confirming a side effect. *Am J Psychiatry* 133:864, 1976

137. Sandison RA, Whitelaw E, Currie JDC: Clinical trails with Mellaril (TP21) in the treatment of schizophrenia. *J Ment Sci* 106:732–741, 1960

138. Freyhan FA: Loss of ejaculation during Mellanil treatment. *Am J Psychiatry* 118:171–172, 1961

139. Haider I: Thioridazine and sexual dysfunctions. *Int J Neuropsychiatry* 2:255–257, 1962

140. Shader RI: Sexual dysfunction associated with thioridazine hydrochloride. *JAMA* 188:1007–1009, 1964

141. Clein L: Thioridazine and ejaculation. *Br Med J* 2:548–549, 1962

142. Datshkovsky J: Mellaril: Ejaculation disorders. *Am J Psychiatry* 118:564, 1961

143. Singh H: A case of inhibition of ejaculation as a side effect of Mellaril. *Am J Psychiatry* 117:1041, 1961

144. Singh H: Therapeutic use of thioridazine in premature ejaculation. *Am J Psychiatry* 119:891, 1963

145. Witton K: Sexual dysfunction secondary to Mellaril. *Dis Nerv Syst* 23:175, 1962

146. Shader RI: Ejaculation disorders, in Shader RI, DiMascio A (eds): *Psychotropic Drug Side Effects.* Baltimore, Williams & Wilkins Co., 1970

147. Mellgren A: Treatment of ejaculatio praecox with thioridazine *Psychother Psychosom* 15:454–460, 1967

148. Money J, Yankowitz, R., The sympathetic-inhibiting effects of the drug Ismelin on human male eroticism, with a note on Mellaril. *J Sex Res* 3:69–82, 1967

149. Taubel DE: Mellaril: Ejaculation disorders. *Am J Psychiatry* 119:87, 1962

150. Greenberg HR, Carrillo C: Thioridazine-induced inhibition of mastubatory ejaculation in an adolescent. *Am J Psychiatry* 124:991–993, 1968

151. Heaton-Ward WA: The present position of the use of tranquilizers in psychiatric patients. *Curr Med Drugs* 6:14–20, 1965

152. Heller J: Another case of inhibition of ejaculation as a side effect of Mellaril. *Am J Psychiatry* 118:173, 1961
153. Green M: Inhibition of ejaculation as a side effect of Mellaril. *Am J Psychiatry* 118:172–173, 1961
154. Shader R, Grinspoon L: Schizophrenia, oligospermia, and the phenothiazines. *Dis Nerv Syst* 28:240–244, 1967
155. Kotin J, Wilbert DE, Verburg D, et al: Thioridazine and sexual dysfunction. *Am J Psychiatry* 133:82–85, 1976
156. Quershi MS: Thioridazine and ejaculation. *Medicus (Kanachi)* 15:39, 1962
157. Dorman BW, Schmidt JD: Association of priapism in phenothiazine therapy. *J Urol* 116:51–53, 1976
158. Dahl DS, Middleton RG: Comparison between cavernoscephenous and cavernospongiosum shunting in the treatment of idiopathic priapism: A report of 5 operations. *J Urol* 112:614, 1974
159. Schmidt JD: Intracorporal shunt procedures for priapism. *Arch Surg* 103:409, 1971
160. Shengy RS: Nocturnal enuresis caused by psychotropic drugs. *Am J Psychiatry* 137:739–740, 1980
161. Greenberg HR: Inhibition of ejaculation by chlorpromazine. *J Nerv Ment Dis* 152:364–366, 1971
162. Bolelovcky Z: Chlorpromazine inhibition of ejaculation. *Act Nerv Super (Praha)* 7:245, 1965
163. Tennett G, Bancroft J, Cass J: The control of deviant sexual behavior by drugs: A double-blind controlled study of benperidol, chlorpromazine and placebo. *Arch Sex Behav* 3:261–271, 1974
164. Dawson-Butterworth K: Idiopathic priapism associated with schizophrenia. *Br J Clin Pract* 23:125–126, 1969
165. Meiraz D, Fishelovitch J: Priaspism and largactil medication. *Isr J Med Sci* 51:1254–1255, 1969
166. Larocque MA, Cosgrove MD: Priapism: A review of 46 cases. *J Urol* 112:770–773, 1974
167. Bastecky J, Gregova L: Priapism as a possible complication of the chlorpromazine treatment. *Activ Nerv Supp* 16:175, 1974
168. Dawson-Butterworth K: Priapism and phenothiazines. *Br Med J* 4:118, 1970
169. Merkin TE: Priapism as a sequela of chlorpromazine therapy. *JACEP* 6:367–368, 1977
170. Ditman KS: Inhibition of ejaculation by chloroprothixine. *Am J Psychiatry* 120:1004–1005, 1964
171. Shader RI: Sexual dysfunction associated with mesoridazine besylate (Serentil). *Psychopharmacologia* 27:293–294, 1972
172. Gottlieb JI, Lustberg T: Phenothiazine-induced priapism: A case report. *Am J Psychiatry* 134:1445–1446, 1977
173. Bartholomew AA: A long-acting phenothiazine as a possible agent to control deviant sexual behavior. *Am J Psychiatry* 124:77–83, 1968
174. Dillon JB, Bates TJN: Fluphenazine enanthate in the maintenance treatment of schizophrenia. *Br Med J* 2:1328, 1966
175. Charalampous KD, Freemesser GF, Malev J, et al: Loxapine succinate: A controlled double-blind study in schizophrenia. *Curr Ther Res* 16:829–837, 1974
176. Goldstein B, Weiner D, Banas F: Clinical evaluation of thiothixine in chronic ambulatory schizophrenic patients, in Lehmann HE, Bann TA (eds): *The Thioxanthenes: Modern Problems in Pharmacopsychiatry*, Volume 2. New York, Kargen, 1969
177. Blair JH, Simpson GM: Effects of antipsychotic drugs on reproductive functions. *Dis Nerv Syst* 27:645–647, 1966
178. Berger SH: Trifluoperazine and haloperidol: Sources of ejaculatory pain. *Am J Psychiatry* 136:350, 1979

179. Bors E, Comarr AE: Neurological disturbances of sexual function with special reference to 529 patients with spinal cord injury. *Urol Rev* 10:191–222, 1960

180. Wyatt RJ, Fram DH, Buchbinder R, et al: Treatment of intractable narcolepsy with a monoamine oxidase inhibitor. *N Eng J Med* 285:987–991, 1971

181. Friedman S, Kantor I, Sobel S, et al: A follow-up study on the chemotherapy of neurodermatitis with a monoamine oxidase inhibitor. *J Nerv Ment Dis* 166:349–357, 1978

182. Hollander MH, Ban TA: Ejaculatio retarda due to phenelzine. *Psychiatr J Univ Ottawa* 4:233–234, 1980

183. Rapp MS: Two cases of ejaculatory impairment related to phenelzine. *Am J Psychiatry* 136:1200–1201, 1979

184. Glass RM: Ejaculatory impairment from both phenelzine and imipramine with tinnitus from phenelzine. *J Clin Psychopharmacol* 1:152–154, 1981

185. Blair JH, Simpson GM, Kline KS: Monoamine oxidase inhibitor and sperm production. *JAMA* 181:182, 1962

186. Davis J, Clyman MJ, Decker A, et al: Effect of phenelzine on semen in infertility: A preliminary report. *Fertil Steril* 17:221–225, 1966

187. Kohn RM: Nocturnal orthostatic syncope in pargyline therapy. *JAMA* 187:229, 1964

188. Simpson GM, Blair JH, Amuso D: Effects of anti-depressants on genitourinary function. *Dis Nerv Syst* 26:787–789, 1965

189. Bennett D: Treatment of ejaculatio praecox with monoamine-oxidase inhibitors. *Lancet* 1:1309, 1961

190. Everett HC: The use of bethanechol chloride with tricyclic antidepressants. *Am J Psychiatry* 132:1202–1204, 1975

191. Couper-Smartt JD, Rodham R: A technique for surveying side-effects of tricyclic drugs with reference to reported sexual effects. *J Int Med Res* 1:473–476, 1973

192. Greenberg HR: Erectile impotence during the course of Tofranil therapy. *Am J Psychiatry* 121:1021, 1965

193. Ruskin DB, Goldner RD: Treatment of depressions in private practice with imipramine. *Dis Nerv Syst* 20:391–399, 1959

194. Kahn MAM: Side effects of amitriptyline. *Br Med J* 3:708, 1975

195. Hekimian LJ, Friedhoft AJ, Deever E: A comparison of the onset of action and therapeutic efficacy of amoxapine and amitriptyline. *J Clin Psychiatry* 39:633–637, 1978

196. Nininger JE: Inhibition of ejaculation by amitriptyline. *Am J Psychiatry* 135:750–751, 1978

197. Beaumont G: Sexual side-effects of clomipramine (Anafranil). *J Int Med Res* 5 (suppl):37–44, 1977

198. Beaumont G: Side-effects of toxicity of clomipramine. *Br J Clin Pract* (suppl 3):51–53, 1979

199. Lasich AJ: Clinical evidence of a new antidepressant. *Med Proc, Mediesae Bydiaes* 14:312–317, 1968

200. Wootten LW, Bailey RI: Experiences with clomipramine (Anafranil) in the treatment of the phobic anxiety states in general practice. *J Int Med Res* 3(suppl 1):101–107, 1975

201. Yassa R: Sexual disorders in the course of clomipramine treatment: A report of three cases. *Can J Psychiatry* 27:148–149, 1982

202. Clarke FC: The treatment of depression in general practice. *S Afr Med J* 43:724–725, 1969

203. Anath J, Pechnold JC, Steern NVD, et al: Double-blind comparative study of chlorimipramine in obsessive nerosis. *Curr Ther Res* 25:703–709, 1979

204. Eaton H: Clomipramine (Anafranil) in the treatment of premature ejaculation. *J Int Med Res* 1:432–434, 1973

205. Waxman DA: A general practitioner trial of clomipramine (Anafranil) in obsessions and phobias. *J Int Med Res* 3(suppl 1):94–100, 1975

206. McLean JD, Forsythe RG, Kapkin IA: Unusual side-effect of clomipramine associated with yawning. *Can J Psychiatry* 28:569–570, 1983

207. Schwarcz G: Case report of inhibition of ejaculation and retrograde ejaculation as side-effects of amoxapine. *Am J Psychiatry* 139:233–234, 1982
208. Kulik FA, Wilbur R: Case report of painful ejaculation as a side effect of amoxapine. *Am J Psychiatry* 139:234–235, 1982
209. Shen WW: Female orgasmic inhibition by amoxapine. *Am J Psychiatry* 139:1221, 1982
210. Getzoff PL: Psychotropic drug induced male infertility: A case report. *Infertility* 1:53–58, 1978
211. Vinarova E, Uhlir O, Stika L, et al: Side-effects of lithium administration. *Activitas Nervosa Supperior (Praha)* 14:105–107, 1972
212. Scher M, Krieger JN, Jvergens S: Trazodone and priapism. *Am J Psychiatry* 140:1362–1363, 1983
213. Blay SL, Ferraz MPT, Calil HM: Lithium-induced male sexual impairment: Two case reports. *J Clin Psychiatry* 43:497–498, 1982
214. Magnus RV, Dean BC, Curry SH: Clorazepate: Double-blind crossover comparison of a single nightly dose with diazepam thrice daily in anxiety. *Dis Nerv Syst* 38:317–321, 1977
215. General Practitioner Research Group: A single-dose anti-anxiety drug. *Practitioner* 215:98–l0l, 1975
216. Usdin GL: Preliminary report on librium, a new psychopharmacologic agent. *J Louisiana State Med Soc* 112:142–147, 1960
217. Hughes JM: Failure to ejaculate with chlordiazepoxide. *Am J Psychiatry* 121:610–611, 1964
218. Biron P: Diminished libido with cimetidine therapy. *Can Med Assoc J* 121:404–405, 1979
219. Gifford LM, Aevgle ME, Myerson RM, et al: Cimetidine postmarket outpatient surveillance program. *JAMA* 243:1532–1536, 1980
220. Wolfe MM: Impotence of cimetidine treatment. *N Engl J Med* 300:94, 1979
221. Peden NR, Cargill JM, Browning MCK, et al: Male sexual dysfunction during treatment with cimetidine. *Br Med J* 1:659, 1979
222. Hall WW: Breast changes in males on cimitidine. *N Engl J Med* 295:841, 1976
223. Carlson HE, Ippoliti AF: Cimetidine, an H_2-antihistamine, stimulates prolactin secretion in man. *J Clin Endocrinol Metab* 45:367–370, 1977
224. Adaikan PG, Karim SMM: Male sexual dysfunction during treatment with cimetidine. *Br Med J* 1:1282, 1283, 1979
225. Neri A, Aygen M, Zuckerman Z, et al: Subjective assessment of sexual dysfunction of patients on long-term administration of digoxin. *Arch Sexual Behav* 9:343–347, 1980
226. Lewinn EB: Gynecomastia during digitalis therapy. *N Engl J Med* 248:316–320, 1953
227. Navab A, Koss LG, LaDue JS: Estrogen-like activity of digitalis. *JAMA* 194:30–32, 1965
228. Stoffer SS, Hynes KM, Jiany NS, et al: Digoxin and abnormal serum hormone levels. *JAMA* 225:1643–1644, 1973
229. Duggan ML, Morgan C: Heparin: A cause of priapism? *South Med J* 63:1131–1134, 1970
230. Schneider J, Kaffarnik H: Impotence in patients treated with clofibrate. *Atherosclerosis* 21:455–457, 1975
231. Coronary Drug Project Research Group: Clofibrate and niacin in coronary heart disease. *JAMA* 231:360–380, 1975
232. McHaffie DJ, Guz A, Johnston A: Impotence in patient on disopyramide. *Lancet* 1:230, 1977
233. Admad S: Disopyramide and impotence. *South Med J* 73:958, 1980
234. Shader RI, Greenblatt DJ: Belladonna alkaloids and synthetic anticholinergic: Uses and

toxicity, in Shader RI (ed): *Psychiatric Complicationa of Medical Drugs*, New York, Raven Press, 1972

235. Schwartz NH, Robinson BD: Impotence due to methantheline bromide. *NY State J Med* 52:1530, 1952

236. Wagner G, Brindley GS: Effects of atropine on erection. Presented at *First Inter Conf Vas Impotence*, New York, 1978

237. Wagner G, Green R: *Impotence: Physiological, Psychological, Surgical diagnosis and treatment*. New York, Plenum Press, 1981.

238. Wagner G, Levin RJ: Effect of atropine and methylatropine on human vaginal blood flow, sexual arousal and climax. *Acta Pharmacol Toxicol* 46:321–325, 1980

239. Lichter PR, Newman LP, Wheeler NC, et al: Patient tolerance to carbonic anhydrase inhibitors. *Am J Opthalmol* 85:495,502, 1978

240. Wallace TR, Fraunfelder FT, Petursson GJ, et al: Decreased libido—a side effect of carbonic anhydrase inhibitor. *Ann Opthalmol* 11:1563–1566, 1979

241. Epstein DL, Grant WM: Carbonic anhydrase inhibitor side effects. *Arch Opthalmol* 95:1378–1382, 1977

242. Hedley DW, Maroun JA, Espir MLE: Evaluation of baclofer (Lioresal) for spasticity in multiple sclerosis. *Postgrad Med J* 51:615–618, 1975

243. Evans BE, Aledort LM: Inhibition of ejaculation due to epsilon aminocaproic acid. *N Engl J Med* 298:166–167, 1978

244. Carney DE, Tweddell ED: Double-blind evaluation of long acting diethylpropian by-drochloride in obese patients from a general practice. *Med J Aust* 1:13–15, 1975

245. Snyder S, Karacan I, Salis PJ: Disulfiram and nocturnal penile tumescence in the chronic alcoholic. *Biol Psychiatry* 16:399–406, 1981

246. Gale AS: Ketamine prevention of penile turgescence. *JAMA* 219:1629, 1972

247. Pietras JR, Cromie WJ, Duckett JW: Ketamine as a detumescence agent during hy-pospadias repair. *J of Urol* 121:654, 1979

248. Chapman RM, Rees LH, Sutcliffe SB, et al: Cyclic combination chemotherapy and gonadal function. *Lancet* 1:285–289, 1979

249. Shalet SM: Effects of cancer chemotherapy on gonadal function of patients. *Cancer Treatment Rev* 7:141–152, 1980

250. Thachil JV, Jewett MAS, Rider WD: The effects of cancer and cancer therapy on male fertility. *J Urol* 126:141–145, 1981

251. Schilsky RL, Lewis BJ, Sherins RJ, et al: Gonadal dysfunction in patients receiving chemotherapy for cancer. *Ann Intern Med* 93:109–114, 1980

252. Greenberg MS, Aisenberg AC, Arky RA: Gynecomastia after chemotherapy. *Clin Res* 27:386A, 1979

253. Buffin J: Pharmacosexology: The effects of drugs on sexual function. A review. *J Psychoactive Drugs* 14:5–44, 1982

254. Pinder RM, Brogden RN, Sawyer PR, et al: Fenfluramine: A review of its pharmacological properties and therapeutic efficacy in obesity. *Drugs* 10:241–323, 1982

255. Howard DJ,Rees JR: Long term perhexiline maleate and liver function. *Br Med J* 1:133, 1976

256. Pilcher J, Chandraseklhar KP, Rees JR, et al: Long-term assessment of perhixiline maleate in angina pectoris. *Postgrad Med J* (April suppl):11–118, 1973

257. Peck AW: Impotence in farm workers. *Br Med J* 1:690, 1970

258. Espir MLE, Hall JW, Schirreffs JG, et al: Impotence in farm workers using toxic chemicals. *Br Med J* 1:423–425, 1970

259. Layzer RB: Myeloneuropathy after prolonged exposure to nitrous oxide. *Lancet* 1:1227–1230, 1978

260. Schiavi RC, White D: Androgens and male sexual function: A review of human studies. *J Sex Marital Ther* 2:214–228, 1976

261. Segraves RT, Schoenberg HW, Ivanoff J: Serum testosterone and prolactin levels in erectile dysfunction. *J Sex Marital Ther* 9:19–26, 1983

262. Rose RM: The psychological effects of androgens and estrogens—A review, in Shader RI (ed): *Psychiatric Complications of Medical Drugs.* New York, Raven Press, 1972

263. Freund K: Therapeutic sex drive reduction. *Acta Psychiatr Scand* (suppl 287):5–38, 1980

264. Laschet U, Laschet L: Three years clinical results with cyproteroneacetate in the inhibiting regulation of male sexuality. *Acta Endocrinol* (suppl):138–183, 1969

265. Jeffcoate WJ, Matthews RW, Edwards CRW, et al: The effect of cyproterone acetate on serum testosterone, Lh, FSH, and prolactin in male sexual offenders. *Clin Endocrinol* 13:189–195, 1980

266. Boas CVE: Cyproteronecetate in sexuological outpatient practice. *Psychiatr Neurol Neurochir* 76:151–154, 1973

267. Bosch JJ: Manipulation of sexual behavior by anti-androgens. *Psychiatr Neurol Neurochir* 76:147–149, 1973

268. Bancroft J, Tennent G, Loucas K, et al: The control of deviant sexual behavior by drugs: 1, Behavioral changes following oestrogens and antiandrogens. *Br J Psychiatry* 125:310–315, 1974

269. Cooper AJ, Ismail AA, Phanjoo AL, et al: Antiandrogen (cyprotone acetate) therapy in deviant hypersexuality. *Br Psychiatry* 120:59–63, 1972

270. Berlin F, Meinecke C: Treatment of sex offenders with antiandrogenic medication. *Am J Psychiatry* 138:601–602, 1981

271. Paulson DF, Kane RP: Medrogestone: A prospective study in the pharmaceutical management of benign prostatic hyperplasia. *J Urol* 113:811–815, 1975

272. Palanca E, Juco W: Conservative treatment of benign prostatic hyperplasia. *Curr Med Res Opinion* 4:513–520, 1977

273. Meiraz D, Margolin Y, Leu-Ran A, et al: Treatment of benign prostatic hyperplasia with hydroxy-progesterone-caprovate: Placebo-controlled study. *Urology* 9:144–148, 1977

274. Hollister LE: The mystique of social drugs and sex, in Sandler M, Gessa GL (eds): *Sexual behavior: Pharmacology and biochemistry* New York, Raven Press, 1975

275. Carter CS, Davis JM: Effects of drugs on sexual arousal and performance, in Meyer JK (ed): *Clinical Management of Sexual Disorders.* Baltimore, Williams & Wilkins Co., 1976

276. Bignani G: Pharmacologic influences on mating behavior in the male rat. *Psychopharmacologia* 10:44–58, 1966

277. Parr D: Sexual aspects of drug abuse in narcotic addicts. *Br J Addiction* 71:261–268, 1976

278. Waud SP: The effects of toxic doses of benzyl methyl carbinamine (Benzedrine) in man. *JAMA* 110:206, 1938

279. Bett WR: Benzedrine sulphate in clinical medicine. *Postgrad Med J* 22:205, 1946

280. Carr RB: Acute psychotic reaction after inhaling methylamphetamine. *Br Med J* 1:1476, 1954

281. Monroe RR, Drell HJ: Oral use of stimulants obtained from inhalers. *JAMA* 135:909, 1947

282. Angrist B, Gershon S: Clinical effects of amphetamine and L-dopa on sexuality and aggression. *Compulsive Psychiatry* 17:715–722, 1976

283. Bell DS, Trethowan WH: Amphetamine addiction and disturbed sexuality. *Arch Gen Psychiatry* 4:74–78, 1961

284. Gossop MR, Connell PH: Drug dependence and sexual dysfunction: A comparison of intravenous users of narcotics and oral users of amphetamines. *Br J Psychiatry* 124:431–434, 1974

285. Ellinwood EH, Rockwell WJK: Effect of drug use on sexual behavior. *Med Aspects Hum Sexuality* 9:10–31, 1975

286. Connell PH: *Amphetamine Psychosis*, Maudsley Monograph No. 5. London, Chapman and Hall, 1958

287. Gay GR, Newmeyer JA, Elion RA, et al: Drug-sex practice in the Haight-Ashbury or "the sensuous hippie," in Sandler M, Gessa GL (eds): *Sexual Behavior: Pharmacology and Biochemistry.* New York, Raven Press, 1975

288. Angtist B, Gershon S: Amphetamine abuse in New York City—1966–1968. *Semin Psychiatry* 1:195–207, 1969

289. Angrist BM, Gershon S: Psychiatric sequelae of amphetamine use, in Shader RI (ed): *Psychiatric Complications of Medical Drugs.* New York, Raven Press, 1972

290. Gay GR, Sheppard CW: Sex in the drug culture. *Med Aspects Hum Sexuality* 6:28–35, 1972

291. Greaves G: Sexual disturbances among chronic amphetamine users. *J Nerv Ment Dis* 155:363–365, 1972

292. Chopra GS: Man and marijuana. *Int J Addictions* 4:215–247, 1969

293. Harmon J, Aliapoulios MA: Gynecomastia in marijuana users. *N Engl J Med* 287:936, 1972

294. Kolodny RC, Masters WH, Kolodner RM, et al: Depression of plasma testosterone levels after chronic intensive marijuana use. *N Engl J Med* 290:872–874, 1974

295. Mendelson JH, Kuehnle J, Ellingboe J, et al: Plasma testosterone levels before, during, and after chronic marijuana smoking. *N Engl J Med* 291:1051–1055, 1974

296. Merari A, Barak A, Plaves M: Effect of $^{1\,(2)}$ - tetra-hydrocannabinol on copulation in the male rat. *Psychopharmacologia* 28:243–246, 1973

297. Siegel RK: Cocaine: Recreational use and intoxication, in Peterson, RC, Stillman RC (eds): *Cocaine 1977, NIDA Research Monograph 13.* Rockville, Maryland, Department of Health, Education, and Welfare, 1977

298. Everett GM: Amylonitrite ("poppers") as an aphrodisiac, in Sandler M, Gessa GL (eds): *Sexual Behavior: Pharmacology and Biochemistry.* New York, Raven Press, 1975

299. Welti RS, Brodsky JB: Treatment of intraoperative penile tumescence. *J Urol* 124:925–926, 1980

300. DeLeon G, Wexler HK: Heroin addiction: Its relation to sexual behavior and sexual experience. *J Abnorm Psychol* 81:36–38, 1973

301. Wieland WF, Yunger M: Sexual effects and side effects of heroin and methadone. *Proceedings of the Third National Conference on Methadone.* Washington, DC, US Government Printing Office, 1971

302. Mathis JL: Sexual aspects of heroin addiction. *Med Aspects Hum Sexuality* 4:98–103, 1970

303. Chambers CD, Brill L, Langrod J: Physiological and psychological side-effects reported during maintenance therapy, in Chambers CD, Brill L (eds): *Methadone: Experience and Issues.* New York, Behavioral Publications, 1973

304. Goldstein A: Blind dosage comparisons and other studies in a large methadone program. *J Psychedelic Drugs* 4:177–181, 1971

305. Goldstein A: Blind controlled dosage comparison with methadone in 200 patients. *Proceedings of the Third National Conference on Methadone Treatment.* Washington, DC, US Government Printing Office, 1971

306. Goldstein A, Judson BA: Efficacy and side effects of 3 widely different methadone doses. *Proceedings of the Fifth National Conference on Methadone Treatment.* Washington DC, US Government Printing Office, 1973

307. Martin WR, Jasinski D.R., Haertzen CA, et al: Methadone—a reevaluation. *Arch Gen Pscyhiatry* 28:286–295, 1973

308. Garbutt G, Goldstein A: Blind comparison of three methadone maintenance dosages in 180 patients. *Proceeding of the Fourth National Conference on Methadone Treatment.* New York, National Association for Prevention of Addiction to Narcotics, 1972

309. Bloom WA, Butcher BT: Methadone side-effects and related symptoms in 200 methadone maintenance patients. *Proceedings of the Third National Conference on Methadone Treatment.* Washington, DC, US Government Printing Office, 1971

310. Crowley TJ, Simpson R: Methadone dose and human sexual behavior. *Int J Addictions* 13:285–295, 1978

311. Cushman P, Dole VP: Detoxification of rehabilitated methadone-maintained patients. *JAMA* 226:747–752, 1973

312. Mintz J, O'Hare K, O'Brien CP, et al: Sexual problems of heroin addicts. *Arch Gen Psychiatry* 31:700–703, 1974

313. Cicero TJ, Bell RD, Wiest WG, et al: Function of the male sex organs in heroin and methadone users. *N Engl J Med* 292:882–887, 1975

314. Cushman P: Sexual behavior in heroin addiction and methadone maintenance. *NY State J Med* 72:1261–1265, 1972

315. Smith DE, Moser C, Wesson DR, et al: A clinical guide to the diagnosis and treatment of heroin-related sexual dysfunction. *J Psychoactive Drugs* 14:91–99, 1982

316. Kneek MJ: Medical safety and side effects of methadone in tolerant individuals. *JAMA* 223:665–668, 1973

317. Espejo R, Hogben G, Stimmel B: Sexual performance of men on methadone maintenance. *Proceeding of the National Conference on Methadone Treatment,* New York, 1973

318. Senay EC, Dorus W, Renault PF: Methadyl acetate and methadone. *JAMA* 237:138–142, 1977

319. Mirin SM, Meyer RE, Mendelson JH, et al: Opiate use and sexual function. *Am J Psychiatry* 137:909–915, 1980

320. Cushman P: Plasma testosterone in narcotic addiction. *Am J Med* 55:452–458, 1973

321. Glick BB, Baughman WL, Jessen JN, et al: Endogenous opiate systems and primate reproduction: Inability of naloxone to induce sexual activity in Rhesus males. *Arch Sexual Behav* 11:267–275, 1982

322. Bors E, Turner RD: Neurologic Urology, in Kaufmen JJ (eds): *Advances in Diagnostic Urology.* Boston, Little Brown, 1964

323. Weiss HD: The physiology of human penile erection. *Ann Intern Med* 76:793–799, 1972

324. Domer F, Wessler G, Brown R, Charles C: Involvement of the sympathetic nervous system in the urinary bladder internal sphincter and in penile erections in the anesthetized cat. *Invest Urol* 15:404–407, 1978

325. Dors LD, Brody MJ: Hemodynamic mechanisms of erections in the canine penis. *Am J Physiol* 213:1526–1531, 1967

326. Melman A, Henry D, Felton D, et al: Alternation of the penile corpora in patients with erectile impotence. *Invest Urol* 17:474–477, 1980

327. Benson G, McConnell J, Lipschultz L, et al: Neuromorphology and neuropharmacology of the human penis: an in vitro study. *J Clin Invest* 65:506–513, 1980

328. Benson GS, McConnell JA, Schmidt WA: Penile polsters: Functional structures or atherosclerotic changes? *J Urol* 125:800–803, 1981

329. Gessa GL, Tagliamonte A: Possible role of brain serotonin and dopamine in controlling male sexual behavior. *Adv Biochem Psychopharmacol* 11:217–228, 1974

330. Ghadiran AM, Chovinard G, Annable L: Sexual dysfunction and plasma prolactin levels in neuroleptic-treated schizophrenic outpatients. *J Nerv Ment Dis* 170:463–467, 1982

331. Gross MD: Reversal by bethanechol of sexual dysfunction caused by anticholinergic antidepressants. *Am J Psychiatry* 139:1193–1194, 1982

332. Shen WW, Mallya AR: Psychotropic-induced sexual inhibition. *Am J Psychiatry* 140:514–515, 1983
333. Nurnberg HG, Ambrosini PJ: Urinary incontinence in patients receiving neuroleptics. *J Clin Psychiatry* 40:271–274, 1979
334. Shenoy RS: Nocturnal enuresis caused by psychotropic drugs. *Am J Psychiatry* 137:739–740, 1980
335. Nakanishi H, Kaneko M: Is thioridazine-induced ejaculation failure peripheral? *Res Commun Clin Pathol Pharmacol* 19:549–552, 1978

3

Sexual Dysfunction in Neurological Disease

ELLIOTT L. MANCALL, ROBERT J. ALONSO, and
WENDY B. MARLOWE

INTRODUCTION

Disorders of sexual function in the human result from a remarkable variety of structural lesions involving the nervous system. Sexual dysfunction is widely recognized as a reflection of disorders of the peripheral nervous system and of the spinal cord; however, it is less widely appreciated that lesions of the cerebral hemispheres may also produce changes in this respect, at times so startling, dramatic, or bizarre as to be regarded, albeit inappropriately, as psychogenic in origin. It is tempting to suggest a simple dichotomy in this respect: lesions in the peripheral nervous system might be expected to induce disorders of potency, involving erection, ejaculation, or both, whereas lesions of the central nervous system, and particularly of the cerebral hemispheres, might be anticipated to result in disorders of libido, i.e., of sexual energy and desire. This division may be valid to a point but, as will be seen, does not really hold up to critical scrutiny, and in general, one cannot determine with certainty, on the basis of the type of sexual disorder alone, the site of neural involvement in any given patient.

The frequency of disorders of sexual function following organic lesions of the nervous system, and particularly of the cerebral hemispheres, cannot be stated with precision. It is, however, interesting to note that in a study

ELLIOTT L. MANCALL, ROBERT J. ALONSO, and WENDY B. MARLOWE • Department of Neurology, Hahnemann University School of Medicine, Philadelphia, Pennsylvania 19102.

devoted to impotence alone, 80% of 1138 men attending a general medical clinic were demonstrated to have an identifiable organic or pharmacological cause for their disorder.[1] The explanation for the gap in our knowledge in this area is in fact not difficult to identify. Detailed information regarding sexual performance is either not sought by physicians or, even in the face of direct inquiry, may be withheld by patients, reflecting in both circumstances the widespread feeling even today that such information is not properly the domain of the neurological physician. Even when pertinent data are provided, the scope is often limited and interpretation rendered difficult because of failure to explore social, emotional, or other nonorganic parameters of potential significance, to say nothing of important biological aspects of reproduction. Conclusions in this neglected area of neurology must then all too often be based on anecdotal material. Nonetheless, a basic consistency can be ascertained in much of the human material which has been reported, as will be reviewed later; not infrequently, parallels can be drawn between such isolated observations in patients and data derived from an ever-growing body of investigations in experimental animals.

It should be clear that a rational assessment of sexual function in the human, or, indeed, in the experimental animal, must then attempt to address specifically a number of diverse biological and psychological factors including, at the very least, libido, defined briefly as sexual energy; potency; frequency and/or duration of intercourse; and choice of sex object. Unfortunately, much of the published data fails to address such individual issues. Thus, although it would be pertinent to try to distinguish among these distinct parameters of sexual function and, indeed, to classify sexual disorders on such a basis, the paucity of suitable information precludes such an approach. One must therefore deal for the most part with less refined data which can be used crudely but nonetheless reasonably accurately to establish at least an anatomically based categorization of these problems. Limited though such an approach may be, it does provide the most suitable use of information now available in the literature.

NEUROANATOMICAL CONSIDERATIONS

It is self-evident that the establishment of a meaningful relationship between lesions of the central and peripheral nervous system and disorders of sexual function must be based initially on an awareness of the neural mechanisms subserving sexual performance. It is only with an appreciation of such basic anatomical features that an understanding of the reported clinical phenomena can be achieved. It is therefore appropriate at this point to provide an overview of pertinent anatomical data in the human.[2-5]

The innervation of the genitalia in both males and females has not been entirely clarified. In males, the testes and epididymis receive sympathetic innervation, primarily vasomotor in nature, from the lower thoracic cord (T9–T10), distributed particularly via the spermatic and hypogastric plexuses. It is not known whether parasympathetic fibers innervate these structures. The prostate gland and the seminal vesicles and related structures receive sympathetic fibers derived from the upper lumbar cord via the inferior mesenteric, hypogastric, and pelvic plexuses; postganglionic fibers are distributed to the smooth muscles of the seminal vesicles, the vas deferens, and ejaculatory ducts, and to the prostate and the erectile tissues. Such sympathetic fibers are primarily vasoconstrictor in function; stimulation also induces contraction of the smooth muscles of the ductal system, causing expulsion of seminal fluid with concomitant contraction of the musculature of the bladder neck, thus preventing retrograde passage of the seminal fluid into the bladder itself. The importance of these mechanisms in the process of ejaculation is clear. These structures also receive parasympathetic innervation from the sacral cord (S2–S4), traveling in the pelvic nerve (the so-called nervi erigentes). Parasympathetic fibers are primarily vasodilator in function and are thus of major significance insofar as erection is concerned; a glandular secretory function is also suggested.

In the female, the ovary receives both sympathetic and parasympathetic innervation, the former derived from the lower thoracic levels (T10–T11), the latter via the vagus nerve with a probable contribution from sacral levels as well. The function of autonomic innervation to the ovary is not clear, since much ovarian function would appear to be hormonally mediated; however, relevance reflecting vasomotor control may be suggested. The uterus derives its most prominent innervation from the sympathetic system, originating in the lower thoracic and upper lumbar levels of the spinal cord, and transmitted via the hypogastric and uterovaginal plexuses; there are probably additional contributions from the lumbar and sacral ganglia of the sympathetic trunks. Although less clearly defined, there would also appear to be parasympathetic supply to the uterus derived from the sacral cord. The function of such autonomic innervation to the uterus, whether sympathetic or parasympathetic, is also enigmatic; again, as with the ovary, vasomotor control may be of central importance. The vagina receives both sympathetic and parasympathetic fibers, the former vasoconstrictor, the latter vasodilator. There is thought to be at least some autonomic innervation to the vaginal musculature as well.

Within the spinal cord, preganglionic neurons of the sympathetic system are found in the medial and intermediolateral columns of the central gray in the thoracic and upper lumbar segments. Preganglionic parasympathetic neurons, on the other hand, are found in the general visceral efferent nuclei of the brainstem and in the sacral cord, particularly in the S2–S4 segments in a zone between the dorsal and ventral gray. The precise distribution of descending, i.e., suprasegmental, autonomic fiber systems within the spinal cord is not well established. It is widely held that such descending fibers travel with, or in close proximity to, the corticospinal tracts.

The central neural connections of these autonomic fibers are found primarily in the hypothalamus, controlled in turn by those portions of the hemispheres loosely referred to as the "limbic system" or "rhinencephalon." Derived at least to a large extent from the primordial olfactory placode, the structures generally included in what might be designated as the "vegetative" or "visceral" brain represent the most primitive portions of the human cerebrum. They may be recognized in the human as richly interconnecting rings of neural tissue deep within each cerebral hemisphere, largely surrounding the foramen of Monro and the corpus callosum. The most primitive of all is the innermost ring, sometimes referred to as the hippocampal–piriform complex, and including, among others, the olfactory striae, hippocampus, amygdala, fasciola cinerea, and indusium griseum. Sometimes referred to as the ento-or archipallium, this phylogenetically ancient gray matter complex is closely encompassed in turn by the meso- or paleopallium, the true "grand limbic lobe" of Broca, comprising the cingulate gyrus, hippocampal gyrus, insula of Reil, entorhinal and prepiriform areas, and septal region. These structures cannot be considered homogeneous in terms of either fine structure or connections; nonetheless, they do appear to be phylogenetically and anatomically interrelated, and despite confusion in terminology and, indeed, a lack of agreement as to precisely which structures in fact belong to these systems, there would seem to be ample justification for considering them a loose functional unit in the present context.

These primitive limbic structures receive abundant *afferent* input from virtually all sensory systems as well as from cortical association areas. A number of *efferent* fiber systems can be identified, including, for example, the diagonal band of Broca, the medial forebrain bundle, the fornix, the stria terminalis, and the habenulointerpeduncular tract. For the most part these efferent pathways terminate within the hypothalamus. From the hypothalamus, impulses are directed to some extent to the thalamus via the mamillothalamic tract (Vicq d'Azyr) but are also and perhaps more importantly relayed caudally to and through the mesencephalic tegmentum to the reticular formation of the lower brainstem and spinal cord, ultimately influencing the autonomic neurons of the sympathetic and parasympathetic systems at segmental, i.e., thoracolumbar and craniosacral, levels. The hypothalamus is, as is well recognized, intimately related to the pituitary gland as well: the supraopticohypophysial tract, derived from the supraoptic and paraventricular nuclei, can be traced to the posterior lobe of the pituitary, the neurohypophysis, whereas the hypophysial portal system transmits hormonal inhibiting and releasing factors from the median eminence to the anterior lobe, or adenohypophysis. In terms of sexual function, the hypothalamus may thus exert meaningful influence in three distinct ways. The first is through direct or indirect descending neural influences on brainstem and spinal autonomic centers via the midbrain tegmentum; the second comprises the neurohypophysial secretions, primarily of the peptides vasopressin and oxytocin, the latter particularly pertinent insofar as mammary and uterine functions are concerned; and the third reflects the rich hormonal activity of the anterior pituitary directed toward gonadal functions.

The hypothalamus may therefore in a very real sense be looked upon broadly as the central regulatory apparatus for the autonomic nervous system as well as for the neuroendocrine apparatus. It is clear, however, on the basis of well-recognized anatomical connections, that the function of the hypothalamus is in turn modulated by the limbic areas already enumerated. Since these primitive cortical areas in their turn receive important input from both sensory and associational cortex, a complex system is provided for autonomic and neuroendocrine regulation and modification in the face of a multitude of ever-changing environmental, somatic, visceral, and psychic forces. On the basis of abundant human and animal data, a number of functions can be assigned, wholly or in part, to this neural network[6-9] including olfaction; regulation of a host of cardiac, respiratory, vasomotor, alimentary, and pulmonary and glandular functions; memory acquisition, storage, and/or retrieval; and, in the psychic sphere, feelings and affective tone and patterns of behavior. There is also ample experimental data relating this anatomical complex to sexual performance; in fact, MacLean has defined this part of the brain as being primarily concerned with preservation of both self and species.[10-14] It is to this latter function that attention will be devoted hereafter. It is worth noting, however, that a number of these seemingly disparate functions are in fact interrelated: thus, the role of olfaction vis-à-vis bodily odors, including, in the human, the use of perfumes, in sexual activity hardly requires comment. For purposes of this presentation, however, we shall attempt to confine reference to sexual functions alone. It may finally be pointed out that psychological influences on sexual behavioral patterns are in all likelihood also mediated through the limbic–hypothalamic axis.

DISEASE OF THE CEREBRAL HEMISPHERES

Alterations in sexual function, in particular reduction in libido, have been recorded on a number of occasions in association with diffuse or poorly localized brain disease.[15-17] Disturbances of sexual function with *focal* lesions of the cerebrum are, however, more meaningful. In this respect, disease of the temporal lobes appears especially important, not surprisingly in light of the importance of mesial temporal structures such as the uncus, amygdala, hippocampus, and hippocampal gyrus in the limbic/rhinence-phalic apparatus. Patients with well-documented temporal lobe (complex partial, psychomotor) seizures provide much pertinent information in this respect.[18] Obvious sexual phenomena are rare but well-recognized features in some patients so afflicted; thus, erotic sensations have been noted as part of the aura, and overt sexual verbalizations or coital movements have been encountered during the course of the seizures themselves, presumably part of the automatisms typical of such attacks.[19-22] Seizures have been observed to be triggered by masturbation and may end in orgasm[23]; conversely, in some patients orgasm may comprise part of the aura of the psychomotor seizure, along with intense genital sensations.[24] Exhibitionism has also been described as part of the automatisms of such temporal lobe seizures.[18,25] Postictal sexual arousal leading at times to sexual assault has also been noted, characteristically associated with amnesia.[26] It should be pointed out, however, that not all seizures with sexual overtones originate in temporal lobe epileptogenic foci. Intense erotic sensations with or without overt sexual movements during seizures have been encountered with lesions of the superior parietal lobule.[27,28] These are remarkably rare occurrences, however, and perhaps not entirely unrelated in any case: the patient described by Erickson[27] had a parasagittal hemangioma in the parietal lobe, adjacent to, if not actually implicating, the cingulate gyrus, and thus at least indirectly related in terms of limbic anatomy.

Sexual dysfunction is commonly encountered in patients with temporal lobe epilepsy during interictal periods as well, far in excess of the frequency of such disorders in epileptics with seizure foci in other portions of the brain. Such alterations may take the form of reduced libido[26,29-31] or of impotence.[32-35] Sexual perversions such as transvestism have been noted not uncommonly.[29,36-38] Careful studies indicate that such functional impairment cannot be attributed to the psychosocial stresses to which epileptics in general are exposed, to the effects of chronic institutionalization, or to the actions of anticonvulsant agents. Interestingly, at least some improvement in sexual performance has been noted after therapeutic intervention, either with drugs or with temporal lobectomy.[39-42] Hill et al.,[43] describing their experience in a large series of individuals undergoing temporal lobectomy for epilepsy, describe changes in sexuality in 16 of 27 cases. One individual became impotent, but for the most part patients postoperatively described both an increased sex drive and increased potency. One patient became decidedly hypersexual, with features of exhibitionism, homosexual tendencies, and almost constant masturbation. Curiously, one such patient who had been sexually promiscuous prior to surgery adopted normal sexual habits after temporal lobectomy, and two others with abnormal sexual tendencies preoperatively developed normal libido and sexual activity thereafter.[44]

In addition to changes in sexual behavior observed in individuals with temporal lobe seizures, that is, with irritative, i.e., epileptogenic lesions involving especially the mesial temporal lobes, alterations in sexual habits and performance, at times dramatic in degree, may also result from *destructive* lesions involving the mesial aspects of the temporal lobes, particularly when such lesions are bilateral. These were first noted following bilateral temporal lobectomy in monkeys by Klüver and Bucy[45,46]; operated animals developed visual agnosia; oral tendencies; hypermetamorphosis (defined as a tendency to attend to every visual stimulus, touching every object in sight); alterations in behavior with the development of remarkable docility; hyperphagia; and striking hypersexuality with the adoption of diverse sexual patterns including heterosexual, homosexual, and autosexual activity. Some species differences have been subsequently observed: thus, Schreiner and Kling[47] noted the development of the Klüver–Bucy syndrome in cats with bilateral lesions involving the amygdala but pointed out that more extensive resection involving the hippocampi would actually prevent these clinical manifestations; such changes could also be abolished by placing an additional lesion in the hypothalamus. Human cases of the Klüver–Bucy syndrome have been infrequently recognized. Tersian and Dalle Ore[48] noted the development of this syndrome in a young man after bilateral temporal lobectomy; postoperatively the patient became an exhibitionist and demonstrated decided homosexual tendencies with almost incessant masturbation. Increased sexual activity was also noted by Green et al.[49] in a patient after bilateral anterior temporal lobectomy. The Klüver–Bucy syndrome has also been noted in the human after viral encephalitis, presumably herpetic in nature and involving with particular severity the mesial temporal structures. The youth reported by Marlowe et al.[50] exhibited a convincing change in sexual preference after recovery from such an acute encephalitis, developing overtly homosexual tendencies, and others[51,52] have described women who manifested remarkable hypersexual behavior during recovery from acute viral encephalitis. Serious craniocerebral trauma has also been followed by the development of the Klüver–Bucy syndrome; the young woman reported by Hooshmand et al.[53] exhibited marked nondiscriminative sexual promiscuity after recovery from acute injury. Hypersexuality as part of a Klüver–Bucy syndrome has been reported in Pick's disease[54] and in Alzheimer's disease.[55] Hypersexuality with frequent erections and ejaculations has also been noted in association with a typical but transient Klüver–Bucy syndrome in an epileptic patient after pneumoencephalography[56]; curiously this individual was seriously disturbed by these sexual manifestations but found he could not overcome an irresistible compulsion to carry out such acts. Finally, male sexual deviation has been noted in association with temporal lobe damage early in life.[57]

In our own experience, and in keeping with the observation of Jelgersma,[55] we have encountered one man of 72 with early features of Alzheimer's disease characterized primarily by a severe disorder of memory who exhibited marked hypersexuality, described as increased libido, but associated with impaired potency. Since the earliest lesions of Alzheimer's disease predominate in the hippocampus, i.e., in the mesial temporal lobes bilaterally, such changes are perhaps not unexpected, and, indeed, brief allusions to increased sexual activity under such circumstances are not uncommon. It is to be admitted, however, that as the dementing process proceeds, patients with Alzheimer's disease become increasingly apathetic and tend to lose all interest in sexual activity. We have also had the opportunity to observe a 57-year-old man who developed a severe amnesic dementia indicative of bilateral mesial temporal lobe destruction after a serious automobile accident. In contrast to the individual reported by Hooshmand,[53] this patient exhibited a striking and abrupt loss of libido, developing, according to his wife, a complete disinterest in sexual activity of any sort, in marked contrast to the vigorously heterosexual pattern of behavior that pertained prior to his head injury.

It must be emphasized that altered patterns of sexual behavior are not universally encountered in patients with temporal lobe disease, even when such lesions are bilateral. Thus, in ten pathologically verified cases of necrotizing encephalitis involving the temporal lobes and limbic areas, Hierons et al.[58] found hypersexual behavior in only one instance and this only to a relatively mild degree. Similarly, Pilleri[59] found no alterations in sexual behavior in two cases of Pick's disease, or in one case of Alzheimer's disease, despite the development of other features of the Klüver–Bucy syndrome in these individuals.

Deviations in sexual activity have been noted infrequently in patients with cerebral lesions outside of the temporal lobes. Freeman,[60] reviewing 35 years' experience with frontal lobotomy, did, however, note increased sexual behavior postoperatively in a number of patients, reflecting perhaps in large part release from debilitating obsessional or ruminative states. In a few cases hypersexuality of alarming proportion was encountered. The development of sexually oriented seizure activity in individuals with superior parietal lobe disease has already been noted.[27,28] Unilateral or bilateral lesions placed in the inferior thalamic peduncle and adjacent deep structures during the performance of ansotomy for relief of movement disorders[61] has been followed by loss of libido in both males and females, as well as impotence; such observations are perhaps not suprising in light of the recognized importance of the septal area, anterior thalamus, thalamus, gyrus rectus, and anterior cingulate gyrus in the production of erection in primates[62–66]; in fact, reduction of sexual activity has been noted in the experimental animal following lesions in the medial preoptic and anterior hypothalamic area.[67] Reduced sexual activity has also been observed in numerous patients with Parkinson's disease. A remarkable increase in sexual performance may follow therapy with levadopa; such an improvement probably is not due to an aphrodisiac action of L-dopa, as has been suggested by some observers but, rather reflects improvement in motility, i.e., restoration of the ability to move about sufficiently to resume more nearly normal sexual activity.

DISEASE OF THE HYPOTHALAMIC–PITUITARY AXIS

In the sexually developed, i.e., postpubertal individual, destructive pituitary lesions are characteristically associated with changes in sexual behavior, with impotence in the male, amenorrhea, at times with galactorrhea, in the female, and reduced libido in both.[68] When pituitary insufficiency appears before puberty, secondary sexual characteristics fail to appear, and the patients will generally exhibit both impotence and minimal or absent sexual interest. Destruction of the tuberal nuclei and tracts usually results in arrest or delay in sexual development, often with associated obesity, a syndrome termed *adiposogenital dystrophy* or Fröhlich's syndrome. A somewhat similar clinical picture is characteristic of the *Prader–Willi* syndrome, with hypotonia, short stature, obesity, hypogonadism, and impotence. In this condition the penis and testes are small; testicular biopsy reveals immature tissue of fibrosis. Long-term administration of gonadotropic hormones may induce puberty and spermatogenesis.[69]

Hypothalamic dysfunction has been implicated in the Laurence–Moon–Bardet–Biedl syndrome,[70] although definite neuropathological studies are lacking. This autosomal recessive condition is characterized by retinitis pigmentosa, mental retardation, polydactyly, and hypogonadism. Impotence and infertility are common in afflicted males.

The term "true isosexual precocious puberty" refers to the phenomenon of normal pubertal development occurring at an earlier-than-expected age. This is to be distinguished from heterosexual precosity or the adrenogenital syndrome. Although the pathophysiology of this disorder is poorly understood, alteration in sleep gonadotropin production or disorder of hypothalamic inhibitory mechanisms has been postulated,[71] and, in fact, tumors of the posterior hypothalamus have been associated with its appearance.

DISEASES OF THE SPINAL CORD

TRAUMA

Sexual disorders following spinal cord injury have been extensively documented.[72-74] The degree of sexual dysfunction in these circumstances is determined by a diversity of factors, perhaps most importantly the level of the spinal cord lesion itself and its completeness. A remarkable preservation of at least some sexual activity is, however, not uncommon, even with severe damage. In a study of 1295 male patients with spinal cord injury at various spinal levels, Tarabulcy noted preservation of erection in 77% of patients; coitus was successfully performed in 35%, although ejaculation was possible in only 10%.[73] The fertility of male paraplegics is diminished even in the presence of successful coitus, owing to low spermatozoa counts and decreased sperm motility.

Male patients with complete or incomplete *upper* motor neuron spinal lesions, i.e., those above the level of T10, often describe spontaneous reflex erections. This type of erection, unwilled by the patient, may be produced by stimulation of body surfaces below the level of the spinal lesion. Despite the relatively high percentage of occurrence of reflex erection, however, lesions of the cervical and thoracic spinal cord when complete are invariably associated with a marked decrease in emission, ejaculation, and orgasm, along with saddle anesthesia and loss of voluntary control of the anal sphincter and pelvic floor musculature.

In patients with complete *lower* motor lesions involving the lumbar spinal cord, Horenstein[75] reported a 25% incidence of psychogenic erection and a 25% incidence of reflex erection; 20% of patients reported ejaculation or orgasm. Ejaculation was quite weak, however, owing to the flaccid pelvic muscles and the absence of sphincter muscle tone and of perineal reflexes.

Patients with lesions of the conus medullaris, the terminal portion of the spinal cord, and of the roots of the cauda equina, often experience profound disturbances of sexual, bladder, and bowel functions. Complete lesions of the conus medullaris or cauda equina are followed by impotence, loss of anal and external urethral sphincter tone, varying degrees of saddle anesthesia, loss of anal and bulbocavernosus reflexes, and loss of voluntary control of the anal sphincter and of the musculature of the floor of the pelvis. Incomplete lesions of the cauda equina alone are often difficult to distinguish from those of the lumbosacral plexus and may present initially with incomplete or asymmetrical findings including paralysis, areflexia, radicular sensory loss, and pain, but with little if any sphincteric or sexual dysfunction.

Sexual problems in females with spinal cord injury differ somewhat from those of men. Prolonged ammenorrhea may follow spinal cord injury. Sensation during intercourse is often lost, although reflex and psychogenic clitoral erection appears to follow the same general principles as those outlined for penile erection in the male. Although the capacity for orgasm appears absent in many paraplegic females, isolated reports of "transfer of erogenous zones"[76] suggest that heightened sexual arousal may be achieved by intense tactile stimulation of body parts above the level of the lesion, specifically the breasts, nipples, lips, ears, and neck. In contrast to male paraplegics in whom fertility is impaired, spinal cord injury in females, whether complete or incomplete, does not effect the ability to conceive. Pregnancy itself ordinarily presents surprisingly few problems in women with spinal cord injury; there have been many cases of female paraplegics becoming pregnant and subsequently delivering normal children. There seems to be a slightly higher incidence of premature births in this patient population, however. Special problems can arise on occasion. For example, respiratory insufficiency may develop in women with high cervical cord lesions in whom breathing is largely diaphragmatic. A curious syndrome known as *autonomic dysreflexia* may appear in the paraplegic in the first and second stages of labor; manifested by headache, labile hypertension, cardiac dysryhthmia, and at times cerebral and retinal ischemia or death,[77-78] this syndrome may be difficult to distinguish from toxemia of pregnancy. It may be interrupted by the use of spinal anesthesia or an autonomic blocking agent. Its appearance demands prompt cesarean section.

MULTIPLE SCLEROSIS

Sexual dysfunction is a frequent symptom of multiple sclerosis. Such alterations may reflect the occurrence of demyelinated plaques in close proximity to cortical and subcortical areas involved in the human sexual response, but in the majority of cases are probably due to involvement of the nerve tracts in the lateral and posterior columns of the spinal cord. Since multiple sclerosis is a disorder of the white matter of the central nervous system, the disorders of sexual function are for the most part those of an upper motor neuron nature.

Partial or total impotence has been observed in nearly 50% of males with an established diagnosis of multiple sclerosis.[79] Those with long-standing disease appear to have a greater incidence of impotence. Studies of autonomic function yield normal responses for the most part, although Vas demonstrated a correlation between impotence and anhidrosis, impaired sweating being observed below the level of T10 in all patients with total impotence. Bulbocavernosus, scrotal, and anal sphincter reflexes are absent in all totally impotent patients, as well as in a majority of those partially impaired. Sexual potency may actually fluctuate in such patients, exhibiting a relapsing and remitting course as found with other manifestations of the disease; this is of course of some clinical importance in counseling patients regarding the prognosis of the sexual disturbance accompanying multiple sclerosis. For reasons not entirely clear, urinary gonadotropin (FSH–LH) excretion is found elevated in all totally impotent men as well as in some of those partially affected.[79] Though not conclusive, these findings suggest a deficiency of circulating testosterone, the administration of which may be therapeutic in value in the management of select patients.

A few studies of female sexual dysfunction in multiple sclerosis[80] indicate that 40–50% of women experience at some time in the course of their disease difficulties involving orgasm, dyspareunia, lack of vaginal lubrication, or diminished libido. All symptoms are more prominent in advanced stages of the disease.

Sexual readjustments including prolonged foreplay, self-stimulation, surgical implantations in cases of organic erectile dysfunction, and formal counseling may all significantly effect sexual performance and marital well-being in patients with multiple sclerosis. The bowel and bladder dysfunction that accompanies the disease in these patients with sexual disorder may be treated by anticipatory planning with diminished fluid intake and bowel and bladder emptying prior to intercourse. Flexor spasms may be troublesome during intercourse and should be controlled with appropriate medication.

Female patients with multiple sclerosis who are only mildly affected continue to menstruate and ovulate normally. Uncomplicated multiple sclerosis has almost no effect on pregnancy. However, the effect of pregnancy on the course of the disease in these patients is less certain. Several authors have found the relapse rates of the disease during pregnancy to be 50–100% higher than during the nonpregnant state, the relapse occurring particularly during the first 3 postpartum months.[81,82]

VASCULAR DISEASE

Acute vascular lesions of the spinal cord, i.e., infarction due to occlusion of either the anterior spinal or the paired posterior spinal arteries or prolonged ischemia due to systemic hypotension, dissecting aortic aneurysm, or prolonged aortic clamping, resemble pathophysiologically those complete or incomplete lesions encountered with spinal cord trauma, and the same patterns of sexual dysfunction may be discerned. The myelopathy associated with collagen vascular disease such as systemic lupus erythematosus or polyarteritis nodosa is probably due to cord ischemia resulting from occlusion of small and medium-sized arteries reflecting the underlying vasculitis. The clinical presentation and resulting sexual dysfunction are also similar to those described with spinal cord injuries.

Impotence may also be a prominent finding in the Leriche syndrome appearing as a result of thrombotic or embolic occlusions of the aorta or of the iliac arteries. Occlusive disease occurs more frequently in the terminal portion of the aorta with variable extension into the iliac and femoral arteries. The hallmark symptom of the disease is intermittent claudication. This symptom is present in the buttock and thigh with proximal occlusions and in the calf muscle with disease of the femoral and popliteal arteries. Localized, segmental, chronic, or slowly progressive occlusions in the aortoiliac or superficial femoral arterial distribution are generally well tolerated, and these patients tend to have extremities that are relatively normal in appearance. Patients with acute occlusions or far-advanced proximal and distal disease demonstrate pallor, rest pain, hair loss, trophic nail changes, dependent rubor, ischemic ulceration, and eventual gangrene. The physical examination is useful in substantiating the diagnosis and localizing the levels of aortoiliac occlusive disease. Auscultation should be performed over the midabdomen and the femoral vessels in the groin as well as the popliteal vessels listening for bruits. Peripheral pulses may be lost or significant attenuation in pulse amplitude may be appreciated. The diagnosis is confirmed by noninvasive vascular imaging or arteriography. Surgical treatment consists of bypass grafting or endarterectomy, though sudden occlusion of the distal aorta is poorly tolerated and requires emergency surgical intervention.

Vascular malformations of the cord, though uncommon, may cause bleeding into the subarachnoid space, or into the substance of the spinal cord itself. Paraparesis, sensory loss, sphincter disturbances, and impotence may result.

MISCELLANEOUS DISEASES OF THE SPINAL CORD

A diverse group of disorders may result in myelopathy with associated sexual dysfunction. Deficiency of vitamin B_{12} (cyanocobalamin) and perhaps of folate may produce the syndrome of subacute combined degeneration of the spinal cord. Initially, symptoms of numbness and paresthesia indicate posterior column involvement, followed by weakness, spasticity, and extensor plantar responses. Impotence may be an early manifestation of the disease and is invariably present during the later stages. Recovery may be complete if treatment with vitamin B_{12} is instituted within the first 3–4 months of onset of symptoms.

Cervical spondylosis with myelopathy presents typically with neck pain and stiffness with radicular pain in the upper extremities and a spastic paraparesis of variable degree. As the myelopathy progresses, impotence follows with loss of bowel and bladder function late in the disease. Additional causes of myelopathy which may produce impotence include radiation injury and spinal arachnoiditis, among others. Indeed, it may fairly be said that any disease of the spinal cord can result in impotence if sufficiently extensive. An interesting exception to this rule concerns disorders that are confined to the gray matter of the anterior horns, such as poliomyelitis or amyotrophic lateral sclerosis; in conditions such as these, the innervation of the sexual organs is generally spared, and sexual dysfunction is related primarily to the degree of weakness experienced by the patient.

DISEASES OF THE PERIPHERAL NERVOUS SYSTEM

SYPHILIS

Spirochetal involvement of the posterior spinal roots produces the syndrome of tabes dorsalis (locomotor ataxia). Impotence occurs due to loss of spinal reflex activity and is found in association with loss of bladder sensation and a hypotonic bladder. Lightning ("tabetic") pains, ataxia, and impaired vibratory and position sense in the legs are found, and degenerative osteoarthropathy (Charcot's joints) is seen in up to 10% of these patients. The impotence and hypotonic bladder are due to deafferentation at the sacral level (S2–S3). Unfortunately, sexual and bladder difficulties may persist despite appropriate and vigorous therapy with penicillin.

DIABETES MELLITUS

The incidence of involvement of the peripheral nervous system in diabetes mellitus ranges from 15 to 50% of all cases. A number of clinical syndromes have been described. The most common is a slowly progressive sensory polyneuropathy manifested by numbness and paresthesias of the feet with associated loss of tendon reflexes. Autonomic neuropathy marked by anhidrosis, nocturnal diarrhea, gastric and bladder atony, postural hypotension, and impotence may coexist or may appear independently.[83]

Acute, asymmetrical, and predominantly motor neuropathies (mononeuropathy multiplex) may also occur in the diabetic, although less commonly; involvement of the bowel and bladder and sexual dysfunction reflect here affection of the nerve roots of the cauda equina or the lumbosacral plexus. This type of neuropathy is probably due to infarction of the nerve due to small-vessel disease and generally has a good prognosis, with recovery of function within months, occasionally years.

Impotence may also appear in the diabetic without other stigmata of autonomic neuropathy or other disease of the peripheral nervous system. When supporting neuropathic features are lacking, other causes of impotence should be sought—psychogenic, Iatrogenic, or vascular.

AMYLOIDOSIS

Amyloid is an amorphous extracellular fibrillar protein substance which may accumulate in the heart, kidney, intestinal, and peripheral nerve. The disease may be familial (familial amyloid polyneuropathy) with an autosomal dominant mode of inheritance or may appear sporadically in association with chronic infections or inflammatory diseases such as tuberculosis or rheumatoid arthritis. The peripheral nervous system is only rarely affected by amyloidosis due to infection or inflammation. Amyloid deposition is also associated with certain malignancies, including medullary carcinoma of the thyroid or multiple myeloma, and with macroglobulinemia. Early symptoms of neural involvement include numbness, paresthesias, and, rarely, pain in the extremities with relative preservation of touch and vibration sense and of tendon reflex activity. Autonomic dysfunction may be profound with vasomotor instability, diarrhea, constipation, anhidrosis, and impotence. Diagnosis is made on the basis of biopsy of skin, rectal mucosa, or other affected organs such as liver, spleen, and gut.

RENAL DISEASE

Polyneuropathy as a complication of chronic renal disease occurs in approximately two thirds of patients beginning dialysis therapy. The course of the neuropathy is slowly progressive with a combination of muscle weakness, atrophy, sensory loss, and areflexia, often with burning dysesthesias. A recent study of home dialysis patients[84] has demonstrated diminished libido and impotence in both males and females with uremia, presumably reflecting this polyneuropathy. Hormonal factors may play a supplemental role in the sexual dysfunction of these patients.[85]

IDIOPATHIC ORTHOSTATIC HYPOTENSION (PRIMARY AUTONOMIC INSUFFICIENCY)

Idiopathic orthostatic hypotension is a degenerative disease of middle and late adult life,[86] involving various parts of the nervous system with primary affection of the postganglionic sympathetic nerves. The parasympathetic system is relatively spared. A similar form of the disease[87] may affect the preganglionic neurons in the intermediolateral cell column of the spinal cord and is usually associated with widespread loss of neurons in the brainstem, e.g., in the substantia nigra and locus ceruleus. Both forms of the disease present with symptoms of autonomic insufficiency, with orthostatic hypotension, syncope, anhidrosis, atonic bladder and bowel, and impotence. Extrapyramidal signs may be seen in the latter disorder.

Familial dysautonomia, the Riley–Day syndrome, is a recessive degenerative disorder of the nervous system occurring predominantly in Jewish children. The clinical presentation is one of widespread autonomic dysfunction with loss of effective temperature control, hyperhidrosis, labile blood pressure, vasomotor skin changes, dysphagia, hyporeflexia, and impairment or loss of pain and temperature sensation in the extremities. Men affected with this disorder are invariably impotent. Neuropathological studies reveal loss of small myelinated and unmyelinated nerve fibers in peripheral nerves as well as cell loss in the sympathetic and parasympathetic ganglia.

OTHER NEUROPATHIES

Other disease states either causing or associated with polyneuropathy or autonomic neuropathy include chronic alcohol use with undernutrition, hypothyroidism, hepatic disease, sarcoidosis, porphyria, heavy-metal intoxication (particularly by lead and arsenic), and collagen vascular disease. In all of these impotence may appear. In addition, trauma to the lumbosacral plexus resulting in bowel and bladder disorder and sexual dysfunction may occur as a complication of major abdominal surgery such as abdominal peroneal resection, lymph node dissection, or abdominal aneurysm repair. Radiation-induced plexopathy may appear as a delayed effect of radiation therapy to the pelvis and retroperitoneum.

NEUROLOGICAL HISTORY AND EXAMINATION IN PATIENTS WITH SEXUAL DYSFUNCTION

As in any other area of medicine, the diagnosis and treatment of patients with sexual dysfunction due to underlying neurological disease proceeds from the information obtained from an orderly history and a systematic complete physical and neurological examination. The neurological history in these individuals should include information regarding the location, nature, and duration of any painful symptoms, especially those present in the low back, lower extremities, and perineal areas. Attention should be given to symptoms of numbness, tingling, and paresthesias in the extremities as possible evidence of a peripheral neuropathy. Questions concerning lightheadedness, syncope, and other symptoms related to orthostasis may be helpful. Bowel and bladder dysfunction including constipation, diarrhea, and incontinence is often seen in association with sexual dysfunction and must be sought after by appropriate questioning.

The neurological examination may follow the general physical examination and proceeds in a systematic fashion with evaluation of higher cortical function and of cranial nerves, tests of motor, sensory, and reflex activity, and tests of the gait and station, followed by an assessment of sphincteric and autonomic nervous system function. The elements of the neurological examination most pertinent to the evaluation of a patient with sexual dysfunction include detailed testing of sensory and motor modalities in the perineal area and lower extremities, with elicitation of the perineal reflexes including the bulbocavernosus reflex. Rectal and pelvic examinations should be routine with particular note made of the rectal tone. Tests of autonomic function including evaluation of skin temperature, vasomotor responses to temperature, response of blood pressure and heart rate to Valsalva maneuvers or change in posture, cold pressor test, and observation of sweating patterns and tearing (Schirmer's test) are all useful in evaluation of the patient with suspected autonomic dysfunction.

Laboratory tests should include routine hematological studies including complete blood counts, renal/liver function tests, fasting blood sugar, and urinalysis. Measurement of specific hormones including thyroid and testosterone may also be indicated. Vaginal (Papanicolaou) smears and cultures of vaginal and/or urethral discharges should be performed. Special studies including glucose tolerance testing and measurement of hypothalamic pituitary hormones including follicle-stimulating hormone, luteinizing hormone, and prolactin may be useful in distinguishing patients with hypogonadotropic hypogonadism. The measurement of nocturnal penile tumescence is of assistance in determining whether impotence is present on an organic or a psychogenic basis, though it is nonspecific insofar as the etiology of organic dysfunction is concerned. Bladder function is best assessed by cystometrogram. Electroencephalography, computerized tomography, and electromyography with nerve conduction studies are reserved for patients with specific findings on the examination.

REFERENCES

1. Slugg MF, Morley JE, Elson MK, et al: Impotence in medical clinic outpatients. *JAMA* 249 (13):1736–1740, 1983
2. Crosby EC, Humphrey T, Lauer EQ, et al: *Correlative Anatomy of the Nervous System.* New York, MacMillan, 1962
3. Appenzeller, O: *The Autonomic Nervous System.* New York, North Holland, 1976
4. Brodal A: *Neurological Anatomy.* New York, Oxford University Press, 1981
5. Yakovlev PI: Motility, behavior and the brain. *J Nerv Ment Dis* 104(4):313–335, 1948
6. Isaacson, RL: *The Limbic System.* New York, Plenum Press, 1974
7. Papez JW: *Limbic Mechanisms.* New York, Plenum Press, 1978
8. Pool JL: The visceral brain of man. *J Neurol* 2:45–63, 1958
9. Wood, CD: Behavioral changes following discrete lesions of temporal lobe structures. *Neurology* 8:215–220, 1958
10. MacLean PD: Psychosomatic disease and the "visceral brain." *Psychosom Med* 11:338–353, 1949
11. MacLean PD: The limbic system ("visceral brain") and emotional behavior. *Arch Neurol* 73:130–134, 1955
12. MacLean PD: Contrasting functions of limbic and neocortical systems of the brain and their relevance to psychophysiological aspects of medicine. *Am J Med* 25(4):611–626, 1958
13. MacLean PD: The limbic system with respect to self-preservation and the preservation of the species. *J Nerv Ment Dis* 127:1–ll, 1958
14. MacLean PD: Man and his animal brains. *Mod Med* 32:95–106, 1964
15. Kalliomaki JL, Markkanen TK, Mustonen VA: Sexual behavior after cerebral vascular accident. *Fertil Steril* 12(2):1961, 1961
16. Weinstein EA: Sexual disturbances after brain injury. *Med Aspects Hum Sexuality* 8(10):10–31, 1974
17. Kosteljanetz M, Jensen TS, Norgard B, et al: Sexual and hypothalamic dysfunction in the postconcussional syndrome: *Acta Neurol Scand 63(3):169–180, 1981*
18. Walker, AE: The libidinous temporal lobe. *Arch Suisses Neurol* 111:473–484, 1972
19. Freemon FR, Nevis AH: Temporal lobe sexual seizures. *Neurology* 19:87–90, 1969
20. Currier RD, Suess JF, Orlando JA: Psychomotor sexual seizures: *Trans Am Neurol Assoc* 94:178–182, 1969
21. Currier RD, Little SC, Seuss JF, et al: Sexual seizures. *Arch Neurol* 25:260–264, 1971
22. Gautier-Smith PC: Cerebral dysfunction and disorders of sexual behavior. *Rev Neurol (Paris)* 136(4):311–319, 1980
23. Bancaud J: Paroxysmal sexual manifestations and temporal epilepsy. *Electroenceph Clin Neurophysiol* 30 (4):371, 1971
24. Van Reeth PC, Oierkens J, Luminet D: Hypersexuality in epilepsy and temporal lobe tumors. *Acta Neurol Psychiatry* 58(2):194, 1958
25. Hooshmand H, Brawley BW: Temporal lobe seizures and exhibitionism. *Neurology* 19:1119–1124, 1969

26. Gastaut H, Callomb H: Etude de compartment sexuel chez les epileptiques psychoma-teurs, *Ann Medicophys* 112:657, 1954
27. Erickson TC: Erotomania (nymphomania) as an expression of cortical epileptiform dis-charge. *Arch Neurol Psych (Chicago)* 53:226–231, 1945
28. Smith BH, Khatri AM: Cortical localization of sexual feeling. *Psychosomatics* 20(2):771–776, 1979
29. Taylor DC: Sexual behavior and epilepsy. *Arch Neurol* 21(5):510–516, 1969
30. Taylor DC: Appetitive inadequacy in the sex behavior of temporal lobe epileptics. *J Neuro-Visc Relations* (suppl 10):486–490, 1971
31. Blumer D: The sexual behaviour of patients with temporal lobe epilepsy before and after surgical treatment. *J Neuro-Visc Relations* (suppl 10):469–476, 1971
32. Johnson J: Sexual impotence and the limbic system. *Br J Psychiatry* 111:300–303, 1965
33. Hierons R: Impotence in patients with temporal lobe lesions. *Lancet* 2(467):761–763, 1966
34. Saunders M, Rawson M: Sexuality in male epileptics. *J Neurol Sci* 10:577–583, 1970
35. Hierons R: Impotence in temporal lobe lesions. *J Neuro-Visc Relations* (suppl 10):477–481, 1971
36. Walinder J: Transvestism, definition and evidence in favor of occasional derivation from cerebral dysfunction. *Int J Neuropsychiatry* 1(6):567–573, 1965
37. Hunter R: Transvestism, impotence and temporal lobe dysfunction. *J Neurol Sci* 4:357–360, 1967
38. Spate HF: Des Limbischen Systems in der Pathogenese des Transvestitismus. *Psychiatr Neurol Med* 22(9):339–344, 1970
39. Blumer D, Walker AE: Sexual behavior in temporal lobe epilepsy. *Arch Neurol* 16:37–43, 1967
40. Blumer D: Hypersexual episodes in temporal lobe epilepsy. *Am J Psychiatry* 126:83–90, 1970
41. Cogen PH, Lobo Antunes J, Correll JW: Reproductive function in temporal lobe epilepsy: The effect of temporal lobectomy. *Surg Neurol* 12:243–246, 1979
42. Hill D, Pond DA, Mitchell W, et al: Personality changes following temporal lobectomy for epilepsy. *J Ment Sci* 103:18–27, 1957
43. Hill D, Pond DA, Mitchell W, et al: Personality changes following temporal lobectomy for epilepsy. *Br J Psychiatry* 103:18–27, 1957
44. Pond DA, Bidwell B: Personality changes following temporal lobectomy for epilepsy. *Br Med J* 2:1520–1523, 1954.
45. Klüver H, Bucy P: An analysis of certain effects of bilateral temporal lobectomy in the rhesus monkey with special reference to psychic blindness. *J Psychiatry* 5:33, 1938
46. Klüver H: "The temporal lobe symdrome": Produced by bilateral ablations, in GE Wol-stenholm and M O'Connor (eds): *Ciba Foundation on the Neurological Basis of Behavior.* Boston, Little, Brown, 1958
47. Schreiner L, Kling A: Behavioral changes following rhinencephalic injury in cat. *J Neu-rophysiol* 16:643–659, 1953
48. Tersian H, Dalle Ore G: Syndrome of Klüver and Bucy. *Neurology* 5(6):373–380, 1955
49. Green JR, Duisberg REG, McGrath WB: Focal epilepsy of psychomotor type: A prelim-inary report of observation on effects of surgical therapy. *J Neurosurg* 8:157–172, 1951
50. Marlowe WB, Mancall EL, Thomas JJ: Complete Klüver–Bucy syndrome in man. *Cortex* 11:53–59, 1975
51. Sanvito WL, Tilbery CP, Ribeiro–Pinto L, et al: Sindrome De Klüver–Bucy Determinada Por Encefalite A Virus. *Arq Neurospiquiatr* 40(3):251–259, 1982
52. Shraberg D, Weisberg L: The Klüver–Bucy syndrome in man. *J Nerv Ment Dis* 166(2):130–134, 1978

53. Hooshmand H, Sepdham T, Vries JK: Klüver–Bucy Syndrome. *JAMA* 229(13):1782, 1974
54. Balajthy B: Symptomatology of the temporal lobe in Pick's convolutional atrophy. *Acta Med Acad Sci Hung* 20:301–316, 1964
55. Jelgersma HC: Ein Fall von Juveniler Hereditarer Demenz vom Alzheimer Typ mit Parkinsonismus und Klüver–Bucy–Syndrom. *Arch Psychiatr Neurol* 205:262–266, 1964
56. Anastasopoulos G, Kokkini D: Transient bulimia–anorexia and hypersexuality following pneumoencephalography in a case of psychomotor epilepsy. *J Neuropsychiatry* 4(3):135–142, 1963
57. Kolarsky A, Freund K, Machek J, et al: Male sexual deviation. *Arch Gen Psychiat* 17:735–743, 1967
58. Hierons R, Janota I, Coresllis JAN: The late effects of necrotizing encephalitis of the temporal lobes and limbic areas: A clinico-pathological study of 10 cases. *Psychol Med* 8:21–42, 1978
59. Pilleri G: The Klüver–Bucy syndrome in man. *Psychiatr Neurol (Basel)* 152:65–103, 1966
60. Freeman W: Sexual behavior and fertility after frontal lobotomy. *Biol Psychiatry* 6(1):97–104, 1973
61. Meyers R: Evidence of a locus of the neural mechanisms for libido and penile potency in the septo-fornico-hypothalamic region of the human brain. *Trans Ann Neurol Assoc* 86:81–85, 1961
62. MacLean PD, Ploog, DW: Cerebral representation of penile erection. *J Neurophysiol* 25:29–55, 1962
63. MacLean PD, Denniston RH, Dua S: Further studies on cerebral representation of penile erection: Caudal thalamus, medbrain, and pons. *J Neurophysiol* 26:273–293, 1963
64. Dua S, MacLean PD: Localization for penile erection in medial frontal lobe. *Am J Physiol* 207(6):1425–1434, 1964
65. Robinson BW, Michkin M: Ejaculation evoked by stimulation of the preoptic area in monkey. *Phsiol Behav* 1:269–272, 1966
66. Perachio AA, Marr LD, Alexander M: Sexual behavior in male rhesus monkeys elicited by electrical stimulation of preoptic and hypothalamic areas. *Brain Res* 177:127–144, 1979
67. Slimp J, Hart BL, Goy RW: Heterosexual, autosexual and social behavior of adult male rhesus monkeys with medial preoptic–anterior hypothalamic lesions. *Brain Res* 142:105–122, 1978
68. Lisk R: Sexual behavior: Hormonal control, in Martini L, Ganong WF (eds): *Neuroendocrinology*, Volume 11. New York, Academic Press, 1967, pp 197–239
69. Hamilton CR, Scully RE, Kliman D: Hypogonadotropism in Prader Willi syndrome, induction of puberty and spermatogenesis by clomiphene citrate. *Am J Med* 52:322, 1972
70. Dekaban AS, Parkes JS, Ross GT, Laurence–Moon syndrome: Evaluation of endocrinological function and phenotypic concordance and report of cases. *Med Ann DC* 41:687, 1972
71. Kinney FM, et al: Radioimmunoassoyable serum LH and FSH in girls with sexual precocity, premature menarche and ardrenarche. *J Clin Endocrinol* 29:1272, 1969
72. Munro D, Horne HW, Paull DP: The effect of injury to the spinal cord and cauda equina on the sexual potency of men. *N Engl J Med* 239(4): 903–911, 1948
73. Tarabulcy E: Sexual functions in the normal and paraplegic. *Paraplegia* 10:201–208, 1972
74. Comarr AE: Sex among patients with spinal cord and cauda equina lesions. *Med Aspects Hum Sexuality* 7(3):222, 1973
75. Horenstein S: Sexual dysfunction in neurologic disease. *Med Aspects Hum Sexuality* 2:31, 1976
76. Kolodney RQ, Masters WH, Johnson VE: *Textbook of Sexual Medicine.* Boston, Little, Brown, 1979

77. P   .er AB, Raffieux M, Ziegler WH: Pregnancy and labor in high traumatic spinal cord
    ⸱ons. *Paraplegia* 7:210–216, 1969
78. Goller H, Paeslock V: Pregnancy damage and birth complication in the children of
    paraplegic women. *Paraplegia* 10:213–217, 1972
79. Vas CJ: Sexual impotence and some autonomic disturbances in men with multiple scle-
    rosis. *Acta Neurol Scand* 45:166–182, 1969
80. Lundberg PO: Sexual dysfunction in multiple sclerosis. *Sexual Disabil* 1:218–222, 1978
81. Millar JS, Alleson RS, Cheeseman EA, et al: Pregnancy as a factor in influencing relapse
    in desseminted sclerosis. *Brain* 82:417–426, 1959
82. Schapira K, Poskanzer DC, Nevel DJ, et al: Marriage, pregnancy and multiple sclerosis.
    Brain 89:419–428, 1966
83. Ewing OJ, Campbell IW, Burt AA, et al: Vascular reflexes in diabetic autonomic neu-
    ropathy. *Lancet* 2:1353–1356, 1973
84. Bailey GL: The sick kidney and sex. *N Engl J Med* 296:1288–1289, 1977
85. Holdsworth S: The pituitary–testicular axis in man with chronic renal failure. *N Engl J
    Med* 296:1245–1249, 1977
86. Bradbury S, Eggleston C: Postural hypotension, a report of three cases. *Am Heart J* 1:72–
    86, 1925
87. Shy GM, Drager GA; A neurological syndrome associated with orthostatic hypotension:
    A clinical pathologic study. *Arch Neurol* 2:511, 1960

4

The Psychological Evaluation and Therapy of Psychogenic Impotence

STEPHEN B. LEVINE

INTRODUCTION

The appreciation of any clinical contribution should be preceded by the caveat "Consider the source." All conclusions are subtly influenced by the author's assumptions, philosophical perspective, and/or other biases. The scientific ideal that the progression from observations to conclusions should be absolutely logical is rarely achieved. In clinical arenas, progress is made when investigators dealing with the same problems from different perspectives reach similar conclusions.

The source of this contribution is a psychiatrist, who could perhaps be most accurately described as developmentally or psychodynamically oriented. This chapter is based on 10 years' experience with clinical sexual problems. I view my continuing conceptual evolution during this period as both encouraging and unsettling. It is encouraging if change is viewed as a sign of maturation; it is unsettling to realize that one has perceived similar phenomena in very different ways. This chapter is a summary of my understanding of the causes of psychological impotence and the means of restoring erectile function. Its ultimate validity and utility await the test of time.

STEPHEN B. LEVINE • Department of Psychiatry, Case Western Reserve University School of Medicine, Cleveland, Ohio 44106.

PATHOGENESIS OF PSYCHOLOGICAL IMPOTENCE

The majority of the literature on psychological impotence focuses on its recognition or treatment. In-depth discussion of the pathogenesis is surprisingly rare. Rather, etiology is usually summarized in terms of competing, seemingly mutually exclusive theories.[1] Although the theoretical constructs applied to this problem—psychodynamic,[2] behavioral,[3] cognitive,[4] and systems theory[5]—may provide an illuminating perspective, each is an attempt to force a symptom into a conceptual framework. Therapists who have seen large numbers of impotent men stress the fact that the symptom has *no* universal pathogenesis.[6-10] It is quite probable that psychogenic impotence is the end product of multiple temperamental, familial, affectual, cognitive, cultural, maturational, *and* biological factors. When one considers the slow evolutionary process of developing causal hypotheses and the difficulty of establishing their validity, one can appreciate the reasons for giving discussions of pathogenesis short shrift.

Performance anxiety is the modern explanation for the final common pathway to psychogenic impotence.[11,12] After an episode of erectile failure, almost any man will become worried, if not preoccupied, about the state of subsequent erections. Performance anxiety can be severe enough to distract the man from the sensual stimuli that ordinarily arouse and maintain excitement. The baffling question about performance anxiety is: Why this man, at this time, with this particular symptom?

The clinician can articulate cogent practical answers to these questions. These answers begin to emerge during the initial contacts with the man and his partner. During these contacts, it is usually helpful to consider the symptom from four perspectives:

1. At what stage of life does the symptom appear?
2. What are the quality and quantity of sexual desire?
3. What role does the partner play?
4. What is the significance of past developmental experiences?

This early phase of psychiatric evaluation enables the clinician to form causal hypotheses that lead to specific, individualized treatment approaches.

ELABORATION OF THE EVALUATION PERSPECTIVES

Perspective One: At What Stage of Life Does the Symptom Appear?

It is useful to separate men with lifelong, or primary, impotence from those whose symptoms follow a long period of aproblematic sexual functioning (i.e., secondary impotence).[11] The causes of these two types of impotence, as well as the response to therapy, are usually quite discrete. Secondary psychological impotence is far more prevalent than primary impotence.

Conceptual models of the causality of these two types of impotence are presented below. Although quite useful, they are too simple for many cases. Complicated cases require a synthesis of concepts derived from both models to adequately explain the symptom.

Model for Secondary Impotence — Unrecognized Affects Stemming from New Life Circumstances

Occasional sexual failures are understandable when one considers the difficulty involved in achieving the three basic requirements of good sexual function—i.e., willingness to make love; capacity to relax; ability to concentrate on sensation.[13] Strong feeling states, such as anger, guilt, shame, disgust, anxiety, and sadness, can induce a temporary unwillingness to make love, inability to relax, or preoccupation with other matters. Although the men are physically present, they are not always psychologically available for lovemaking. In addition, substance abuse may cause a physiological inability to erect. The vast majority of erectile failures are followed by sexual encounters under better psychological and physiological conditions. The performance anxiety initially evoked by impotence fades away after one or more successful experiences.

Persistent impotence usually means that the initial failure was not due to an incident of minor personal significance. Curiously, these men often consider their dysfunctions inexplicable, despite recent major transitions in their lives—e.g., changes involving the quality of long-standing relationships, partners, or work. It is hard to avoid relating such problems to the widespread male belief that sex should be possible anytime, anywhere, with anybody. Secondary psychogenic impotence is a reminder that the penis is not a machine. The unrecognized affects that cause impotence are products of meaningful changes in personal life. Several such changes are illustrated in the following case reports.

CASE 1: HOSTILE, UNRECEPTIVE PARTNER

A 50-year-old hard-working, religious, devoted father was married to a woman who prided herself on her worldliness and was contemptuous of his limitations. She had a series of affairs and was disinterested in having sexual contact with her husband. He did not seem to realize that his wife's blatant derision was relevant to his years of deteriorating potency.

CASE 2: LINGERING DISTRUST OF WOMEN; FEAR OF BEING HURT AGAIN

A mild-mannered air traffic controller claimed that his wife's decision to divorce him was a complete surprise. For 6 months after being "thrown out of his home," he visited his children, worked, and drank heavily in his lonely apartment. His deep sense of loss and bitterness was gradually modified by an increasingly intimate relationship with the woman he eventually married. He was totally baffled by his erectile failure with his fiancée.

CASE 3: INADEQUATELY RESOLVED GRIEF; GUILT OVER PREMATURE INTIMACY

Three months after his wife's death, a 58-year-old man began dating. He sought help for impotence after sexual failures with three partners. When asked if thoughts of his wife intruded upon him during sexual intimacies, he replied, "Never! My children have been very supportive of my dating. Logically, there is no reason for me not to date. Life must go on!" He then cried throughout his lengthy description of their many beautiful years of marriage and the horror of her slow, painful death. Leaving the interview, he said, "Maybe I did feel strange with other women."

CASE 4: DISPLACED ANXIETY OVER JOB FUNCTION

A middle-aged man developed impotence the night after his boss urged him to assume a supervisory position. He was quite worried about his competence—"panicked, in fact"—because this position had previously been held only by engineers. He never related his worries about inadequacy in his new career role to his new sexual anxiety.

These men failed to appreciate the presence and significance of unpleasant affects during sexual intimacy. Patient 1 was unable to face the reality of his painful position as a cuckold. Patient 2 was unable to account for his tension whenever he engaged in sexual activity with a woman he loved. Patient 3 almost succeeded in isolating the painful past from his new intimacies with other women. Patient 4 tried to use sex for a respite from his mental preoccupation with job problems. Prior to entering their new life circumstances, none of these men had any erectile difficulties.

Any list of the psychological causes of secondary impotence could be extended to great length. Its exact contents are less important than the recognition of the patient's inability to deal with the affects (e.g., anxiety, anger, fear, guilt) behind the "causes"—e.g., marital deterioration, extramarital affair, job failure. These feelings may be avoided with defense mechanisms, but are ultimately expressed as performance anxiety.

Model for Primary Psychogenic Impotence — Developmental Failure to Overcome Fear of Women

First coital opportunities are typically accompanied by considerable anxiety. This anxiety is manifested as nervousness rather than a discrete fear and detracts from the pleasure of this important rite of passage. Once coital success begins to dispel this nervousness, subsequent experiences can be more leisurely and pleasurable.

It is likely that clinicians see only a fraction of those who are initially impotent. Most impotent beginners achieve success in subsequent experiences with the same partners. Some, however, are so humiliated that they avoid intimacy for a long time. The few who seek help are likely to present as young, panicky heterosexuals. The clinician's warmth, sympathy, and reassurance usually relieve their anxiety and enable them to try again. Although such cases are gratifying to the clinician, they offer little insight into the sources of the anxiety.

Most men with long-standing primary impotence have other obvious psychiatric difficulties. An appreciation of these other difficulties places their sexual symptom in perspective. Associated disorders fall into five categories: gender identity problems—e.g., transsexualism, transvestism; perversions—e.g., sadism, pedophilia, masochism; homosexuality—e.g., homoerotic male trying to be a heterosexual; character neurosis—e.g., obsessive–compulsive disorder, passive–dependent character; psychosis—e.g., schizophrenia or borderline disorders.

CASE 5: GENDER IDENTITY DISORDER

A man who eventually had sex reassignment surgery was married for 20 years without having intercourse. After failing in his initial coital attempts, he was only rarely able to participate in mutual genital play; such activity was always accompanied by the fantasy that his partner's body was his body. He had been secretly cross-dressing since early childhood and often lapsed into a fantasy of being a girl. He had neither the desire nor the self-confidence necessary for intercourse.

CASE 6: MASOCHISTIC PERVERSION

A socially isolated, 63-year-old schoolteacher wanted to be put in touch with a sexual surrogate in order to have intercourse once before he died. His autoerotic life was dominated by a spanking scenario. A few times a year he hired a prostitute. Pretending that he had been naughty, she would put him over her knees and spank him. He usually achieved orgasm with masturbation immediately afterward. He had never been able to maintain an erection for intercourse and had given up trying. He was too fearful and ashamed of himself to attempt any sexual intimacies with the few women he had ever dated.

CASE 7: EGO–DYSTONIC HOMOSEXUALITY

A passive, effeminate musician and his devoted wife were referred for help in consummating their 16-year marriage. Their two children were adopted. Their mutual masturbatory sexual pattern caused them periodic distress. His weak desire for sex with his wife contrasted with his strong homoerotic interests. Although he had experienced these attractions since adolescence, he had not had any actual homosexual experiences. He fled from a religious order at age 20 when faced with an opportunity for homosexual behavior. For 2 years thereafter, constant anxiety prevented his going to school and work. He was embarrassed by his fear of being swallowed up in his wife's vagina.

CASE 8: CHARACTER NEUROSIS

A passive, obsessive–compulsive, heterosexual 28-year-old man had been unable to have intercourse with his wife of 4 years. Their verbal communication had dwindled considerably, and there had been no physical contact for more than 3 years. Prior to having cardiac surgery at age 8, the patient had been chronically ill. He continued to be a quiet, socially isolated child. He dated only one girl. His future in-laws made their disappointment with their daughter's choice painfully obvious. Although he petted eagerly prior to marriage, he claimed that religious beliefs prevented him from attempting intercourse. After the wedding, however, he could not get excited with his wife.

Despite diverse etiologies, a defective sense of self generally precedes primary impotence. It is a serious error to attribute doubts about masculinity only to the initial sexual failure. The issues involved in the therapy of such men are not usually as simple and discrete as those in cases of pure secondary impotence. The success rates achieved with any approach to primary impotence are always much lower than those achieved with men who have had a great deal of successful coital experience. Men with long-standing primary impotence (e.g., patient 8) may achieve coital success; more often than not, however, both the patient and the therapist become concerned about matters more basic than potency—e.g., identity, inability to form close relationships, fear of loss of psychological integrity through physical union with a woman, or pervasive passivity. Such men are basically frightened of women. The sources of their fears are not readily accessible. Short-term therapies for impotent men with obvious psychiatric difficulties—especially those without supportive partners—are unlikely to effect *lasting* potency.

Some elemental fear of women is normal, even among potent young men. Many men are unable to acknowledge this fear, and most cannot account for it. The fear may derive from unconscious sources that are qualitatively similar to those that cause impotence—e.g., fear of losing their separate masculine identity by merging with a woman, anger over real or imagined past maternal injustices, guilt over past excitement and sexual desires for both parents, sense of inadequate masculinity stemming from limited paternal involvement. The vital differences, however, lie in the degree of unconscious fear, the fear-suppressing capacity, or the ability to be excited by their partners.

On rare occasions, a relatively normal young man seeks help for the persistent inability to achieve intercourse. Although this masculine heterosexual without perverse tendencies may be socially at ease, successful in his work sphere, and lacking in neurotic symptoms, an inexplicable anxiety prevents him from having intercourse. The presence of such ego strengths generally indicates that the focal problem will be quite amenable to treatment.

The first perspective can now be refocused: "What developmental task was in progress when the erectile problem began?" For most men, the answer involves dealing with a new life challenge; for some, however, the task was establishing an initial heterosexual relationship. The refocused perspective enables conceptualization of the ultimate therapeutic task.

PERSPECTIVE TWO: WHAT ARE THE QUALITY AND QUANTITY OF SEXUAL DESIRE? IS IT INHIBITED, DEFICIENT, OR INTACT?

Despite their expressed desire for intercourse and their repeated coital attempts, many psychologically impotent men lack genuine sexual drive. What seems like sexual drive is only an expression of their wish to be capable of having coitus. As such, it should be considered cognitive desire and contrasted with somatically experienced visceral desire. The latter can be evaluated by asking about the presence of spontaneous sexual excitement and the length of time that elapses between perceived feelings about needing a sexual outlet.[14] These questions usually enable the clinician to make the useful distinction between cognitive and visceral desire.

DSM–III sexual dysfunction categories divide psychologically impotent men into two groups. Psychogenic impotence per se is no longer a diagnosis. Rather, these men are divided into those with deficient desire (desire inhibition) and those who have sexual drive but cannot maintain excitement (excitement inhibition).[15] Since excitement inhibitions are the most easily treated forms of secondary impotence, this distinction is quite important. Men with excitement inhibitions are trapped by their fears of sexual failure and vigilant preoccupation with their erections during lovemaking. When their pernicious performance anxiety stems from largely resolved psychological dilemmas, they can be significantly helped by simple interventions. The therapist needs to explain the origin and maintenance of the problem in a way that makes sense to the patient—i.e., label the original interfering affects and explain the destructive features of performance anxiety. The patient needs to be reassured that the symptom is neither rare nor permanent. Lovemaking without intercourse—i.e., sensate focus[11]—is usually prescribed. This procedure enables the man to relax, concentrate on sensation, and become aroused. Some patients report being cured by the following visit. It is far more common for the underlying psychological dilemma to be ongoing; in such cases, the therapeutic focus should be on its resolution. Once the dilemma is resolved, interventions aimed at excitement inhibitions can be employed.

Unfortunately, most psychologically impotent men cannot be rapidly and effectively treated because, in DSM–III terminology, they have "desire inhibitions." The differential diagnosis of "desire inhibitions" can be quite complicated.[16] Desire *deficiency* states, such as those found among patients with unrecognized depressions, systemic illnesses, drug effects, and other biogenic low-libido states, e.g., Klinefelter's syndrome, may be erroneously diagnosed as inhibitions. In patients with true inhibitions, the drive is present but deflected or hidden from the conscious self. Questions concerning masturbatory activity and imagery, dream imagery, nocturnal emissions, and sex with other partners are useful in recognizing the distinctions between drive deficiencies and true inhibitions. This decision is vital because therapy for a deficiency is quite different from that for an inhibition. This dilemma is especially common in physically normal older men with weakened libidos.[14]

Although there is little knowledge about the physiological basis for libido, a number of clinically useful phenomena have been observed. Viscerally experienced drive often disappears under the following conditions: preoccupation with life crises; grief; depression; partner unavailability due to illness, sexual disinterest, separation, or death; "falling out of love"; aging; psychosis. Easily recognized inhibitions commonly occur as a result of fear of death or injury following physical illness (e.g., myocardial infarction or cardiac surgery); persistent erectile, ejaculatory, or partner dysfunction; or suppressed anger at partner. Inhibitions that are more difficult to recognize can occur in men who have a maternal transference to their sexual partners; enter into heterosexual relationships in an attempt to conceal gender identity disorders, paraphilias, or homosexuality; or demonstrate a characteristic inability to express anger.

The psychological cause of the desire problem is, of course, the determining factor in its treatment. Problems stemming from either a deficiency or inhibition of drive do not respond to techniques that effectively alleviate excitement inhibition. Sensate focus exercises will not help men who have a cognitive desire for sex but lack any genuine sexual interest in their partners. The patient's attention needs to be focused on the underlying problem, rather than the sexual failure per se. Mental health professionals are quite familiar with such problems. The fact that sex therapists have been able to help these men indicates their competence in treating communication problems, interpersonal conflicts, and intrapsychic inhibition of affect expression. Both sex therapists and mental health professionals soon learn, however, that many desire problems cannot be resolved with current therapeutic techniques.[16]

PERSPECTIVE THREE: IS THE PARTNER A VICTIM OR A SABOTEUR?

When a woman maintains a warm, receptive, supportive attitude prior to and during her partner's impotence, she may be viewed as a victim of his intrapsychic conflicts and performance anxiety. Many partners deal with their new sexual deprivation and narcissistic worries in a noncritical, unpressured interpersonal manner. In such relationships, impotence is a product of intrapsychic dynamics—e.g., previous unresolved marital entanglements, unconscious maternal cathexis.

When a partner deliberately or inadvertently, consciously or unconsciously functions as saboteur, the etiology and therapy of the problem are very different. Although the impotence in such relationships is associated with male intrapsychic conflict, it is more accurately assessed as a response to intuitively experienced partner unreceptivity. Conjoint therapy employing sensate focus exercises can quickly unmask the saboteur. When potency begins to return, the woman ceases to cooperate, develops a new symptom, or launches a vitriolic attack on her partner. The various motives behind such sabotage must be understood and resolved before a viable, sexually and emotionally gratifying relationship can be established.

Evaluation of the wives of psychogenically impotent men is almost always helpful. The wife–victim of a man with secondary impotence may know more about the problem than does her husband; the wife–saboteur reveals her critical attitudes and conflicting motives in her discussions with the clinician. Some wives begin as victims. They inadvertently become saboteurs in response to their anger at the man's withdrawal. Probably the most common treatment mistake with secondarily impotent married men is the failure to appreciate the current interpersonal milieu. The man's conflicts, however neurotically expressed in the past, never previously prevented intercourse.

PERSPECTIVE FOUR: WHAT IS THE SIGNIFICANCE OF PAST DEVELOPMENTAL EXPERIENCES?

Unconscious processes are probably involved in every case of psychogenic impotence. Even in cases with obvious precipitants, symptoms may be attributed to both the immediate antecedents and the unconscious conflicts and affects they provoke. For example, guilt over being unfaithful to his hopelessly demented wife caused a very proper, 60-year-old man to become impotent. However, much of his new sexual anxiety was generated by his experiences coping with his mother's promiscuity when he was 12.

Treatment planning is largely dependent on the answers to two questions about unconscious determinants:

1. *Are unmastered developmental processes the most significant contributors to an individual's vulnerability to impotence?* Certain patterns of erectile dysfunction indicate a serious vulnerability to sexual failure: persistent primary impotence; potency only with derogated women; frequent, recurring impotence throughout adulthood; potency occurring only when the needs of the partner are ignored. (The latter three are sometimes classified imprecisely as "situational" impotence.) Treatment aimed at mastery of the remote forces responsible for the man's constriction is usually indicated. Unless the partner is especially supportive and intuitive, her involvement ceases once the underlying vulnerability is diagnosed.

2. *Are the significant unconscious determinants accessible to exploration?* Kaplan has categorized the sources of unconscious anxiety that produce inhibited desire and excitement into three levels.[16] Mild sources include performance anxiety, guilt over sexual activity and pleasure, overconcern with the partner's pleasure, and response to partner dysfunction. These problems are often quickly resolved with conjoint or individual therapy. Midlevel sources include angry inhibitions due to interpersonal conflict and fears of success and intimacy. Deeper sources include severe relationship problems, castration anxiety associated with oedipal conflicts or preoedipal pathological introjects. Many midlevel and most deep problems do not generally respond to brief and/or conjoint approaches; the results achieved with classic analytical therapies are also frequently disappointing.

The issue of accessibility is not limited to the depth of the underlying problem; the nature of the man's defensive structure is also involved. Those who employ primitive or immature defensive patterns complicate any therapeutic endeavor. A very passive factory worker who had been unable to consummate his 8-year marriage also suffered from almost complete amnesia about his childhood. His emotional poverty and repression provide a striking contrast to patient 8, the meek, obsessive–compulsive man who was at least capable of recalling and discussing his life. He achieved lasting potency after 4 months of weekly conjoint therapy. The amnesic man is incapable of even thinking about his present or past problem.

Accessibility of the underlying problem is also a function of the therapist's proficiency in, and willingness to use, various therapeutic techniques. On the basis of the experiences of sex therapists of various theoretical orientations, it is apparently possible to restore or effect potency without resolving all of the patient's character and developmental problems. Considerable empirical evidence suggests that a variety of approaches may help impotent patients as long as the problem is carefully diagnosed.[17-19] It is just as important for clinicians to recognize deeply rooted intrapsychicproblems that require intensive individual therapy as it is to recognize those that can be handled with any number of briefer approaches.

TREATMENT GUIDELINES

1. *Diagnostic assessment is the first step.* The initial medical–psychiatric assessment requires considerable clinical judgment. It is likely that many treatment failures are rooted in assessment errors. Three discrete topics must be assessed:

   a. Recognition of the relative contribution of organic factors. The process whereby this is accomplished is discussed elsewhere in this book. Controversy persists between those who favor complete laboratory evaluations for all patients[20] and those who prefer a slow evaluation of the psychological contributions in those whose symptom patterns suggest psychogenic or mixed psychogenic–organic etiologies (S. B. Levine, unpublished observations).
   b. Delineation of specific psychological causes. (See previous section.)
   c. Ascertainment of man's (couple's) willingness and ability to use available therapeutic modalities.

2. *Carefully decide who will be the patient—the man or the couple.*

   a. Married man—The wife's presence in therapy presents opportunities and limitations. With the woman present, the issues tend to initially focus on the interpersonal dimension of life—both sexual and nonsexual. The wife's presence usually implies a commitment to the immediate continuation of the marriage. Her presence limits discussion of his ambivalent love and/or commitment to her. It also has a tendency to prevent an intensive, psychotherapeutically meaningful review of his childhood development, confusion about his sexual orientation, gender identity, or perverse sexual fantasies.

      The couple's wish to be seen together is usually prompted by their sense that the problem lies in their nonsexual relationship, or that each partner is contributing something to the maintenance of the impotence. Conjoint therapy is useful whenever the therapist perceives marital deterioration or feels that a sexually anxious, rejecting spouse is involved in the pathogenesis. Should the wife refuse the recommendation, the therapist, husband, and wife should all question the decision. Sometimes the wife knows she is not interested in helping her husband have sexual relations with her. Sometimes she is afraid her secret will be discovered—e.g., that she does not love her husband or that she has a lover. Sometimes the wife is inexplicably frightened of the unknown therapeutic process.

      The therapist should pay close attention to the feelings of those who are initially frightened. Sometimes undue nervousness stems from unrealistic fantasies about having sex in front of the therapist. Dealing directly with the nervousness enables it to dissipate. Conjoint therapy is a shared intimacy that tends to strengthen the marital bond even before marital conflicts are fully understood and resolved.

Many married men will not enter therapy with their wives. They know they are dealing with issues that would harm their marriages or their wives. They often have lovers, are thinking about divorce, or have perverse sexual preoccupations their wives know nothing about. Their wishes should be respected. Therapy should be individual.

b. Unmarried man living with a woman—Although it is tempting to treat such couples as though they were married, the situations are not quite the same. Many unmarried men will not share their emotional lives fully because they fear losing their partners. With only occasional exceptions, all unmarried men should be given individual therapy. Their girl friends can, however, be very important during the evaluation.

c. Unmarried man without partner—The choice here is between individual and group therapy. Telling a man to find a partner and then return for sex therapy is not a viable option. The recommendation of surrogate therapy, whether it is with a woman who earns her living in this role or an interested friend, is based on the assumption that the basic problem involves sexual technique or stems from anxiety which can be easily overcome after a few positive experiences. Clinicians are likely to have different perspectives and opinions about this approach.

d. Homosexual man and male partner—The choice is between individual and conjoint therapy; the latter is usually restricted to large homosexual communities or therapists known for working with gay couples. Institutions such as the Masters and Johnson Research Institute have had a great deal of experience with homosexual couples.[21] Individual therapy with an impotent homosexual man is not a rare experience for most therapists.

3. *Therapist and patient should be able to agree on at least one psychological causal hypothesis.* The initial evaluation often helps the patient realize that his impotence is probably related to something he overlooked—death of his twin brother, business failure, wife's cancer surgery. If the patient cannot tolerate the idea that the impotence is psychogenic, it is probably best to delay treatment until he changes his mind. Most impotent men first seek

help from a primary-care physician, internist, or urologist. The vast majority of patients who are referred for psychological therapy do not accept the referral.[22] Successful treatment requires a willing patient.

4. *The process of effective therapy, however mysterious, must make mastery possible.* Regardless of its format—psychoanalytic, behavioral, marital—effective therapy effects important changes. For example, it teaches the man how to relax and allow his partner to stimulate him; it strengthens the marital bond; it decreases his resentment and depression; it frees him from transferential confusion of his partner with women of his past. These accomplishments are the work of therapy; potency is the by-product.

Impotence is usually a mystery to the patient and his partner. Effective therapy removes some of the mystery and enables the man to do better in a specific aspect of his life. The therapist listens, talks, makes suggestions, reassures, encourages. The patient (couple) thinks, feels, understands. Frequently potency emerges. The process is usually enigmatic to the patient, who may say "I am not sure what you did, doctor," and somewhat less so to the clinician. The therapist knowingly or unwittingly is helping with the mastery of some personal task that was previously overwhelming.

5. *Therapeutic suggestions are vital diagnostic opportunities.* When Masters and Johnson reported their positive results with sensate focus exercises, many laymen and professionals misunderstood. They thought the instructions to sensually explore the nongenital areas of the body effected the cure. Although these instructions are ingenious, most of the time they cannot be immediately followed by the man or his partner. The resistances to the instructions reveal the feelings, attitudes, or past experiences that prevent healthy sexual function; these impediments must then be dealt with in therapy. The accomplishment of this goal may involve education, ventilation of feelings, discussion of the past, assertiveness training, and/or medication. The therapist's timing and tact are certainly important.

The use of sensate focus exercises and other "techniques" has declined considerably over the years. Most therapists do not believe there is one specific treatment for all types of psychogenic impotence. The diagnostic perceptions previously based on resistances to sensate focus exercises now emerge during prolonged evaluation. Sensate focus is now used as a therapeutic, rather than a diagnostic, procedure. This technique is applicable to relatively few couples.

6. *Some psychogenic impotence, especially secondary varieties, improves spontaneously.* Many studies have found a 15% waiting-list improvement rate. A similar percentage of men get better as soon as therapy begins. Such spontaneous

improvement is probably related to changes in attitude and relationships. It is tempting to consider the concept of "flight into health" as a means of not dealing with the relationship of the symptom to some painful part of one's life.

7. *Beware of the concept of "cure."* Some psychogenic impotence is episodic. For many men, however, a prolonged period of impotence marks the end of sexual life. However reassuring they may be, statements such as "My cases have a 70% cure rate" are misleading. Individual sexual health is reflected by motivation for sexual contact, as well as by the ability to remain tumescent for its duration, have a pleasurable orgasm, and enjoy the entire experience. It is possible to regain potency but not desire; have a new or old orgasmic problem; or rush the experience so much that it is not pleasurable. The improvement must be lasting or the patient is not "cured." When the sexual adaptation of both partners is the criterion for health, "cure" rates invariably fall.[23] Published success rates are rare; those that do exist should be carefully scrutinized for the criteria of success.

Clinicians should not discharge patients too quickly.[24] Patients who are hesitant to stop therapy after initial successes are very wise. Their hesitance should be respected as an indication that the problem is not completely resolved. People who have been successfully treated often ask to come back.

8. *It is not possible for all impotent men to get better.* Sometimes men with extremely chaotic social and emotional lives, hostile wives, or severe early-life traumas cannot be helped. Therapists should be sure that these failures are not due to the treatment format per se. Some formats do not provide sufficient time for resolving psychological dilemmas or sufficient opportunities for considering past or present contributions. Even the most careful, thoughtful, and experienced therapist cannot improve *every* man's erectile function. Therapeutic failures tend to demonstrate at least one of these characteristics:

a. Cognitive but no genuine or visceral desire for the current partner.
b. Inability to find and maintain an intimate relationship.
c. Man who refuses to consider the possibility of his wife's current infidelity.
d. Gender identity confusion or well-developed perversion.

Faced with a therapeutic failure, the clinician needs to reexamine two issues: (1) whether the original assessment of the problem as largely psychogenic was correct, and (2) whether the causal hypotheses provide a cogent explanation for the man's persistent sexual anxiety. The following is an explanation which I accepted:

A post office employee had been rescued from a "life of alcoholic dissipation" by his evangelical minister–wife who heard the word of God. He was potent for 12 years of their marriage, in spite of her three psychotic breakdowns. Shortly after he became the object of her paranoia, his erectile capacity diminished. With increasing frequency and vehemence, this phenothiazine–noncompliant woman threatens to murder him. Twice she has attacked him with a knife in bed.

9. *Sexual arousal and potency are products of three current attributes:*

a. Willingness to make love to the partner.
b. Capacity to achieve relaxation.
c. Capacity to develop a preoccupation with sensation.

One or more deficiencies of these attributes preclude the impotent man's secure erection. If any therapy is going to help, it will do so by increasing willingness, relaxation, and concentration on sensation.

Many men express the psychology of regained potency in terms such as, "I got my confidence back." Performance anxiety is a mixture of the anticipation of failure, which begins when the man contemplates having sex, and the preoccupation with the state of the penis during sexual play. When confidence is regained, the anticipation of failure diminishes, allowing for more relaxation and concentration on sensation.

10. *The therapist should offer considerable hope for recovery.* I have been told by many formerly impotent men (couples) that the single most important thing I said was that I thought they would get better. This enabled them to confront the unmastered parts of their lives. If the therapist has no hope or expectation of improvement, the gloom can become contagious. However, some situations are so deteriorated that the best I can muster is "I don't know. We'll see." I offered this man a lot of hope:

A 50-year-old successful executive was potent during 22 years of marriage. He immediately lost his desire for sex when his wife told him she wanted to marry the man with whom she had been having an affair. In his characteristic anger-suppressing style, he complied with her wishes and made sure she was financially comfortable. After a year of social isolation, he met a woman and quickly grew to love her "beyond his dreams." In spite of his great desire for her, his considerable performance anxiety precluded his erection. Although he was a very good thinker, he had only a modest awareness of his feelings. He was aware of wanting to please his fiancée a great deal. He was also afraid that he might suddenly lose another greatly loved person. At age 8, he had been rescued from the Nazis and sent to America through a foster child program; his parents had perished.

During 15 individual sessions, we discussed his grave childhood losses, his suppressed anger at his ex-wife, and his need to allow his fiancée to give him pleasure. The expectation of potency was continually offered. He gradually became more relaxed and allowed himself to experience her caresses more fully. He regained the capacity to have intercourse but could not overcome his lifelong problem of rapid ejaculation.

11. *Do not lead the patient to believe there is one best treatment for impotence.* First, it is not true. Therapists with radically different assumptions, interests, and formats have helped impotent men recover. Second, if your treatment is unsuccessful, someone else may be able to help him. It is reasonable to say, "This is what I think is reasonable for your situation. I'm sure other therapists may have other ideas." Prolonged working through of grief, maturation, partner change, death of a parent, a child's leaving home, or other situations may eventually enable a "treatment failure" to regain his sexual abilities. The proper therapeutic attitude is characterized by curiosity and eagerness to learn and help—not dogmatic authority.

ESSENCE OF SENSATE FOCUS

John Hunter first prescribed "six amatory experiences without coital connexion" in 1788.[25] Sensate focus as a treatment for impotence was quickly adopted by other therapists after 1970. Prohibiting intercourse reduces the man's vigilant preoccupation with his erectile state. Following instructions to neck and pet as he did during his teen-age years enables him to relax and concentrate on sensation. He is able to become aroused and erect. Masters and Johnson emphasize the fact that sex is a natural function—i.e., if one can remove the acquired inhibition, the body and mind will automatically cooperate to produce erection. These concepts can be taught quite easily. Sensate focus can be formalized into highly specific instructions; each new direction is outlined after the couple masters the previous step.

Step 1—Lying together naked, holding each other and breathing together.

Step 2—Body exploration, excluding breasts and genitals. Take turns being giver and receiver; goal: relax, enjoy, feel a new variety of pleasures, and become aroused.

Step 3—Add breast caressing.

Step 4—Add genital caressing; goal: not erection or orgasm, but pleasurable education and exploration.

Step 5—Genital caressing with orgasm.

Step 6—Vaginal containment with minimum thrusting; intercourse, usually with man supine.

Step 7—Intercourse with thrusting to orgasm.

Step 8—Intercourse with woman supine.

Therapists modify these instructions to meet patients' apparent needs. Since sex is a natural function, the removal of the interfering inhibition is usually more effective than giving directions for actual sexual behavior.

CONCLUSION

Psychogenic impotence is simply the inability to become and stay aroused. The question of why the man does not become aroused when he consciously desires sexual activity is never quite resolved. Dealing with large numbers of impotent men may enable the clinician to more effectively help individual patients. Experience tends to convince the therapist of the possibility that the origin, or at least the maintenance, of the symptom can involve such subtle factors as cruel remarks, emotional indifference, or vague perceptions of not being loved. Psychological impotence presents a great therapeutic challenge—not only because the associated problems are so diverse, but because a hopeful, knowledgeable, kind, patient therapist can make a difference.

ACKNOWLEDGMENT: The author thanks Barbara Juknialis, of the Center for the Critically Ill at University Hospitals of Cleveland, for her editorial assistance in the preparation of this manuscript.

REFERENCES

1. Wagner G, Green R: *Impotence: Physiological, Psychological, Surgical Diagnosis and Treatment.* New York, Plenum Press, 1981
2. Freud S: On the universal tendency to debasement in the sphere of love (1912), in Strachey J (ed): *The Standard Edition of the Complete Psychological Works of Sigmund Freud*, Volume XI. London, The Hogarth Press, 1957, pp 117–190
3. LoPiccolo J, LoPiccolo L (eds): *Handbook of Sex Therapy*. New York, Plenum Press, 1978
4. Gagnon JH, Rosen RC, Lieblum SR: Cognitive and social aspects of sexual dysfunction: Sexual scripts in sex therapy. *J Sex Marital Ther* 8:44–56, 1982
5. Cole CM, Blaheney PE: The myth of the symptomatic vs. asymptomatic partner in conjoint treatment of sexual dysfunction. *J Sex Marital Ther* 5:79–89, 1979
6. Kolodny RC, Masters WH, Johnson VE: *Textbook of Sexual Medicine*. Boston, Little, Brown, 1979
7. Kaplan HS: *The New Sex Therapy*. New York, Brunner/Mazel, 1974
8. Munjack DJ, Oziel J, Kanno PH, et al: Psychological characteristics of males with secondary erectile failure. *Arch Sex Behav* 10:123–132, 1981
9. Derogatis LR, Meyer JK: A psychologic profile of the sexual dysfunctions. *Arch Sex Behav* 8:201–224, 1979
10. Stekel W: *Sexual Impotence in the Male* Volume 2. New York, Liveright, 1927
11. Masters WH, Johnson VE: *Human Sexual Inadequacy*. Boston, Little, Brown, 1970
12. Quadland MC: Private self consciousness, attribution of responsibility, perfectionistic thinking and secondary erectile dysfunction. *J Sex Marital Ther* 6:47–55, 1980

13. Levine SB: Marital sexual dysfunction: Introductory concepts. *Ann Intern Med* 84:448–453, 1976
14. Martin CE: Factors affecting sexual functioning in 60-79-year-old married males. *Arch Sex Behav* 10:399–420, 1981
15. American Psychiatric Association: *DSM-III*. Washington, DC, American Psychiatric Association, 1980
16. Kaplan HS: *Disorders of Sexual Desire*. New York, Simon and Schuster, 1979
17. Wright J, Perrault R, Mathiew M: The treatment of sexual dysfunction. *Arch Gen Psychiatry* 34:881–890, 1977
18. Killman PR, Auerback R: Treatments of premature ejaculation and psychogenic impotence: A critical review of the literature. *Arch Sex Behav* 8:81–100, 1979
19. Karacan I: The treatment of erectile dysfunction. *Direc Psychiatry* 1:Lesson 13, 1981
20. Karacan I: Nocturnal penile tumescence as a biologic marker in assessing erectile dysfunction. *Psychosomatics* 23:349–360, 1982
21. Masters WH, Johnson VE: *Homosexuality in Perspective*. Boston, Little, Brown, 1979
22. Segraves RT, Schoenberg HW, Zarins CK, et al: Referral of impotent patients to a sexual dysfunction clinic. *Arch Sex Behav* 11:521–528, 1982
23. Levine SB: Conceptual suggestions for outcome research in sex therapy. *J Sex Marital Ther* 6:102–108, 1980
24. Dickes R, Strauss D: Countertransference as a factor in premature termination of apparently successful cases. *J Sex Marital Ther* 5:22–27, 1979
25. Hunter J: *Treatise on the Venereal Disease*. London, Mr. G. Nicol and Mr. J. Johnson, 1788, pp 203–204

5

Vasculogenic Impotence

BRUCE L. GEWERTZ and CHRISTOPHER K. ZARINS

INTRODUCTION

In 1923, Leriche first associated atherosclerotic occlusion of the infrarenal abdominal aorta with erectile dysfunction and buttock atrophy.[1] Although great advances have been made in the treatment of lower-extremity ischemia by direct reconstruction, only recently have vascular surgeons specifically addressed the identification and correction of arterial lesions causing impotence. As the public becomes increasingly aware that sexual function can be extended to the extremes of age, appropriate diagnosis and treatment of this syndrome will assume even more importance. This chapter begins with a review of the vascular anatomy of the penis and the commonly available noninvasive methods of assessing penile perfusion. Options in operative and nonoperative treatment will also be discussed.

VASCULAR ANATOMY

Penile blood supply is derived from the left and right internal pudendal arteries, which are major branches of the internal iliac or hypogastric arteries (Figure 1). As the internal pudendal arteries exit from the perineum, they arborize into three paired vessels: the *superficial perineal branch* on the inferior aspect of the penis, the *dorsal penile artery* traveling superficially on

---

BRUCE L. GEWERTZ and CHRISTOPHER K. ZARINS • Department of Surgery, University of Chicago, Chicago, Illinois 60637.

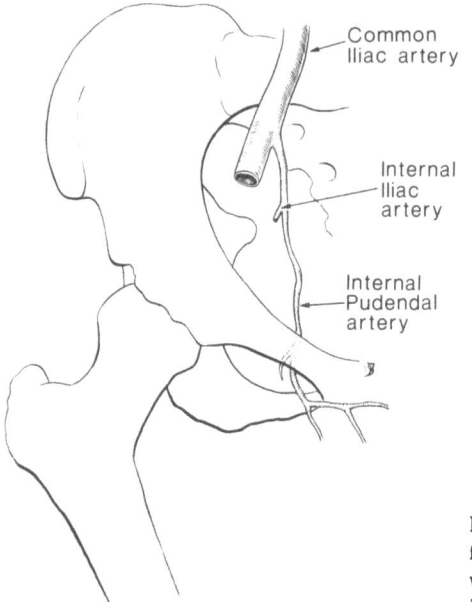

Figure 1. Penile blood supply is derived from the paired internal pudendal arteries which are major branches of the internal iliac (hypogastric) arteries.

the dorsum of the penis, and the *deep penile artery* lying almost entirely within the corpus cavernosum (Figure 2).

Although arterial obstruction can occur at any level, the most common lesions responsible for reduction in penile arterial flow are atherosclerotic occlusions or stenoses in the terminal aorta, the common iliac arteries, or the orifices of the internal iliac arteries. It is important to note that patients

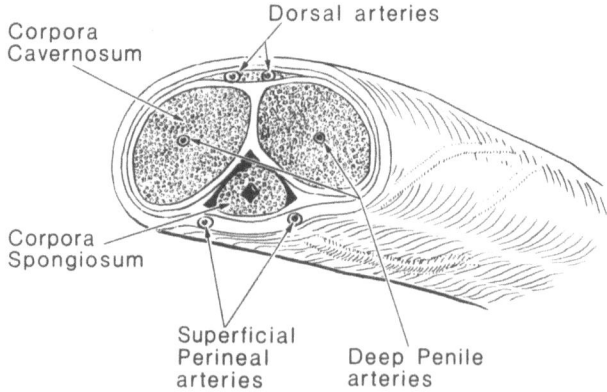

Figure 2. Cross section of the midshaft of the penis demonstrating the major arterial supply including the dorsal, deep penile, and superficial perineal arteries.

with such proximal obstructive lesions may be otherwise asymptomatic depending on their level of physical activity. Distal arterial obstruction in the internal pudental or the penile vessels proper may result from arteriosclerosis or embolization of atherosclerotic debris. Diabetics can also experience periarterial fibrosis in the corpora cavernosa. It is noteworthy that unilateral occlusions of the internal iliac arteries are generally well tolerated because of the paired blood supply through the internal pudendal arteries and the plentiful pelvic collaterals which allow normal perfusion of all six deep penile vessels.

PHYSIOLOGY OF ERECTION

Erection is achieved by a threefold increase in blood flow through the penile arteries. This increased arterial inflow is shunted by physiology valves ("polsters") into the vascular spaces of the corpora cavernosa to produce penile erection. The penis becomes flaccid when the valves redirect blood flow through normal venous drainage patterns through the plexus of Santorini to the hypogastric veins. Recent studies have focused on the role of the bulbocavernosus and ischiocavernosus muscles in this process. It is now thought that muscular contraction can enhance erection by compressing the veins of the corpora against the ischial arch.[2] However, venous outflow obstruction alone is insufficient to produce erection without a simultaneous increase in arterial flow.

Michal and associates measured penile blood flow required to achieve and maintain erection; a wide range of values was documented (45 to 180 ml/min).[3] The average blood flow required to achieve erection was 119 ml/min. A slightly lower rate of flow (72 ml/min) was required to sustain erection. Since increased arterial inflow is essential in achieving and maintaining an erection, any obstruction in the feeding arteries from the level of the aorta to the penis or any dysfunction in the arterial polsters can result in erectile impotence.

HISTORY

Certain features of a patient's history of erectile dysfunction suggest a vascular etiology. Patients frequently describe a gradual onset of impotence characterized by intermittent erectile failure during intercourse progressing to complete inability to obtain an erection. This process is often characterized as a gradual loss of firmness of the penis. Patients with vasculogenic impotence may be able to sustain erections long enough to achieve orgasm by masturbation but not be able to achieve the firmness required for vaginal penetration. On occasion, an adequate erection may be obtained, but when the patient initiates pelvic and lower-extremity movement, arterial blood is diverted to other collateral pathways and erection is not maintained (pelvic "steal"). In general, patients with firm nocturnal erections or episodic erectile failure are unlikely to have vasculogenic impotence.

It is important to note that vasculogenic impotence due to internal iliac or pudendal artery atherosclerosis may predate other symptoms of peripheral vascular occlusive disease such as claudication or buttock atrophy. Unfortunately, patients with generalized peripheral atherosclerosis all too often are not adequately questioned about sexual performance or erectile dysfunction. Even when suspected, impotence is often inappropriately attributed to antihypertensive medication, adrenergic blocking agents, or psychogenic causes without objective documentation of vascular status. The true incidence of vasculogenic impotence is becoming more evident with wider use of objective noninvasive measurements of penile perfusion.[4]

NONINVASIVE ASSESSMENT OF PENILE PERFUSION

Penile:Brachial Systolic Pressure Index

The simplest and most reliable assessment of penile perfusion is the measurement of arterial pressure in the corpora cavernosa perfused by the deep penile arteries. Such measurements may be obtained using a 10-kHz Doppler velocity detector which is positioned directly over one of the six penile arteries. A small pneumatic cuff is positioned proximal to the Doppler probe. The cuff is first inflated until arterial flow is abolished and is then allowed to slowly deflate; the point at which arterial flow returns is defined as the penile systolic pressure. Although individual measurements can be made for each of the six penile arteries, recording pressure in two of the vessels is usually sufficient.

Such absolute pressure measurements are helpful, but it is even more useful to correlate penile perfusion pressure with that obtained simultaneously in a brachial artery. The penile systolic pressure divided by the brachial systolic pressure yields the penile:brachial index (PBI) (Figure 3). A PBI of 1.0 ± 0.1 is normal. A PBI in the range of 0.75–0.9 may indicate some occlusive disease, but this level of perfusion is adequate to achieve and maintain erection. Patients with indices in the midrange (0.60–0.75) *may* have vascular contributions to erectile dysfunction although such values are not *diagnostic* of vasculogenic impotence. Patients with indices less than 0.6 are very likely to have vascular occlusive disease as the cause of their impotence.

Penile : brachial index (PBI)	$=$	$\dfrac{\text{Penile systolic pressure}}{\text{Brachial systolic pressure}}$
> 0.75		Vasculogenic impotence unlikely
0.60–0.75		Vascular causes possible
< 0.60		Highly suggestive of vasculogenic impotence

Figure 3. Comparing penile systolic pressure with brachial systolic pressure (PBI) allows assessment of the degree of vascular compromise.

VELOCITY WAVE FORMS/PLETHYSMOGRAPHY

Some investigators have found it useful to record Doppler velocity wave forms of penile blood flow or penile blood volume.[5-7] Flow wave forms can be obtained with a strip chart recorder directly connected to the Doppler probe. Normal arterial wave forms are triphasic and become progressively damped with occlusive disease (Figure 4). Volume wave forms can be obtained by classic phlethysmographic techniques. Patients with vascular obstruction demonstrate decreased volume amplitude and a flattening artifact of the wave form.

NOCTURNAL PENILE TUMESCENCE

It has been well recognized that normal men have periodic erections during sleep which can be correlated with episodes of rapid eye movement activity. By attaching mercury strain gages around the base and tip of the penis and observing the patient through an entire evening, a temporal record of erections can be correlated with simultaneous electroencephalographic tracings. The number of erections varies widely although norms have been tabulated for each age group. This test is perhaps most useful in patients with penile:brachial indices in the nondiagnostic but suggestive range (0.60–0.75). In general, the presence of normal nocturnal erections eliminates the diagnosis of vasculogenic impotence.[8]

DIRECT ASSESSMENT OF PENILE BLOOD FLOW

During the routine angiographic evaluation of patients with aortoiliac occlusive disease it is appropriate to obtain oblique pelvic views, allowing full visualization of the common iliac arteries and the origins of both internal iliac arteries. In this manner, much of the distal internal iliac circulation can be precisely outlined. Any suspected occlusive lesions can

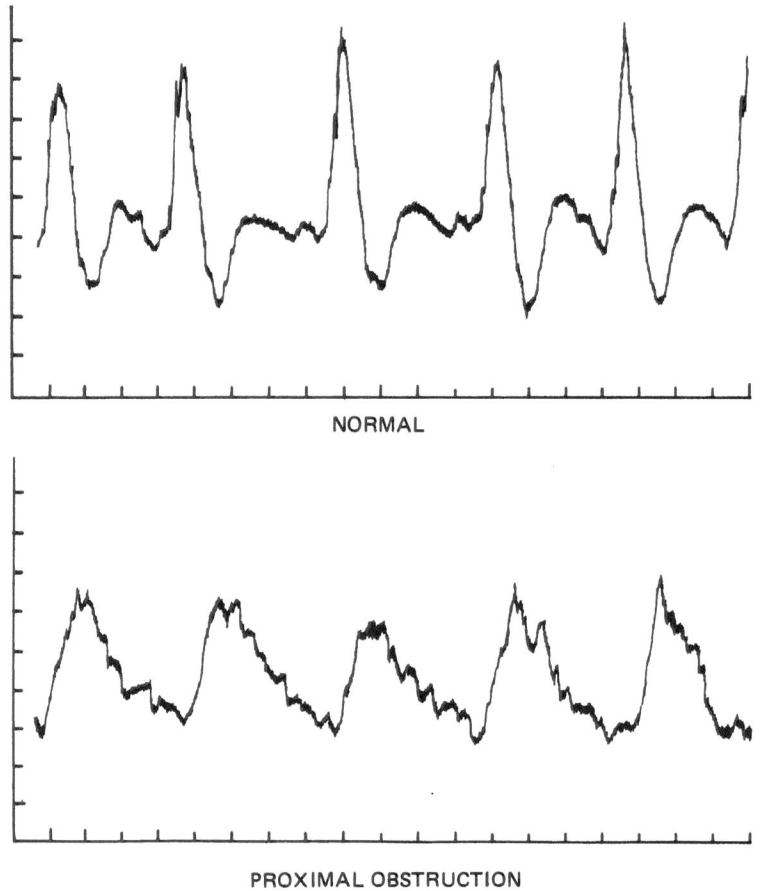

NORMAL

PROXIMAL OBSTRUCTION

Figure 4. Representative arterial wave forms from deep penile arteries using a 10-kHz doppler probe. Normal wave forms are triphasic; with proximal obstruction wave forms are damped becoming biphasic or monophasic.

be further defined by additional selective common or internal iliac injections.

As noted earlier, the most common atherosclerotic lesions limiting penile blood flow occur at the origin of the internal iliac from the common iliac artery and at the exit of the internal pudendal artery from the pelvis. Direct phalloarteriography has been advocated for more precise evaluation of the corpora cavernosa and deep penile artery. This study is rarely used at our institution since more distal reconstructions of penile vessels have proved to be ineffective at this time.

PATIENT SELECTION

Following the diagnosis of vasculogenic impotence the patient and physician must reach a decision regarding the need for therapy. Usually, patients seek medical care for impotence only if correction of sexual dysfunction is important to them. However, on occasion, when a patient understands that more invasive procedures may be required, enthusiasm for therapy begins to wane. There are very real risks associated with vascular reconstruction in patients with advanced atherosclerosis. It is the obligation of the surgeon to make this clear before beginning treatment. Certainly there are other less invasive surgical options including penile prostheses (described in Chapter 10) which allow the patient to resume sexual activity.

TREATMENT

In many patients, operative treatment of vasculogenic impotence is a secondary benefit of the treatment of peripheral vascular occlusive disease.[9,10] Most of these patients present with claudication (exercise-related symptoms) or rest pain of the lower extremities. The proper operative approach to these patients is guided by arteriographic studies, documenting the distribution and severity of aortoiliac disease. The most widely used procedure is an aortobifemoral bypass with a bifurcated Dacron vascular graft (Figure 5). This can be performed with an end-to-end proximal an-

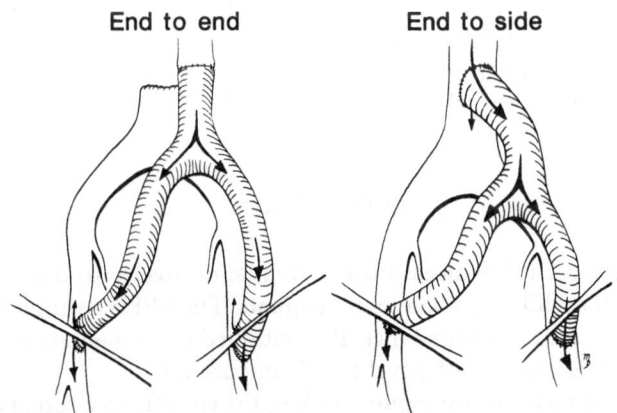

Figure 5. Following end-to-end aortobifemoral bypass, internal iliac perfusion depends on retrograde flow by both common femoral vessels. End-to-side anastomosis maintains antegrade flow in the terminal aorta and internal iliac vessels.

astomosis (which allows retrograde perfusion of the internal iliac arteries via both external iliac arteries) or an end-to-side proximal anstomosis (maintaining antegrade distal aortic and iliac flow). If the latter anastomotic technique is used and both internal iliac arteries are severely involved with atherosclerosis at their origins from the common iliac arteries, localized "eversion" endarterectomies may be required to restore adequate arterial inflow to the pudendal arteries. With this technique short occluding plaques can be removed with a minimum of dissection avoiding injury to autonomic nerves crossing the left iliac artery bifurcation. As noted earlier, revascularization of only one internal iliac is usually sufficient owing to the plentiful collateral circulation.[11]

If such orifice stenoses are isolated lesions unassociated with severe aortoiliac occlusive disease, percutaneous transluminal angioplasty is an attractive treatment option. One or both internal iliacs may be nonoperatively dilated using a specially designed balloon catheter which "fractures" the plaque and restores a large lumen. The physiological result of such dilatations can be objectively assessed by pre- and posttreatment penile:brachial indices; a successful dilation should return the PBI to the normal range.

If the most significant occlusive lesions involve the internal pudendal arteries, direct reconstruction can be performed by (1) reimplantation of one internal pudendal artery into a major branch of the inferior epigastric artery or (2) saphenous vein bypass to the internal pudendal from a proximal patent vessel. Experimental procedures have been attempted for more distal "small-vessel" disease. These have utilized direct microsurgical anastomoses or vein grafts between inferior epigastric vessels and the deep penile artery in the corpus cavernosum. Although arterial inflow is transiently improved, significant complications of these procedures have included priapism, periarterial fibrosis, and occlusion at the anastomotic site with worsening of vascular insufficiency.[12,13]

CONCLUSION

Vascular occlusive disease is too frequently overlooked as a cause of impotence in middle-aged and older patients. The PBI is a simple screening study for vasculogenic impotence. Its continued implementation can avoid inappropriate diagnoses of psychogenic impotence.

With complete arteriographic studies, the specific location of occlusive lesions can be delineated. Operative reconstruction or percutaneous transluminal angioplasty of isolated internal iliac lesions have been reliable in restoring penile arterial supply. At this time, microsurgical anastomoses and bypasses have been largely unsuccessful in treatment of distal arterial obstruction within the penis. However, additional experimental work may change the outlook for such lesions.

REFERENCES

1. Leriche R, Morel A: The syndrome of thrombotic obliteration of the aortic bifurcation. *Ann Surg* 127:193, 1948
2. Doherty JA, Gerhardt HC: Erectile mechanisms in man. *Science* 220:1080, 1982
3. Michal V, Kamar R, Hejhal L: Revascularization procedures of the cavernous bodies, in Zorgniotti AW, Rossi G (eds): *Vasculogeni Impotence.* Springfield, Illinois, Charles C Thomas, 1980, pp 239–255
4. Nath RL, Menzoian JO, and Kaplan KH: The multidisciplinary approach to vasculogenic impotence. *Surgery* 89:124, 1981
5. Abelson D: Diagnostic value of the penile pulse and blood pressure: A Doppler study of impotence in diabetics. *J Urol* 113:636, 1975
6. Britt DB, Kremmerer WT, Robison JR: Penile blood flow determination by mercury strain-guage plethysmography. *Invest Urol* 8:673, 1970
7. Kempczinski RF: Role of the vascular diagnostic laboratory in the evaluation of male impotence. *Am J Surg* 138:138–278, 1979
8. DePalma RG: Impotence in vascular disease: Relationship to vascular surgery. *Br J Surg* 69:514, 1982
9. DePalma RG, Kedia K, Persky L: Surgical options in the correction of vasculogenic impotence. *Vasc Surg* 14:92, 1980
10. Merchant RF Jr, DePalma RG: Effects of femorofemoral grafts on postoperative sexual function; Correlation with penile pulse volume recordings. *Surgery* 90:962, 1981
11. Queral LA, Whitehouse WM, and Flinn WR: Pelvic hemodynamics after aortoiliac reconstruction. *Surgery* 86:799, 1979
12. Casey WC: Revascularization of corpus cavernosus for erectile failure. *Urology* 14:135, 1979
13. Michal V, Kramer R, Bartak V: Femoro-pudendal bypass in the treatment of sexual impotence. *J Cardiovasc Surg* 15:356, 1974

6

Hormonal Considerations in the Evaluation and Treatment of Erectile Dysfunction

THOMAS M. JONES

INTRODUCTION

The concept that hormonal imbalances can account for sexual dysfunction has both rational and irrational bases. The association of absence of the testes with marked diminution of male copulatory behavior was made in antiquity. In this century, the isolation and actual synthesis of the active testicular factors that could restore phenotypic virilization in castrated men should have paved the way for more refined investigations of the effects of testicular steroids and their analogues on sexual behavior. Furthermore, the rather recently acquired ability to accurately measure blood and tissue levels of most of the hormones known to regulate reproduction should have allowed us to discover any and all causal links between documented sexual dysfunction and hormonal deficits and/or excesses. It is not widely acknowledged that these have been established, and I wish to devote space to understanding why wishful thinking still persists in both patients and practitioners before I outline what I consider to be the proper, modest hormonal evaluation of a man with a chief complaint of erectile dysfunction.

THOMAS M. JONES • Department of Medicine, University of Chicago, Chicago, Illinois 60637.

EFFECTS OF ANDROGENS ON THE MATURING MAMMALIAN BRAIN

Although we have accepted our mammalian heritage when we consider other types of hormonal actions such as the regulation of glucose metabolism by insulin, we tend to pick and choose when we relate our sexual behavior to that of other mammals. Nonetheless, a measured review of the development of reproductive behavior in male mammals should develop a useful perspective for considering aspects of human sexual behavior. A variety of reproductive behaviors in mammals are mediated by gonadal steroids. It is useful to consider these behaviors as being imprinted in the developing brain and elicited in the mature brain. To begin this brief overview of relationships between androgens and the central nervous system I shall first consider the sexually dimorphic regulation of gonadotropin release.

PATTERNING OF GONADOTROPIN RELEASE

Along with stereotypic copulatory behaviors (discussed later), the development of noncyclical (versus cyclical) gonadotropin release is dramatically affected by the presence or absence of androgens.[1-3] In our own species, ovulation is assured in endocrinologically intact women by cyclical surges of follicle-stimulating hormone and luteinizing hormone (FSH and LH) from the anterior pituitary gland which occur in a setting of minute-to-minute oscillations in the release of these two hormones.[4] The integration of this aspect of pituitary function with the hypothalamus began to be effectively elucidated over more than 30 years ago[5,6] and continues to be the focus of many aspects of studies of hormones and behavior. The pattern of gonadotropin release in endocrinologically intact adult men is markedly different and is comparatively constant.[7,8] This pattern is also reflected in the release of mature spermatozoa, which is more constant than the release of mature ova. Because of the tight relationship between patterns of gonadotropin release from the pituitary and hypothalamic release of gonadotropin-releasing hormone (GnRH), patterns of gonadotropin release are, in fact, neuroendocrine patterns which originate in purely neural pathways in the brain.

The distinctions between the rhythms of spermatogenesis and of ovulation are present, to a large extent, in all mammals. Studies performed in the rat demonstrate that sexually dimorphic patterns of gonadotropin release are established during a critical period of development and that androgens are critical for establishing the "male" pattern which is manifested in the adult.[9] In a very early study, Pfeiffer[10] showed that implanting a testis in a neonatal female rat led to the abolition of ovulation in the adult and to the development of constant estrus (Figure 1). Later investigators demonstrated that this phenomenon could be induced both by administering testosterone systemically and by implanting small amounts of testosterone in the hypothalamus (Figure 2).[11] However, the effects of testosterone administration can be blunted and even abolished if the experimental animals are pretreated with a variety of pharmacological agents active in the central nervous system; the barbiturates are particularly effective in blocking the virilization of the neural pathways (Figures 3 and 4).[12,13] This latter interaction should lead one to speculate about the po-

Survey of types of operations and hypophyseal reaction in the positive cases

EXPERI-MENT NO.	NUMBER OF ANIMALS	TYPE OF OPERATION		HYPOPHYSEAL POTENTIALITIES
		At birth	About puberty	
I	11 ♂	Castration	Ovary in eye	F & L*
II	10 ♂	Castration, testes in neck	Ovary in eye	F
III	28 ♂	Castration, ovaries in neck	Ovary in eye	F & L*
IV	10 ♀	Castration	Ovary in eye	F & L
V	14 ♀	Castration, ovaries in neck	. . . .	F & L
VI	16 ♀	Castration, testes in neck	Ovary in eye	F**
VII	50 ♂	Ovaries in body cavity	. . . .	F
VIII	22 ♂	Ovaries in neck	Ovary in eye	F
IX	39 ♀	Testis under skin	. . . .	F & L
X	117 ♀	Testes in body cavity	. . . .	F**
XI	69 ♀	Testes in neck	. . . .	F**
XII	12 ♀	. . . .	Adult testis in neck	F & L
XIII	12 ♀	. . . .	Testes of newborn in neck	F & L
XIV	12 ♀	. . . .	Testes in kidney	F & L
XV	12 ♀	. . . .	Testes in liver	F & L
XVI	12 ♀	. . . .	Testes dorsal to ovary	F & L
XVII	27 ♀	Testes in liver	. . . .	F & L
XVIII	22 ♀	Testes in neck	Injection of hormones	F**
Total	495			

(F) follicle stimulator. (L) luteinizer. * Experimentally caused maintenance of L potentiality. ** Experimental suppression of L potentiality.

Figure 1. Sexual differentiation of the hypophysis (really the hypothalamus).[10] This early study opened up the field of critical periods for sexual differentiation of the brain. Although it is clear from Pfeiffer's discussion that he thought that sexual differentiation of the pituitary was being described, we now tend to think of the pituitary as being relatively unsexually differentiated. Thus the finding of both "follicle stimulator" and "luteinizer" activity implies to us that the hypothalamus maintained its ability to secrete cyclical levels of LH and FSH. The important groups for purposes of this discussion are groups I, X, and XIV which show that cyclical versus noncyclical gonadotropin secretion can be altered by hormonal treatment at the time of birth but not by hormonal treatments in puberty.

Effects of testosterone on age at vaginal opening and on estrous cycles						
Treatment group	Experiment 1 6 μg TP			Experiment 2 2 μg TP		
	No. rats	Age at vaginal opening‡	PVE†	No. rats	Age at vaginal opening	PVE
A. Controls	18	38 ±1*	0	10	40 ±2	0
B. "Blank" paraffin pellets, brain	17	37 ±1	0	11	38 ±1	0
C. Testosterone-paraffin pellets, sc	15	36 ±1	7	10	36 ±2	4
D. Testosterone-paraffin pellets, brain	19	34 ±1	16	20	36 ±1	16
E. Testosterone in oil, sc (10.0 μg)	17	33 ±1	7	11	36 ±1	8

* Mean ±standard error.
† Persistent vaginal estrus.
‡ Results of multiple range test of Duncan; differences with p >0.05 not included. Age at vaginal opening, Experiment 1: A vs. C, p <0.05; A vs. D, p <0.01; A vs. E, p <0.01; B vs. D, p <0.01; B vs. E, p <0.01; C vs. D, p <0.05; C vs. E, p <0.05. Experiment 2: A vs. D, p <0.05.

Figure 2. Androgen sterilization of the brain.[11] It is not even necessary to administer systemic androgens to young female rats in order to induce androgen sterilization of the brain. One can simply place the testosterone directly into the brain and induce loss of ovarian cyclicity in most of the animals. In addition to showing a very high rate of persistent vaginal estrus, such androgen-treated females also tend to have earlier timing of vaginal opening (a classical sign of progression into puberty in rats).

tential role that endogenous compounds such as endorphins or enkephalins[14] might play in altering neonatal androgen imprinting.

There are two important points to underscore in these and many similar studies: the timing of neuronal imprinting is both critical and rather precise, and the investigations have not studied subtle or graded responses to varying levels of androgens. Moreover, although the critical period has been clearly demonstrated to be in the immediate postnatal period in the rat, it is not only possible but likely that, in many species, the critical period is partly or entirely prenatal. If this should prove to be the case in humans, then the hormonal environment of the mother might well be decisive. Finally, the imprinting of the neural pathways is not solely under the direction of androgens but also involves possible alterations by at least exogenous and perhaps endogenous compounds with central nervous system effects ranging from barbiturates and phenothiazines to endorphins and a variety of neurotransmitters.

Thus, a cautious interpretation of such studies is that the presence of significant amounts of androgens at a critical period in early life can obliterate the development of cyclical gonadotropin release in adult mammals. In addition, the absence of significant amounts of testosterone at this critical period permits the development of cyclical gonadotropin release

	Protection by tranquilizers against androgenization								
Injection(s) on day 5 of age	Incidence of sterility # anovulatory/ # injected				Autopsy data				
	at 60 days of age¹	%	at 120 days of age	%	Condition of ovaries	# of rats	Body wt (g)	Ovarian wt (mg)	Uterine wt (mg)
30 µg TP³	7/8	88	8/8	100	Polyfollicular	8	270±5²	34.2±4.5	398±29
30 µg TP+10 µg Reserpine⁴	6/16	37	11/16	69	Normal	5	266±6	78.8±3.0	462±15
					Polyfollicular⁵	11	266±6	41.3±8.4	519±17
30 µg TP+500 µg Chlorpromazine	5/12	42	9/12	75	Normal	3	273	89.9	483
					Polyfollicular⁵	9	266±4	40.6±2.2	524±32
10 µg Reserpine	0/5	0	0/5	0	Normal	5	263±9	89.4±2.9	413±29
500 µg Chlorpromazine	0/6	0	0/6	0	Normal	6	262±7	82.9±3.9	425±34

1 Incidence of sterility ascertained by laparotomy.
2 Mean ± standard error.
3 In 0.02 ml peanut oil; plus reserpine vehicle.
4 In 0.05 ml.
5 Including ovaries with old CL.

	Protection by barbiturates against androgenization								
Injection(s) on day 5 of age	Incidence of sterility # anovulatory/ # injected				Autopsy data				
	At 45 days of age¹	%	At 90 days of age	%	Condition of ovaries	# of rats	Body wt (g)	Ovarian wt (mg)	Uterine wt (mg)
30 µg TP²+Saline	13/16	81	15/16	94	Normal	1	265	78.6	503
					Polyfollicular	15	286±4	32.9±3.0	418±21
30 µg TP+PB⁴	0/15	0	4/15	27	Normal	11	288±3	92.9±6.0	535±20
					Polyfollicular⁶	4	260±10	56.2±6.9	505±22
30 µg TP+PhB⁵	2/17	12	4/17	23	Normal	13	271±8	108.0±3.0	432±23
					Polyfollicular⁶	7	274±7	61.0±4.1	484±21
30 µg TP+PB+ Metrazol³	18/25	72	7/10	70	Normal	3	253	74.9	354
					Polyfollicular⁶	7	254±7	33.3±1.9	347±13
PB	0/12	0	0/12	0	Normal	12	286±4	93.7±2.5	535±17
PhB	0/9	0	0/9	0	Normal	9	270±12	87.2±1.5	410±30

1 Incidence of sterility ascertained by laparotomy.
2 In 0.02 ml peanut oil.
3 Two injections (0.3 mg/0.05 ml/rat) given 4–5 hr apart.
4 Single injection of 0.5 mg/0.05 ml/rat.
5 Two injections of 2 mg/rat given with PB.
6 Including ovaries with old CL.

Figure 3. Androgen sterilization of brain: effects of tranquilizers.[12] Administering testosterone to 5-day-old female rats renders many of the rats anovulatory at puberty. The ovary shows multiple follicles in such "androgen-sterilized" rats. Simultaneous injection of either chlorpromazine or reserpine blocks a substantial number of testosterone-treated rats from developing polyfollicular ovaries and chronic anovulation. Simultaneous injection of barbiturates is even more effective. Treatment with any of those powerful central-nervous-system-active agents at day 5 without testosterone administration is not shown to have an effect on later reproductive function.

in adult mammals. As an aside, it must be noted that a substantial literature demonstrates that testosterone is converted to estradiol in the hypothalamus as well as in other areas of the brain and that it is the intracellular estradiol that actually "virilizes" the neuronal pathways.[15] In fact, some authors have shown that administration of high levels of estrogens at the critical period can "virilize" the pathways.[16]

Critical exposure time for androgenization of the five-day-old rat as determined by phenobarbital (PhB) injection					
Steroid at time zero on day 5	Time of PhB* injection (hr after steroid)	Incidence of sterility (no. anovulatory/no. injected)			
		At 45 days of age	%	At 90 days of age	%
30 μg TP	None	32/37	86.5	15/16	93.8
30 μg TP	Zero	4/31	12.9	4/17	23.5
30 μg TP	3	14/28	50.0	7/11	63.6
30 μg TP	6	22/30	73.3	13/17	76.5
30 μg TP	9	13/15	86.7	—	—
30 μg TP	12	21/23	91.4	13/14	92.9
30 μg TP	24	20/27	74.1	14/15	93.3

* Single injection of 0.5 mg phenobarbital/00.5 ml/rat.

Figure 4. Androgen sterilization of brain: critical period.[13] Androgen sterilization apparently occurs in a matter of hours in the rat. If phenobarbital is injected at varying time intervals after testosterone treatment, it can be seen that the effect of testosterone is permanent within 12 hr. Investigations of comparable rigor have never been carried out in humans, and thus the entire field of prenatal and neonatal hormonal influences on later sexual behavior is wildly speculative.

There is, then, no claim that high doses of androgens given to adult females can permanently suppress cyclical gonadotropin release or that high doses of estrogens given to adult males can induce cyclical gonadotropin release. More important, there is literally no reason whatsoever to believe that subtle alterations in the androgen/estrogen ratio in adulthood have any influence on imprinting either cyclical or noncyclical gonadotropin release.

Of course, patients complaining of erectile dysfunction have no concern about cyclical versus noncyclical gonadotropin release, and my brief review of this area is meant to sensitize the reader to the limitations that ought to be placed on interpretations of animal data even when the neurohormonal relationships are exceedingly clear. Moreover, I have introduced an important speculative theme that will recur later: the possible roles that powerful compounds synthesized in the central nervous system could play in interfering with androgen-mediated behavioral pathways. I shall now move to a discussion of a more relevant neurohormonal relationship: the one between hormonal milieus and sterotypical precopulatory and copulatory behavior.

IMPRINTING STEREOTYPICAL COPULATORY BEHAVIOR

In virtually all mammals, copulatory and courtship behavior can be dissected into various components, most of which are not only rather rigidly sterotyped but are also species-specific (Figure 5).[17] In most species

ORDER & SPECIES	LOCK?	THRUSTING?	MULTIPLE INTROMISSIONS?	MULTIPLE EJACULATIONS	REFERENCES
Order Lagomorpha					
Oryctolagus cuniculus	no	no	no	yes	Denenberg et al. (1969); Rubin & Azrin (1967)
Lepus californicus	—	—	—	yes	Pontrelli (1968)
Order Chiroptera					
Myotis subulatus	—	no	—	—	Wimsatt (1945)
M. nigricans	yes?	yes	—	—	Wilson (1971)
Nyctalus noctula	—	no?	no?	yes?	Kleiman & Racey (1969)
Order Primates					
Lemur catta	no	yes	no	yes	Jolly (1966)
Galago senegalensis	no?	no	no?	yes?	Lowther (1940); Doyle et al. (1967)
G. demidovi	—	—	no	yes	Blackwell (1969)
Alouatta palliata	no	yes	no?	yes?	Carpenter (1934, 1965)
Saimiri sciureus	no	yes	yes	yes	Clewe (1968); Latta et al. (1967)
Macaca mulatta	no	yes	yes	yes	Carpenter (1942); Kuehn & Young (1965); Michael & Saayman (1967a, b)
M. fuscata	no	yes	yes	yes	Tokuda (1961)
M. nemestrina	no	yes	yes	yes	Tokuda et al. (1968)
M. radiata	no	yes	no	yes	Nadler & Rosenblum (1969); Simonds (1965)
M. arctoides	?	yes	no	yes	Blurton Jones & Trollope (1968)
Cercocebus albigena	no?	yes	yes?	—	Chalmers (1968)
Papio (S. Africa Cape)	no	yes	yes	yes	Hall & DeVore (1965), Saayman (1970)
Papio (Nairobi Park)	no	yes	no	yes	Hall & DeVore (1965)
Papio hamadryas	no	yes	yes	yes?	Kummer (1968)
Cercopithecus aethiops	no	yes	no	no	Struhsaker (1967a); Gartlan (1969)
Cercopithecus spp.	no?	yes?	no	—	Booth (1962)
Hylobates lar	no?	yes	—	—	Coolidge (1933); Carpenter (1940); Berkson & Chaicumpa (1969)
Pan troglodytes	no	yes	no	no?	Yerkes (1939); Goodall (1965, 1969); Reynolds & Reynolds (1965); Kollar et al. (1968)
Gorilla gorilla	no	yes	—	no	Schaller (1963)
Homo sapiens	no	yes	no	yes?	Ford & Beach (1951)
Family Tupaiidae					
Tupaia longipes	—	yes	—	—	Conaway & Sorenson (1966)
T. belangeri	no?	yes?	yes?	—	Martin (1968)
T. glis	no?	yes?	yes?	—	Kaufmann (1965b)
Order Cetacea					
Tursiops truncatus	—	yes	—	—	Tavolga & Essapian (1957)
Order Carnivora					
Canis lupus	yes	yes	no	yes	Yadav (1968)
C. latrans	yes	yes?	no?	yes	Kleiman (1968)
C. familiaris	yes	yes	no	yes	Hart (1967); Fuller & Fox (1969)
Alopex lagopus	yes	yes?	no?	—	Kleiman (1968)
Vulpes vulpes	yes	—	—	—	Kleiman (1967)
Nyctereutes procyonoides	yes	yes?	no?	—	Kleiman (1968)
Chrysocyon brachyurus	yes	—	—	—	Kleiman (1967)
Speothos venaticus	yes	yes?	no?	—	Kleiman (1968)
Cuon alpinus	yes	—	—	—	Sosnovskii (1967); Kleiman (1967)
Lycaon pictus	no	yes	no?	yes?	Cade (1967)
Otocyon megalotis	yes	—	—	—	Kleiman (1968)
Ursus arctos	—	—	no	—	Craighead et al. (1969)
Mustela vison	no	yes	no	—	Enders (1952)
M. furo	no?	no?	no	yes	Hammond & Marshall (1930); Murr (1931)
M. frenata	—	—	—	yes	Wright (1948)
Mephitis mephitis	no?	yes	—	—	Wight (1931); Verts (1967)
Felis catus	no	no	no	yes	Michael (1961); Whalen (1963a); Kling et al. (1969)
Panthera tigris	no	—	no	yes	Sankhala (1967); Gowda (1966)

Figure 5. Components of copulation.[17] This is just a portion of a large table from Dewsbury's scheme to break copulatory behavior into components that can be compared across species. In terms of just the four basic categories covered in this table, it can be seen that our own species is rather boring. Nonetheless, more subtle variations in patterning of copulatory behavior may be of critical importance in sexual encounters in humans.

studied, deviation from this patterned behavior is frequently associated either with onset of aggressive activity between the male and female or with sterile copulations.[18] Stereotyped courtship and copulatory patterns serve to identify species members to one another and prevent, to a great extent, copulatory activity between members of different species. The development of correct behaviors is so important to each species member that little is left to chance; these behaviors can be displayed in the adult only as a consequence of neurological imprinting as reliable as that imprinting which leads to patterned gonadotropin release.[19] For example, Harris and Levine[20] (Figure 6) were able to show that testosterone given to female rats within 4 days of birth abolished the development of female copulatory behavior in the adult (specifically, the lordosis response). In the same study, females given testosterone within the first 4 days, then ovariectomized and given testosterone as adults, developed male copulatory behavior. Finally, males given small doses of estrogen during the first 4 days of birth were shown to have marked diminution in male copulatory behavior as adults (Figure 7). Not surprisingly, pretreatment with barbiturates can obliterate all these effects.[3] A principle emerges: at a critical period of development, neural patterns are imprinted under the influence

The proportion of female rats showing partial or complete female behaviour, or aggressive and repulsive behaviour, when tested with a vigorous normal male

Group	Treatment Neonatal	Adult	No. of rats	No. showing partial female behaviour: hopping, darting, lordosis	No. showing full receptivity	No. showing only aggressive or repulsive behaviour
a	Testosterone	—	18/16	0/0	0/0	18/16*
b	Testosterone	Ovariect. O+P	10	0	0	10
c	Oil	Ovariect. O+P	17	2	15	0
d	Oestradiol	Ovariect. O+P	12	5	7	0
e	Testosterone	Ovariect. T	10	0	0	10
f	Oil	Ovariect. T	7	2	5	0

* The double figures in this row represent the results obtained during two different test sessions.

Ovariect., ovariectomy; O+P, oestrogen and progesterone replacement therapy; T, testosterone administration.

Figure 6. Sexual differentiation of the brain: behavioral consequences in females.[20] Not only are patterns of gonadotropin release subject to sexual differentiation at critical periods, but patterns of stereotyped copulatory behavior are as well. The genetic females in group a lost all of their female copulatory behavior when treated with testosterone early in life. Even administration of ovarian hormones in adulthood (group b) could not restore female copulatory behavior.

The behaviour patterns observed in the various groups of male
rats when tested with an oestrous female

Group	Treatment Neonatal	Adult	No. in group	No male behaviour	Partial behavioural pattern	Full male behavioural pattern
g	Oestradiol	—	31	17	13	1
h	Testosterone	—	10	0	0	10
i	Oil	—	25	2	6	17
j	Oestradiol	Castration testosterone	10	4	4	2
k	Oil	Castration testosterone	5	0	0	5

Figure 7. Sexual differentiation of the brain: behavioral consequences in males.[20] One can also blunt the appearance of male-patterned copulatory behavior by treating genetic males with estradiol after birth. The failure of neonatal estradiol to completely obliterate imprinting of masculine copulatory behavior is of great interest in light of a body of studies demonstrating that intracellular estradiol (normally derived from conversion of testosterone in neural tissue) is an effective "masculine" organizer.

of gonadal steroids which facilitate the display of stereotyped sexual behaviors in adults under the influence of adult levels of the same gonadal steroids. The evocation of these stereotypical behaviors is complicated. A fuller appreciation of this complexity is gained from the following sample of studies describing associations between gonadal steroids and brain.

EFFECTS OF ANDROGENS ON THE MATURE MAMMALIAN BRAIN

It has been shown that castration is followed by clearly demonstrable changes in several areas of the brain, particularly the hypothalamus.[21] On the other hand, administration of exogenous gonadal steroids leads to different, but equally distinct histological changes.[22] Virtually the same areas of the brain show significant and preferential uptake of radioactively labeled testosterone.[23] Administration of testosterone causes changes in patterns of neurological activity,[24] and castration is followed by changes in neurotransmitter levels in various regions of the hypothalamus.[25] Such findings have led quite naturally to the conclusion that there are androgen receptors in the brain which at the very least play an important role in feedback regulation of GnRH release.

A further role is illustrated by Lisk's[26] study of localized testosterone implants in castrated male rats. Lisk found that placing small amounts of testosterone propionate in the preoptic anterior hypothalamic area led to restoration of complete male copulatory response patterns. Implants in other hypothalamic areas produced either no response or a markedly weaker response. Implants in the mamillary region were followed by "hyperexcitability" in the presence of females but not by mounting behavior. Interestingly, this is one of the few studies that has come to my attention which could be construed as uncoupling the link between "libido" and "performance" in mammals although clinicians see this uncoupling in patients with monotonous regularity. In animals treated with hypothalamic implants, no significant stimulation of accessory glands occurs, underlining the fact that the amount of androgens reaching the systemic circulation is trivial.

Lesions in the preoptic anterior hypothalamic areas have been shown to eliminate copulatory behavior in rats despite normal circulating androgens.[27] Electrical stimulation of this same area is followed by stereotypical copulatory activity even in rats with no testes.[28,29]

The studies cited are just a sample from a large literature which provides compelling evidence that stereotypical copulatory behavior in mammals results from activation of gonadal steroid-sensitive pathways with one or more areas of clear localization in the brain.[2,3,19,30] In undisturbed mammals, activation requires the presence of a critical amount of circulating hormones although other types of activation are theoretically possible. Although research to date has focused on the localized brain centers, other studies may be expected to show steroid-sensitive tracts or networks which may defy localization by traditional techniques. At any rate, testosterone deprivation and subsequent replacement in otherwise intact adult male mammals are followed, respectively, by reduction and restoration of male-patterned copulatory behavior.[31] In a very narrow sense, the testicular production of adult male levels of androgens merely serves to ensure binding of a critical level of androgens to appropriate neurons so that copulatory behavior can be elicited.

EFFECTS ON COPULATORY BEHAVIOR

Circannual Rhythms

Most mammals do not display copulatory behavior during the entire year. In fact, display is often limited to rather short spans of time.[32–35] The synchronous display of copulatory behavior in mammalian populations is clearly under the influence of alterations in the amount of daylight to which the mammals are exposed.[36–39] Information about daylight is relayed to the hypothalamus by pathways extending from the retina through the pineal gland.[40,41]

This neuroendocrine system results in marked changes in androgen levels in male mammals (Figure 8) so that during the height of the copulatory season males have dramatically higher testosterone levels than during the quieter part of the year.[42-45] The androgen dependence of a mammal's ability to display copulatory behavior is eloquently demonstrated in a study of the Scottish red deer.[46] If a red-deer stag is castrated, he fails to exhibit copulatory behavior regardless of the time of year. If, however, a castrated stag is given testosterone after his fellow stags have ceased exhibiting copulatory behavior, he begins to display all the behaviors typically seen in the rutting season.

Despite the suggestion that men may have an annual rhythm of testosterone production (Figure 9),[47] the breadth of the excursions in no way approaches that of other mammals. Attempts to document an annual rhythm of reproduction in man have met with almost no success at all.[48,49] Other types of cyclical variations in testosterone levels in humans have been seen (Figure 10), but the authors go out of their way to point out both the limited extent of the excursions and the absolute lack of behavioral correlates.

Thus, humans are, in a sense, disengaged from the physical environment insofar as reproductive behavior is concerned. Even statistically significant changes in plasma testosterone levels may not have any implication for human copulatory behavior unless the levels drop to castrate values. The sense that there is a distinction between humans and other mammals has been shared for some time; one can note the hedging in a statement from Young's classic monograph *Sex and Internal Secretions:* "... in all *subhuman* mammals... the strength or vigor of male behavior is related to the gonadal hormones."[51; p 1222] The disengagement of the neuroendocrine regulation of reproduction from the physical environment as far as annual rhythms are concerned may have a more general implication: alterations in human reproduction may have less to do with environmentally mediated hormonal changes than with endogenous events in the central nervous system. We shall now explore a body of studies that supports this conclusion in another way.

Modification by Exteroceptive Stimuli: Pheromones and Social Stress

Although I have thus far portrayed the relationship between testosterone lack and loss of copulatory behavior as being a simple one in subhuman mammals, it is not. Clegg and his co-workers[52] (Figure 11) compared the effects of testosterone replacement in castrated male sheep. The authors emphasized the difference in responsiveness between rams castrated between 7 and 14 days and rams castrated after puberty. All the prepubertal

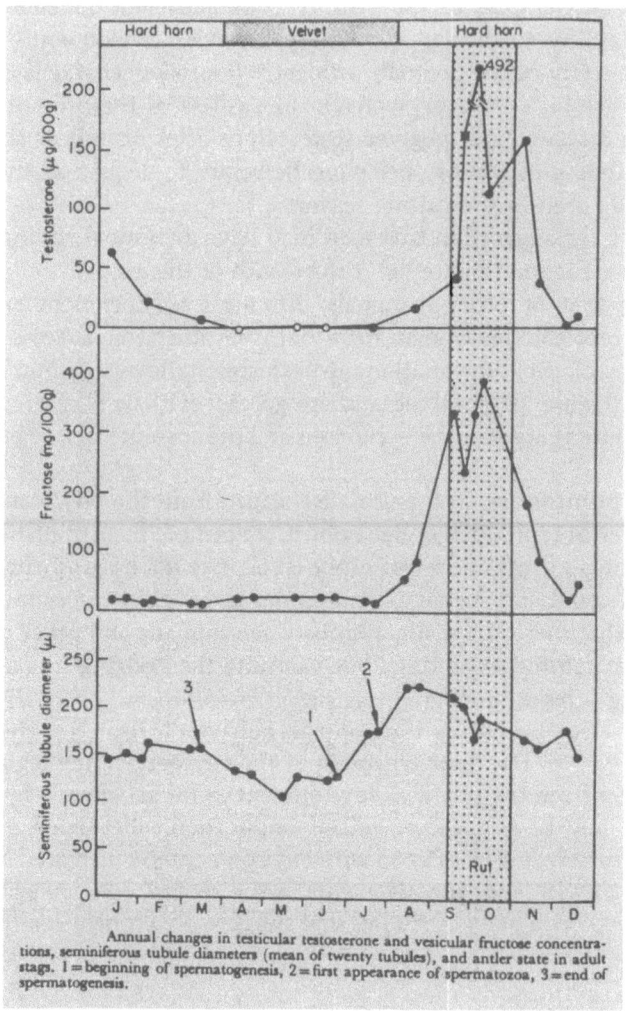

Annual changes in testicular testosterone and vesicular fructose concentrations, seminiferous tubule diameters (mean of twenty tubules), and antler state in adult stags. 1 = beginning of spermatogenesis, 2 = first appearance of spermatozoa, 3 = end of spermatogenesis.

Figure 8. An example of an annual cycle.[42] Seasonally breeding mammals have remarkable changes in gonadal function. This study of Scottish red deer shows dramatic elevations in testosterone levels around the time of the mating season and also shows the waxing and waning of spermatogenesis during the year. In mammals, then, the concentration of copulatory behavior in one season of the year has an easily documentable hormonal basis.

		PLASMA TESTOSTERONE (ng/100ml)				
		April 1974	July 1974	Oct. 1974	Jan. 1975	April 1975
subject no	age (yrs)					
1	44	615	720	729	560	526
2	32	380	441	481	376	435
3	32	723	642	604	552	570
4	45	478	562	543	477	707
5	39	706	844	788	803	689
6	30	861	803	618	750	681
7	24	979	1293	1179	1269	719
8	29	586	650	698	689	611
9	30	659	704	732	539	516
10	41	627	722	1029	746	796
11	34	738	848	734	654	741
12	31	753	790	883	669	635
13	28	471	407	496	613	326
14	36	645	653	771	687	734
15	26	781	1084	1144	586	778
mean	33.5	666	744*	762*	665	631
± SD	5.9	154	225	216	201	133

* values significantly different from April 1974, January 1975 and April 1975 (P_w < 0.01 - < 0.05).

CIRCANNUAL VARIATION IN PLASMA TESTOSTERONE IN MAN.

Figure 9. Is there an annual cycle in humans?[47] Unlike seasonally breeding mammals, humans do not have dramatic annual alterations in plasma testosterone levels. Even studies that report some detectable differences fail to show declines in testosterone sufficient to induce changes in secondary sex characteristics. This unlinking of Leydig cell function from circannual light rhythms may explain why Leydig cell plasticity in humans is virtually impossible to document. In a sense, the establishment of human reproduction as an activity independent of the physical environment may also have resulted in its independence from the social environment.

castrates acquired the full range of copulatory behavior after several weeks of testosterone therapy, implying that the critical imprinting period had been passed. They lost all copulatory behavior after hormonal withdrawal. The postpubertal castrates had a wider range of reactions. Although copulatory behavior decreased, in some rams it was still evident. Furthermore, there was a substantial amount of individual variation in responsiveness. A given level of copulatory activity could be elicited by 50 mg of testosterone propionate in one animal but might not be elicited in another until twice as much hormone was given.

Aside from such apparently unpredictable differences among individuals, certain factors in a mammal's environment can lead to predictable changes. Differences in display of sexual behavior are commonplace in both captive and free-ranging mammalian groups. Frank absence of sexual behavior was observed by Mattner et al.[53] in a proportion of young rams. The authors speculated that rearing rams in large monosexual groups may have contributed to this aberration. Such speculation raises serious doubts about the simplicity of imprinting and eliciting copulatory behavior. Hard and Larsson[54] found that exposing inexperienced male rats to a pair of copulating rats markedly facilitated the development of full copulatory behavior in the inexperienced males. Aside from adult male levels of plasma

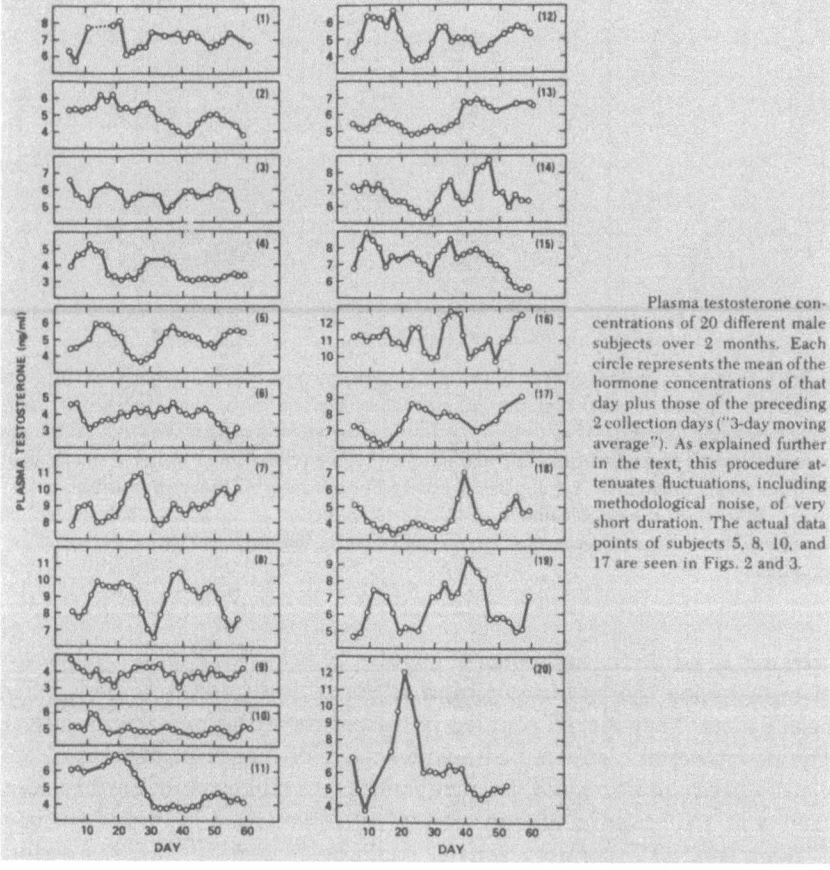

Plasma testosterone concentrations of 20 different male subjects over 2 months. Each circle represents the mean of the hormone concentrations of that day plus those of the preceding 2 collection days ("3-day moving average"). As explained further in the text, this procedure attenuates fluctuations, including methodological noise, of very short duration. The actual data points of subjects 5, 8, 10, and 17 are seen in Figs. 2 and 3.

Figure 10. Other testosterone cycles in humans.[50] Because of the readily documented fluctuations in plasma testosterone levels in normal males, it is unwise to begin a full-scale investigation of the hypothalamopituitary axis until more than one abnormal testosterone level is obtained. In addition, it is somewhat difficult to attribute copulatory performance problems to modestly low testosterone levels when one realizes that, in this group of men, there were no detectable behavioral correlates with the plasma testosterone fluctuations.

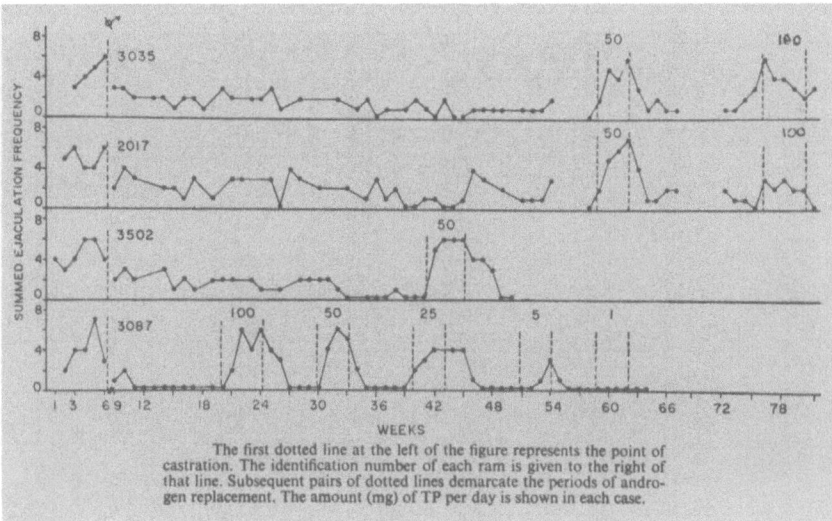

The first dotted line at the left of the figure represents the point of castration. The identification number of each ram is given to the right of that line. Subsequent pairs of dotted lines demarcate the periods of androgen replacement. The amount (mg) of TP per day is shown in each case.

Figure 11. Individual differences in response to androgen manipulation.[52] Too little attention has been paid to individual differences in subhuman mammals. Although I have referred to studies showing how copulatory performance can be altered by changes in testosterone levels, it is important to realize that individual mammals still can differ in their response to the same hormonal stimuli. In this figure, rams castrated at week 6 are given various doses of testosterone propionate. Although it is clear that ejaculation frequency is increased by giving testosterone, it is equally remarkable that certain rams maintain some degree of ejaculation with no testosterone whereas others maintain none. Moreover, ram 2017 has less response to 100 mg of testosterone than do others in the study.

testosterone, there are clearly other factors that facilitate the elicitation of patterned copulatory behavior. Chief among these are olfactory stimuli originating in reproductively active females and tactile factors experienced in precopulatory activity.

Carlsson and Larsson[55] anesthetized the glans penis of male rats and discovered that such treatment inhibited erection in the males and abolished intromission. In support of this is an observation by Kang et al.,[24] who noted that genital stimulation heightened the spindle activity and slow-wave formation which they observed in the preoptic area of the hypothalamus following testosterone treatment of castrate monkeys. One is led to believe that both peripheral neural input and hormonal input are integrated in the brain to trigger the neural messages that coordinate even such seemingly simple responses as penile tumescence. It is also possible that peripheral neural input enhances testosterone levels in intact animals. Saginor and Horton[56] (Figure 12) measured circulating testosterone levels in male rabbits. They found that within 30 min of copulation plasma

Peripheral plasma androstenedione and testosterone in the adult male rabbit		
Rabbit no.	Androstenedione	Testosterone
	mμg/100 ml*	
1	22	64
2	28	46
3	18	12
4	44	38
5	0	43
6	31	61
7	18	22
8	23	77
Mean	23 ± 5.1	45 ± 7.7

* Corrected for mean blank of the methods.

Effect of copulation on plasma androstenedione and testosterone in the male rabbit		
Rabbit no.	Androstenedione	Testosterone
	mμg/100 ml*	
Copulation		
5	0	266
8	24	434
11	17	262
13	0	112
Mean	10	268
Precoital behavior		
12	16	91
13	20	363
14	14	145
Mean	17	200

* Corrected for mean blank of the methods.

Figure 12. Exteroceptive stimuli leading to increased testosterone levels.[56] Placing male rabbits on a table with receptive females (group labeled "precoital behavior") leads to substantial increases in circulating testosterone levels. Even more effective in inducing testosterone rises is copulation itself. The increased circulating testosterone levels probably trigger patterned copulatory activity in male but are by no means the only way in which such activity can be elicited. There is no evidence that Leydig cell output in humans is as responsive to exteroceptive stimuli as is that of the rabbit. Even the most careful studies of normal men have never uncovered a paradigm whereby mean testosterone levels could be raised to 5–6 times control values by a manipulation.

testosterone levels rose significantly. Furthermore, levels also rose simply following exposure to a female.

That such exposure is really a matter of transmitting olfactory stimuli has been well documented. Removal of the olfactory bulb in male mammals leads to a dramatic decrease in all parameters of precopulatory and copulatory behavior (Figure 13).[57-59] Lesions placed in the olfactory area of the brain are equally effective.[27,60] Primates are just as sensitive to such stimuli as are other mammals. Male monkeys invariably manipulate the female's genitalia and then smell their hands immediately following contact.[61] In addition, males sniff female urine as well as the places where females have

Postoperative Mating Behavior in Gonadally Intact Male Mice[1]

Surgical Group	n	Percent Mounting	Mean Latency to First Mount (Min.) ± 1 S.E.M.	Mean Latency to First Ejaculation (Min.) ± 1 S.E.M.	Mean Percent of Tests Resulting in Ejaculation ± 1 S.E.M.
Sham + Normal	11	100	5.4 ± 1.33	39.9 ± 7.61	88 ± 9.90
Unilateral	5	100	5.0 ± 2.08	38.9 ± 11.97	78 ± 12.0
Bilateral	9	22*	-- --	-- --	-- --

[1]Mean latencies to first mount and first ejaculation were calculated from the values that were obtained on the last two postoperative tests.

*Indicated significantly different from Sham + Normal group at beyond the 0.05 level by Chi-square analysis of frequencies employed in calculating percentages.

Mean Body Weight and Testes and Seminal Vesicles Weights

Surgical Group	n	Body Weight ± 1 S.E.M. (g)	Testes Weight ± 1 S.E.M. (mg)	Seminal Vesicles Weight ± 1 S.E.M. (mg)
Sham + Normal	11	41.3 ± 0.94	237.2 ± 7.16	74.2 ± 5.66
Unilateral	5	38.0 ± 0.64	222.7 ± 14.63	79.0 ± 4.23
Bilateral	9	42.1 ± 1.20	228.3 ± 7.84	69.2 ± 4.60

Figure 13. Olfaction and copulation.[57] The role of olfaction in reproductive behavior is critical in most (if not all) mammals. When only one olfactory bulb is removed in the male mouse, there is no significant impairment of copulatory activity. However, removing both olfactory bulbs, rendering the mouse completely anosmic, causes cessation of effective copulation. This cessation is completely independent of alterations in testicular size and, more important, of alterations in testosterone-dependent organs (the seminal vesicles). With studies of this type, we are able to move away from the notion that successful copulatory behavior is completely dependent on testosterone levels. Olfaction, of course, is the essential modality for receiving pheromonal information. Although the role of pheromones in human reproduction is largely speculative, their pervasiveness in other mammals continues to inspire investigation.

been seated. Male copulatory behavior is more frequent and more vigorous when females are in the follicular phase of the estrous cycle than when they are in the luteal phase.[62] Males are more eager to gain access to estrogenized castrated females than to castrated females without estrogen replacement, and once they are with females, copulatory behavior is more vigorous with the estrogenized females.[63,64] Castration of males eliminates their preference for female companionship.[65]

Exposure to estrogenized females has been shown to lead to increases in testicular size in males in the nonbreeding season,[66] whereas exposure to male-only groups was associated with inhibition of male sexual development in immature mammals (Figure 14).[67] Finally, ether extracts of vaginal secretions of estrogenized females were applied to castrated females with the result that males suddenly found these treated castrated females attractive (Figure 15).[68] The elicitation of copulatory behavior by treated females was dramatic in onset. However, extinction of this behavior when the extracts evaporated was quite leisurely, again allowing for a significant contribution of "learning" to behavioral elicitation. Individual differences in the power of this manipulation are also remarkable (Figure 16).

The process of triggering neuroendocrine reflexes in the mammal following receipt of olfactory messages released by another mammal of the same species has aroused considerable interest among workers in reproductive physiology. Such chemical messengers are called pheromones.[69–71] Evidence for pheromonal communication among humans is limited but provocative (Figures 17 and 18).[72,73] However, the role of pheromones in mammalian reproduction is well established, and it is quite clear that the olfactory perception of an estrogenized (receptive) female is one of the strongest triggers for the elicitation of precopulatory and copulatory behaviors in males. Once the female is within tactile range, further facilitation of complete copulation occurs via processing of neural messages from stimulated genitalia. The cumulative effects of such tactile and olfactory stimuli may include both elevations of plasma testosterone and altered activity of areas in the central nervous system known to be critical for triggering patterned copulatory behavior.

Just as such behavior can be facilitated, it can also be subject to inhibition. Koranyi and co-workers[74] (Figure 19) studied sexually experienced male rabbits in an avoidance-conditioning paradigm. They discovered that presentation of the conditioning signal (a buzzer) could easily interrupt or prevent copulatory activity. Although the disruption is of such an immediate nature that it seems to preclude the possibility that it is caused by a change in plasma testosterone, exogenous testosterone administration overcomes the interference (Figure 20).

Disruption of copulation is a common feature of reproduction in mammals either in laboratory populations or in the wild. Le Boeuf and Peterson[75]

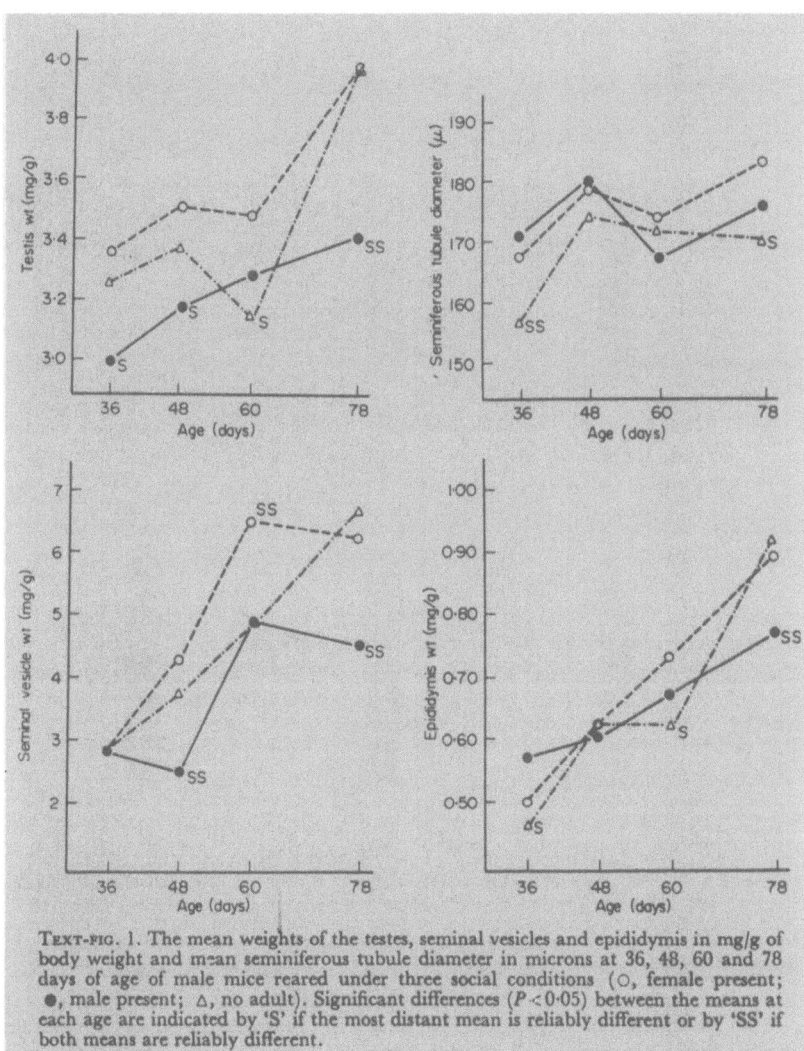

TEXT-FIG. 1. The mean weights of the testes, seminal vesicles and epididymis in mg/g of body weight and mean seminiferous tubule diameter in microns at 36, 48, 60 and 78 days of age of male mice reared under three social conditions (○, female present; ●, male present; △, no adult). Significant differences ($P < 0.05$) between the means at each age are indicated by 'S' if the most distant mean is reliably different or by 'SS' if both means are reliably different.

Figure 14. Pheromones and sexual maturation.[67] As mammals mature, the social environment assumes some importance as a variable influencing the reproductive system. Male mice raised in cages with adult females have heavier testes and larger seminal vesicles than male mice raised with adult males. This difference is thought to be due to pheromones and exemplifies gonadal plasticity vis-à-vis the social environment.

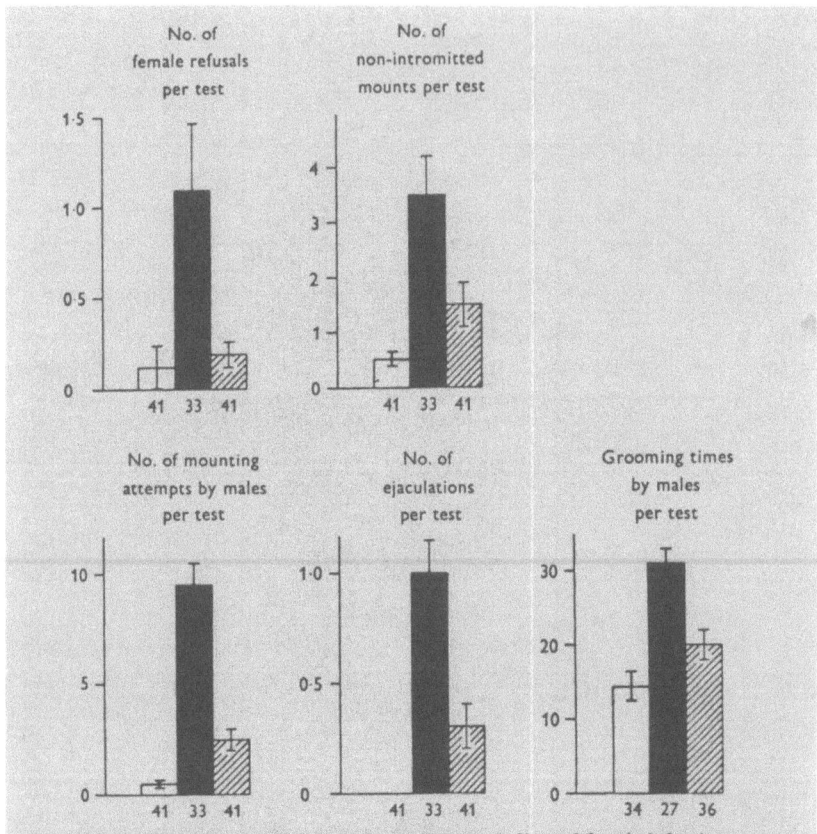

Effects of ether extracts of vaginal secretions on indices of female behaviour (upper part) and of male behaviour (lower part) in rhesus monkeys. Means ± s.e.m. for all five pairs. For the five behavioural measures, the treatment condition was significantly greater than both pre-treatment and withdrawal conditions (upper two measures $P < 0.01$; lower three measures $P < 0.001$). White columns, pre-treatment; black columns, during treatment; hatched columns, after withdrawal of treatment. The numbers at the base of the columns are the number of tests.

Figure 15. Pheromones and copulation.[68] An early effort to isolate the actual chemicals that bear pheromonal information utilized ether extracts of vaginal secretions from estrogenized females. Such studies have led to costly and innovative applied research in the cosmetic industry which has resulted in perfumes with names alluding to "pheromones." Although this has had its comic side, it is not entirely unreasonable to wonder if "pheromonal perfumes" might not be useful in treatment of erectile dysfunction, particularly in men whose partners are postmenopausal. An additional point of interest in this study is the persistence of copulatory behavior by males when the pheromonal stimulus has been withdrawn. Again, there appears to be a role for learning or for other forms of stimulus imprinting.

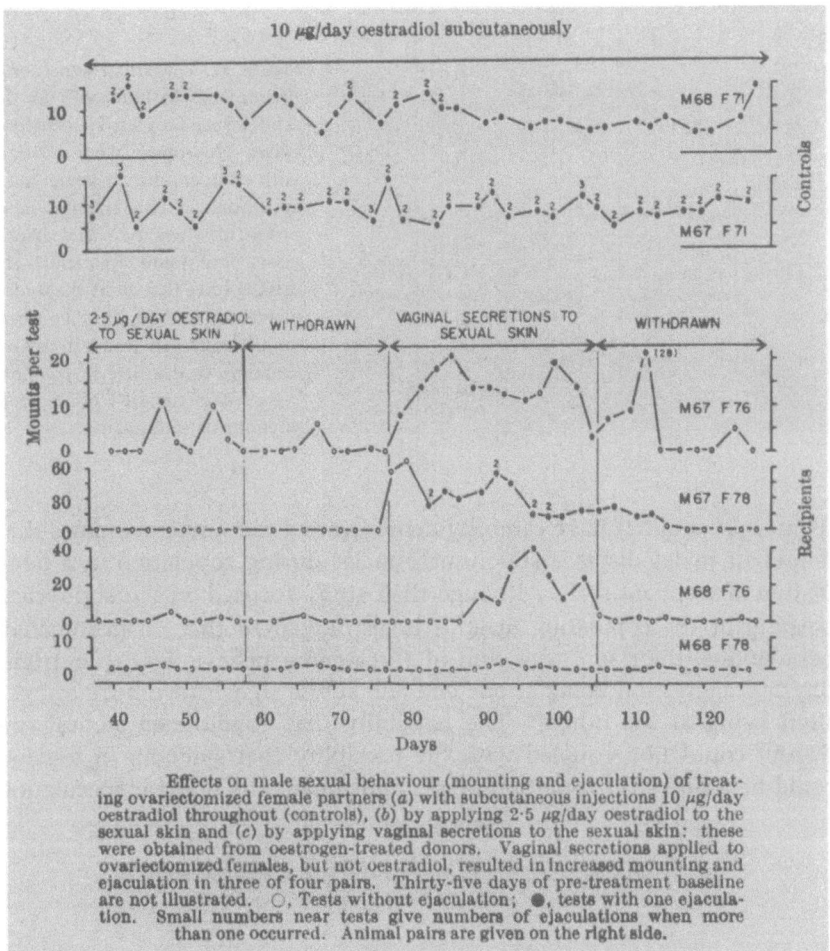

Effects on male sexual behaviour (mounting and ejaculation) of treating ovariectomized female partners (a) with subcutaneous injections 10 μg/day
oestradiol throughout (controls), (b) by applying 2·5 μg/day oestradiol to the
sexual skin and (c) by applying vaginal secretions to the sexual skin: these
were obtained from oestrogen-treated donors. Vaginal secretions applied to
ovariectomized females, but not oestradiol, resulted in increased mounting and
ejaculation in three of four pairs. Thirty-five days of pre-treatment baseline
are not illustrated. ○, Tests without ejaculation; ●, tests with one ejaculation. Small numbers near tests give numbers of ejaculations when more
than one occurred. Animal pairs are given on the right side.

Figure 16. Individual differences in response to pheromones.[63] The same hormonal (and
pheromonal) manipulations affect rhesus monkeys differently. Although it is clear that applying vaginal secretions (containing pheromones) obtained from estrogenized females to the
sexual skin of ovariectomized females increases copulatory behavior in males, it is apparent
that female 76 inspires more copulatory activity than female 78. It also appears that male
67 is more active in this experimental paradigm than male 68. The pheromonal nature of
this communication is emphasized by the lack of significant effect of applying estradiol to
the sexual skin. This study both emphasizes the potential importance of pheromonal communication among primates and underscores the failure of any single explanation of differences in copulatory behavior based on hormonal (or pheromonal) considerations alone.

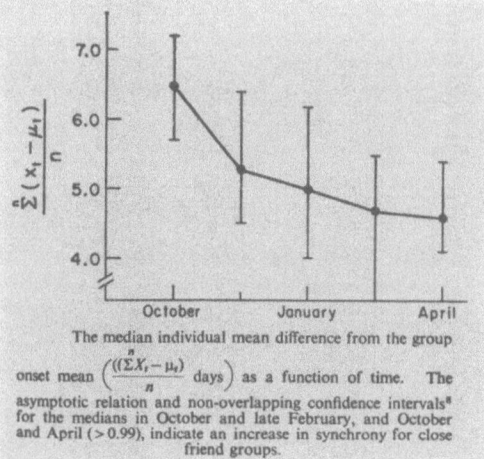

Figure 17. Menstrual synchrony: pheromones in humans.[72] As the school year progresses, menstrual cycles of women who associate with one another become more synchronous. This effect is more powerful when the social associations are more frequent. The driving force that alters the timing of menses is thought to be pheromonal, and this study, in my estimation, is the first to convincingly demonstrate pheromonal phenomena in humans.

The median individual mean difference from the group onset mean $\left(\frac{((\Sigma X_t - \mu_t)}{n}\ \text{days}\right)$ as a function of time. The asymptotic relation and non-overlapping confidence intervals[8] for the medians in October and late February, and October and April (> 0.99), indicate an increase in synchrony for close friend groups.

(Figures 21 and 22) have carefully demonstrated the numerous times that dominant males displace subordinate males during copulation in a population of elephant seals. Although their study focused on actual physical pushing of the copulating male, it is also apparent that, in mammalian populations, there is a spectrum of threatening behaviors with outright physical aggression being at one end and subtle signals (symbolic aggression) being at the other.[76] The possiblity that conditioned stimuli can disrupt copulation coupled with the possiblity that symbolic aggression could be a powerful conditioning stimulus opens the way for speculation

Mean Cycle Lengths and Duration of Menstruation		
Estimated exposure to male (days/week)	Length of cycle (days)	Duration (days)
0–2 N = 56	30.0 ± 3.9	5.0 ± 1.1
3–7 N = 31	28.5 ± 2.9	4.8 ± 1.2
P	≤ 0.03	N.S. ≤ 0.2

Figure 18. Alteration in menstrual cycle length: another probable pheromonal phenomenon.[72] Another fascinating aspect of McClintock's study which is also thought to be under pheromonal control is the observation that menstrual cycles were shorter in women who reported more frequent associations with men than in women who reported infrequent associations with men. Fortunately this study was performed in a women's college where such distinctions could probably be meaningfully made.

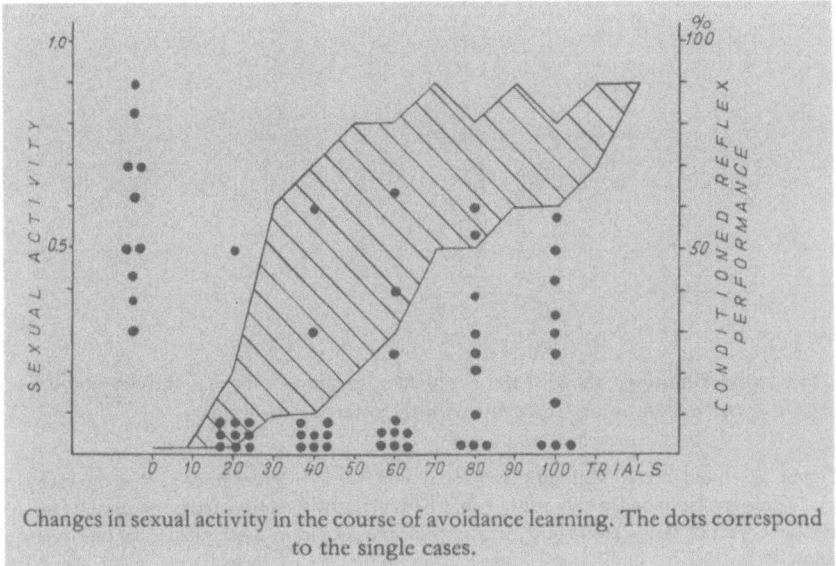

Changes in sexual activity in the course of avoidance learning. The dots correspond to the single cases.

Figure 19. Avoidance conditioning and copulation.[74] In this study, male rabbits with proven vigorous sexual activity in novel situations were conditioned to hop over a barrier when they heard a buzzer in order to avoid an electric shock. Reductions in sexual activity were seen when the conditioned rabbits heard the buzzer in other settings. If one can extrapolate from such a study, it might mean that internalized conflict or stress can inhibit sexual activity. It also clearly indicates that distracting stimuli can be linked by conditioning so that theoretically "neutral" stimuli can assume all the potential for distraction which clearly "negative" stimuli can.

about how the wear and tear of everyday life can ultimately lead to erectile dysfunction in humans in a way that need not have its basis in detectable differences in hormonal production.

In subhuman mammals, males who are at the bottom of the social hierarchy generally fail to achieve any degree of reproductive success and, in fact, exhibit greatly curtailed copulatory behavior.[77-81] This failure to participate in normal copulatory activity is said to be due to the phenomenon of "behavioral castration" and involves measurable decreases in testicular function. One of the most meticulous documentations of behavioral castration has been reported by von Holst[82] (Figures 23 and 24), who has developed a simple method for quantifying social stress in the tree shrew. For our purposes, it is important to emphasize that symbolic aggression in the form of postured confrontation was the most commonly observed form of social stress. Social stress was more characteristically seen in subordinate tree shrews. The anatomical vertification of the extent of behav-

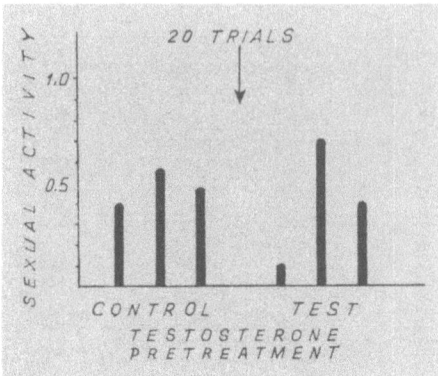

The initial inhibitory effect of the avoidance learning on sexual activity could be prevented by pretreatment with testosterone propionate.

Figure 20. Avoidance conditioning and copulation.[74] It is of great interest that the effect of avoidance conditioning in this study could be reversed by administering exogenous testosterone. Levels of testosterone in plasma were not measured in these rabbits, so one does not know if avoidance conditioning caused drops in circulating testosterone levels. Thus one cannot be certain whether exogenous testosterone restored "normal" testosterone levels or induced higher-than-normal levels. I expect that, in keeping with other studies discussed in this section, Leydig cell function is hampered by avoidance conditioning.

ioral castration in this species is dramatic with testes observed to involute to the point of disappearance of spermatogenesis.

The plasticity of this phenomenon has been observed in other primate species. Male rhesus monkeys have been noted to undergo a fascinating rise and fall in plasma testosterone levels depending on their social environment. If the males are subjected to defeat by being placed in cages with hostile males, their testosterone levels plunge; when they are removed from the hostile environment and placed with receptive females, the testosterone levels rise (Figure 25).[83]

DISPLAYING STEREOTYPICAL AGGRESSION

In the broadest sense, reproductive behavior in mammals also includes intraspecific aggression. Fighting among males of the same species can be seen to have the same seasonal pattern as does copulation.[32,84–86] Within a few years of the synthesis of testosterone, observers reported that testosterone enhanced aggression in primates,[87] which has since been seen in a number of species.[46,88] The availability of sensitive testosterone assays permitted observations that dominant males had higher testosterone levels than did subordinates.[89] Like copulatory behavior, aggression consists of a series of stereotyped patterns[90] which are imprinted in mammals under the influence of androgens at a critical period[91] but which can be elicited by central nervous system stimulation in the adult in the absence of androgens.[92] Moreover, they can be elicited in the adult male more easily than in the adult female when suitable androgen levels are supplied.[88]

Modification by Exteroceptive Stimuli

Like copulatory behavior, aggression takes place in a social context, and its expression is greatly modified by such factors as numbers of the

Social rank and copulation frequency of highest ranking males on area 17. Each male dominates those listed below it; deviations from a linear hierarchy are indicated by arrows. Dotted arrows denote a change in relation which occurred toward the end of the 10-day period. Copulation frequencies are in parentheses.

21 Dec. to 30 Dec.	30 Dec. to 8 Jan.	9 Jan. to 18 Jan.	19 Jan. to 28 Jan.	29 Jan. to 7 Feb.	8 Feb. to 17 Feb.	18 Feb. to 27 Feb.	28 Feb. to 8 Mar.	Total copulations (No.)
NIC	NIC	CLS°	→NIC(1)	GL(6)	GL(15)	GL(19)	GL(5)	46
→UG	→UG↱	NIC	GL(1)	→CLS(13)	→CLS(7)	→CLS(9)	CLS(1)	31
GL	GL- -	GL°	↱CLS(2)	NIC‡	GLS(4)	GLS(8)	GLS(1)	15
WN	WN	GLS	GLS(1)	GLS(5)	└TWO(2)↰	PIN	PIN	8
HSN	└TWO	TWO	└TWO(2)	└TWO(1)	PIN(3)- -¹	YLN(3)	YLN	9
└TWO	YDB	PIN	PIN	PIN	YLN(3)	└TWO‡	BLB	3
BRS	PIN	YLN	YLN	YLN(1)	BO	BLB(2)	BO	3

			Copulations (No.)					
0	0	0	7	26	34	41§	7	

			Females present (range)					
0–2	2–21	24–58	66–102	70–89	54–79	19–51	6–15	

			Males present (range)					
15–27	19–26	19–28	22–29	24–34	24–34	23–35	24–31	

* Indeterminate relation during period despite two bloody fights. † Moved to area 3 after losing fight to YLN at end of period. ‡ Left island during period and did not return. § Three other copulations were observed during this period; two by BO, one by WN.

Figure 21. Dominance and copulatory success.[75] The elephant seal seasonally migrates to selected islands. One can see that the arrival of the males has already started in mid-December followed by the arrival of the females. Territory is staked out by the males, and such territories are well established by the time the maximum number of females is present in late January. The skewing of successful copulation among the males is dramatic, with the three top males in the hierarchy accounting for more than one half of the copulations in the breeding group. Studies such as this reinforce the notion that sexual performance is linked with social success and aggression in mammals. Although there are certainly examples of this sort of skewing in tribal societies (both historical and contemporary), there is little evidence to support this linkage in contemporary Western societies. Yet the failure of sexual performance on the part of a patient often raises issues of social success and self-worth.

Correlates of social rank in four males on area 17 during the period when GL was the alpha male.

Males (in order of rank)	Times other males moved by threats (No.)	Mounts prevented by male (No.)	Copulations interrupted by male (No.)[a]	Mounts prevented by others (%)	Copulations interrupted by others (%)
GL	726	213	15	0	0
CLS	332	52	5	24	15
GLS	332	23	1	71	47
YLN	215	9	0	83	57

[a] Taken from all copulations observed, a total of 152.

Figure 22. Disruption of copulation: effect of social rank.[75] Looking at one subgroup of elephant seals during the breeding, one can see the ways in which copulatory success is experienced by dominant males. The more dominant the male, the more likely he is to displace other males during copulation and the less likely is his own displacement. This phenomenon occurs in virtually all subhuman mammals that have been carefully studied, yet it is my contention that it has no applicability to men in our society.

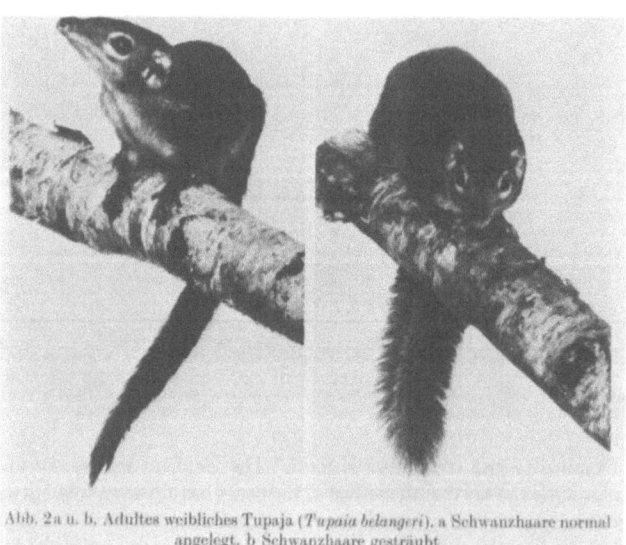

Abb. 2 a u. b, Adultes weibliches Tupaja (*Tupaia belangeri*). a Schwanzhaare normal angelegt. b Schwanzhaare gesträubt

Figure 23. Tail bushing as a sign of social stress in the tree shrew.[82] The tree shrew (often classified as a primitive primate) has a very characteristic response to stress. If placed in a strange environment or if subjected to loud noises or if placed in a cage with more aggressive bullies, the tree shrew ruffles his tail. One can monitor the amount of time a given animal maintains a ruffled tail to estimate a stress rating.

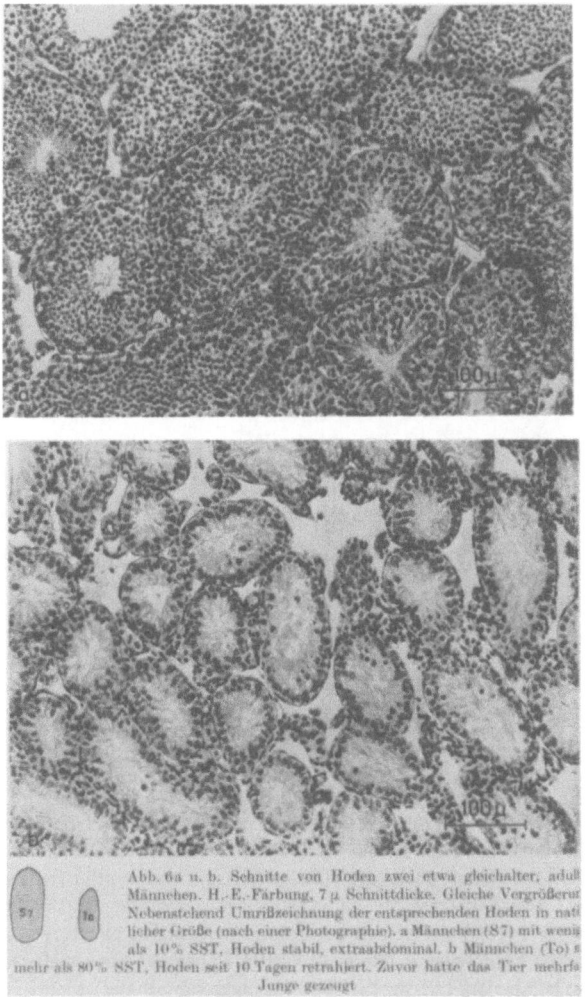

Abb. 6a u. b. Schnitte von Hoden zwei etwa gleichalter, adult Männchen. H.-E.-Färbung, 7 μ Schnittdicke. Gleiche Vergrößerung Nebenstehend Umrißzeichnung der entsprechenden Hoden in natürlicher Größe (nach einer Photographie). a Männchen (S7) mit weniger als 10% SST, Hoden stabil, extraabdominal. b Männchen (To) mit mehr als 80% SST, Hoden seit 10 Tagen retrahiert. Zuvor hatte das Tier mehrere Junge gezeugt

Figure 24. Effects of social stress on testes of tree shrews.[82] If male tree shrews are subjected to such intense social stress that they are observed to have ruffled tails more than 80% of the time, their testes ascend into the abdominal cavity and undergo remarkable involution. This figure illustrates the difference in seminiferous tubule size and Leydig cell mass in unstressed (top) and stressed (bottom) tree shrews. Testicular involution secondary to social stress is actually frequently encountered in male mammals of a variety of species and is called "behavioral castration."

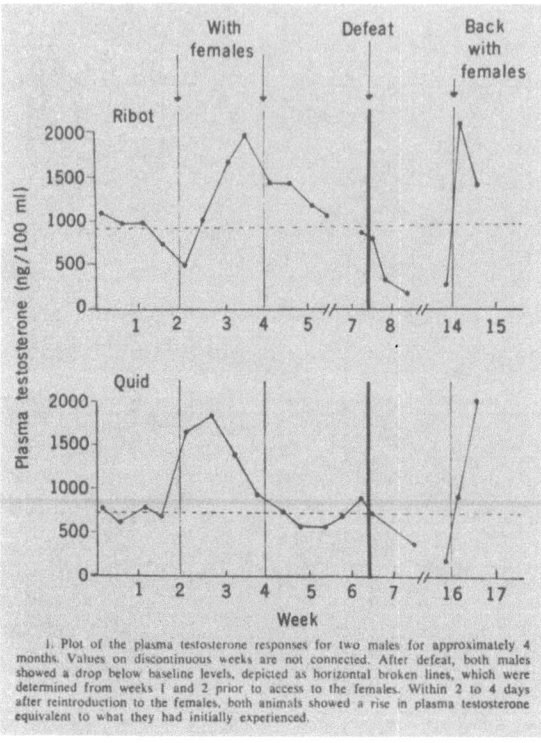

1. Plot of the plasma testosterone responses for two males for approximately 4 months. Values on discontinuous weeks are not connected. After defeat, both males showed a drop below baseline levels, depicted as horizontal broken lines, which were determined from weeks 1 and 2 prior to access to the females. Within 2 to 4 days after reintroduction to the females, both animals showed a rise in plasma testosterone equivalent to what they had initially experienced.

Figure 25. Plasticity of testosterone production in primates.[83] The relationship between hormones and behavior is complex. In this study, plasma testosterone levels in male monkeys actually rise when the solitary males are placed in cages with receptive females. It is thought that the triggers for such increases in Leydig cell output are estrogen-dependent pheromones excreted by receptive females which are processed by the male's olfactory system and translated into increased hypothalamic release of GnRH. When the same males are subjected to aggression (after being placed in cages with strong, aggressive males), their testosterone levels drop. This plasticity of Leydig cell function has never been demonstrated in humans. Efforts to detect reduced testosterone levels in stressed males in prison or in military training camps have failed. At the same time, almost no attention has been paid to the other phenomenon shown in this study: heightening of Leydig cell output by exposure to receptive females. One might persuasively argue that as female partners age and lose endogenous ovarian function, their partners lose a substantial portion of the pheromonal stimulation for Leydig cell function leading to the well-documented decline in testosterone levels with age.

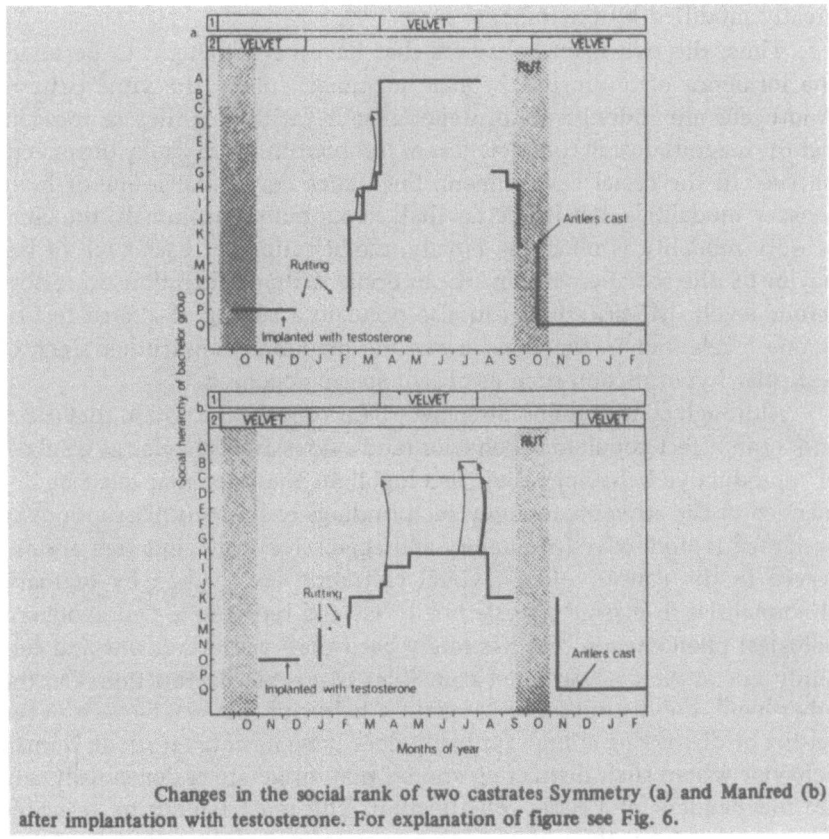

Changes in the social rank of two castrates Symmetry (a) and Manfred (b) after implantation with testosterone. For explanation of figure see Fig. 6.

Figure 26. Influence of testosterone on social rank.[46] In the red deer, the season of greatest reproductive activity (the rut) occurs in late September and October. After the rut, testosterone levels begin to decline and the antlers are shed in winter. Resurgence of testosterone levels in the spring is accompanied by new antler growth (velvet). When testosterone is implanted in castrate males so that their testosterone levels are out of phase with the rest of the breeding group, dramatic shifts in the existing social structure occur. It is important to realize the extent of the differences in testosterone levels between the two experimental stags and the rest of the breeding group (see Figure 8).

same species within a given social space, relatedness of individuals, and hormonal status of group members (Figure 26). Crowding is known to influence the exhibition of aggression regardless of the hormonal status of the aggressor.[77,93–95] Less aggression occurs among littermates as compared to unrelated members of the group.[96–98] Aggressive males are much more likely to attack other males than to attack females.[99,100] Like the cues that trigger patterned copulatory behavior, expression of aggression is greatly modified by pheromonal cues.[101-105]

Thus, the two main behaviors that have been thought to be under the influence of androgens in male mammals follow the same pattern. Androgens are undoubtedly of importance in facilitating their expression, but the magnitude and completeness of the exhibition are vitally dependent on cues in the social environment. Such cues may involve one or more sensory modalities, but it is clear that, in subhuman mammals, the chief sensory modality is olfaction. Finally, modifications of each type of behavior by the social environment can occur without alterations in testosterone levels. Modifications can also occur in a setting of altered testosterone levels, but in these instances, the mammal shows other signs of testicular hypofunction such as absent spermatogenesis.

Although all the studies discussed so far support the notion that social stress can affect copulatory behavior (and aggressive behavior as a subset of reproductive behavior), they also highlight the rigor that must be demanded of the attempts to apply such findings to humans. Disruptions of patterned reproductive (copulatory and aggressive) behaviors that are observed in the context of behavioral castration are marked by dramatic abnormalities in plasma testosterone levels and represent a neuroendocrinological phenomenon that has rarely been observed in humans and certainly not in men whose chief complaint is erectile dysfunction. On the other hand, the disruption of copulatory behavior that can be seen in the setting of distracting stimuli probably does have its counterpart in human behavior where such distracting stimuli may originate endogenously and are independent of Leydig cell function. The most tantalizing principle that emerges from these data is that sensory cues from other mammals are potent modifiers of expression of androgen-facilitated behaviors.

The discussion to this point has set the stage for more accurately considering human behavior as an example of mammalian behavior. It can be easily seen why the links between copulatory behavior, aggression, virility, and androgens have been forged in the minds of so many patients and practitioners. The leap from observing that androgens are essential for the expression of reproductive behaviors to deciding that the failure of complete expression of copulatory behavior is due to lack of androgens has led to routine measurement of plasma testosterone in males complaining of erectile dysfunction. I shall now examine just a few additional problems with this leap.

EFFECTS OF ANDROGENS ON HUMAN BEHAVIOR

The control of erection and ejaculation in humans is complicated, involving elements of both the central and peripheral nervous system.[106-108] If we can correctly extrapolate from the mammalian literature, the central component is most clearly influenced by androgens. The potential for androgens to affect the psyche in a positive way was eloquently expressed by the eminent physiologist Brown-Séquard nearly 100 years ago:

> The day after the first subcutaneous injection [of testicular extract] and still more after the two succeeding ones, a radical change took place in me and I had ample reason to say and to write that I had regained at least all the strength I possessed a good many years ago.[109]

THE PROBLEM OF AGING

Brown-Séquard's testimony perhaps illustrates one reason for the persistence of the illusory promise of androgen therapy. As one after another investigator has pursued this promise, each ought to have been reminded that Brown-Séquard was an old man at the time he wrote this article. Extensive data now exist which demonstrate the very common decline in plasma testosterone levels with age. Some have reported a decline at age 40.[110] Others do not find a decline until age 50.[111] Stearns et al.[112] found that free testosterone levels decreased before total testosterone levels. This decrease in Leydig cell function is clearly a reflection of primary testicular failure because plasma gonadotropin levels are either unchanged or actually elevated (Figure 27).[113] Failure to accurately describe patient populations in relationship to age can lead to a gross overestimate of pathogical hypogonadism in men with impotence.[114]

There exists, then, a considerable justification for more eagerly considering androgen deficit when faced with the complaint of erectile dysfunction in the older patient, for, in this setting, the physician probably has a chance of finding plasma testosterone levels below the "normal" range.

ANDROGENS AND COPULATORY BEHAVIOR: ANDROGENS IN MEN WITH ERECTILE DYSFUNCTION AND ANDROGENS FOR MEN WITH ERECTILE DYSFUNCTION

I shall now address the problem of the relationship between "low–normal" plasma testosterone levels and erectile dysfunction in younger patients. Despite an occasional study,[115,116] most investigators fail to find significantly reduced androgen levels in impotent males when compared with controls whether the impotence occurs without intercurrent illness (Figure 28)[117] or with such illness as diabetes[118] or paraplegia.[119]

Basal plasma hormone levels in young (<50 yr) and elderly (>65 yr) males

Male adults	LH (mIU/ml)	FSH (mIU/ml)	T (ng/100 ml)	E_1 (ng/100 ml)	E_2 (ng/100 ml)	100 E_2/T
<50 yr (n = 30)						
$\bar{m}$	13.0	5.6	492	4.3	1.4	0.32
$\bar{m}$ ± 2 SEM	11–14.5	4.5–7.0	440–550	3.7–4.9	1.1–1.7	0.26–0.40
>65 yr (n = 30)						
$\bar{m}$	24.1	15.8	281	5.2	2.1	0.73
$\bar{m}$ ± 2 SEM	18.9–30.6	11.4–21.8	247–320	4.4–6.1	1.7–2.6	0.54–0.96
Level of sign. of difference p	0.001	0.001	0.001	0.05	0.02	0.001

Figure 27. Testosterone levels decline with age.[113] The most likely association between sexual dysfunction and hormonal abnormalities is found in men over the age of 60. The gradual reduction of circulating testosterone levels which statistically characterizes this group of men is accompanied by elevations of plasma gonadotropin levels, implying that this is a problem of primary testicular involution rather than of Leydig cell dysfunction induced by dampening of signals from the brain. Whether or not decreased exposure to reproductively active females also contributes to the well-documented reduction in copulatory activity in older men is entirely speculative. Nonetheless, exogenous testosterone supplementation will not reliably improve copulatory performance in all men with low testosterones in the later decades of life.

A number of studies have convincingly demonstrated the futility of attempting to treat unselected men with uncomplicated erectile dysfunction with androgens. Testosterone has been administered orally and parenterally.[120] Endogenous testosterone production has been stimulated by human chorionic gonadotropin[119] by gonadotropin-releasing hormone[121] and by clomiphene citrate.[122] None of these therapies has been shown to have a consistent effect when compared to placebo.

One has to assume that a certain critical level of plasma testosterone must be achieved in most men before complete copulatory behavior can be displayed, but beyond that level, further elevations in plasma testosterone do not elicit copulatory behavior more readily. Certainly men without a complaint of erectile dysfunction experience no dramatic increase in copulatory behavior when testosterone levels are raised.[123] Although some investigators have reported measurable changes induced by shifts of androgens within this "normal" range, scrutiny of the reported data raises serious questions about its significance (Figure 29).[124] There is no evidence of changes in the central nervous system components of patterned copulatory behavior in humans induced by such modest variations.[30] This is in marked contrast to demonstrable changes in central components induced by androgen replacement in frankly hypogonadal men.[125]

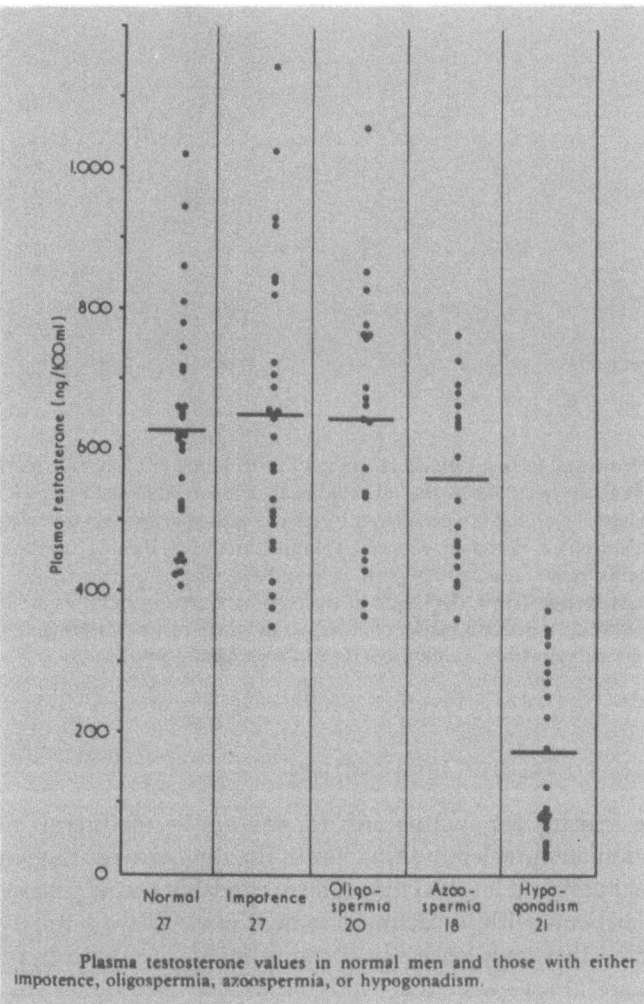

Plasma testosterone values in normal men and those with either impotence, oligospermia, azoospermia, or hypogonadism.

Figure 28. Normal testosterone levels in men with erectile dysfunction.[117] There is very little justification for assuming that men with erectile dysfunction have reductions in plasma testosterone levels when compared to age-matched controls. This does not mean that an occasional patient with erectile dysfunction might not have an endocrine problem, but the hormonal evaluation is parsimonious.

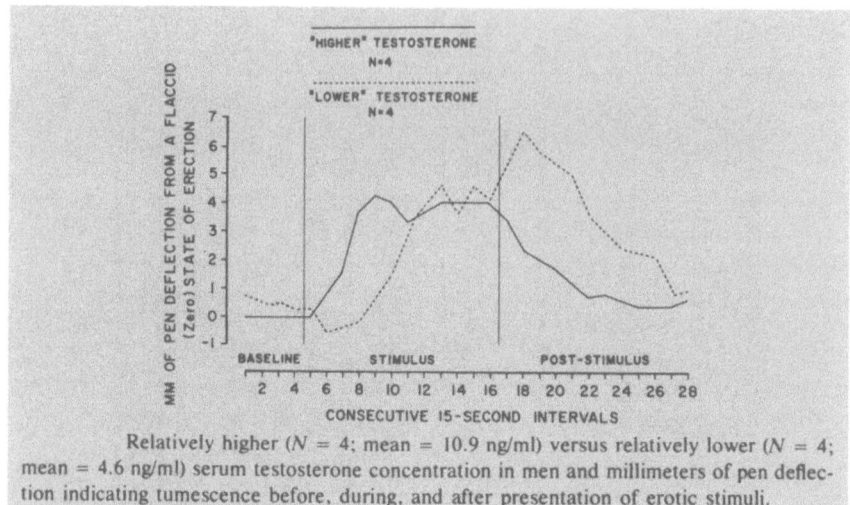

Relatively higher (N = 4; mean = 10.9 ng/ml) versus relatively lower (N = 4; mean = 4.6 ng/ml) serum testosterone concentration in men and millimeters of pen deflection indicating tumescence before, during, and after presentation of erotic stimuli.

Figure 29. An attempt to find behavioral changes due to subtle differences in testosterone.[124] This figure is taken from one of the few studies that reportedly demonstrate a detectable reduction in sexual performance parameters correlated with lower plasma testosterone levels. In this paradigm, men are exposed to pornographic pictures while they are attached to devices measuring penile tumescence. Although there may be a delay in erection detection in men with lower testosterone levels, the height of the erection is greater and the duration may be longer. It would be, I suspect, a matter of choice as to which sort of performance one would choose, but probably neither would drive men to seek clinical advice.

PROLACTIN AND ERECTILE DYSFUNCTION

There remains yet another area for caution in interpreting hormonal studies in impotent males and that lies in the literature relating impotence to abnormal prolactin levels. This problem probably has its genesis in early studies of patients with prolactin-secreting tumors of the pituitary. Besser et al.[126] noted that impotence was a complaint in men with hyperprolactinemia. Careful review of that study as well as subsequent studies[127-130] demonstrates that the majority of these patients had both hyperprolactinemia and evidence of reduced Leydig cell function (Figure 30). There are two possibilities for the Leydig cell failure: either the prolactinomas were of sufficient size to interfere with gonadotropin secretion or the high prolactin levels interfered with gonadotropin receptors.[131-133]

If one studies men with more modest elevations in prolactin without reduced testosterone levels, one need not discover any complaints referable to sexual dysfunction.[134] Furthermore, agents that lower prolactin levels have not been shown to be effective in correcting impotence in men without prolactinomas.[121]

We have, then, only two groups of men in whom there is a great likelihood of accounting for erectile dysfunction on the basis of a hormonal cause: older men and men with acquired hypogonadism of pituitary or hypothalamic origin. Clinical evaluation may not effectively delineate regression of virilization in the first group but clearly ought to do so in

					Serum prolactin (mU/l)		Serum thyroxine (nmol/l)		Plasma testosterone (nmol/l)		Peak plasma cortisol during hypoglycaemia (nmol/l)		Peak plasma growth hormone during hypoglycaemia (nmol/l)	
Case	Duration of therapy (mo)	Clinical change	Pituitary fossa on skull X-ray	CAT ± metrizamide cisternography	Before	After	Before	After	Before	After	Before	After	Before	After
1	3	Potency restored	No change	No suprasellar extension, position of diaphragma sellae normal	1770	<500	100	76	6·6	9·2	690	720	28	62
2	6	Potency restored	Smaller (2100 mm²) still pronounced asymmetry	No suprasellar extension—slightly empty sella (5 mm)	>4600	<100	45	68	7·0	12·0	520	644	2	11
3	10	Facial pain resolved, potency restored	No change	No suprasellar extension—moderately empty sella	3387	166	95	90	5·3	19·0	760	670		
4	9	Headache and galactorrhoea resolved, gynaecomastia improved	ND	ND	>13 000	200	63		9·1	30·2	290	850	1	6
5	6	Headache resolved, potency restored	No change	No suprasellar extension—position of diaphragma sellae normal	>13 000	282	77	70	11·4	7·3	660	720		
6	10	Potency improved	Sella better defined but still huge	Much of extrasellar extension gone (residual tumour on L esp), and small empty sella centrally	>13 000	1050	49	62	7·4	15·5	870	640		31
7	8	Potency restored	No change		1450	122	75	97	11·4	21·3	950	920	26	84
8	11	Impotence persists	Smaller (3700²) and better defined	Extrasellar extension almost gone, with development of a large empty sella	>13 000	220	88	80	6·7	16·4	830	660	15	34
Reference Range					<450		60–150		8·5–27·5		>600		>20	

RESULTS OF BROMOCRIPTINE THERAPY IN MALE HYPERPROLACTINAEMIC PATIENTS

ND = not done

Figure 30. Impotence in hyperprolactinemic men: the confounding variable of reduced Leydig cell function.[129] The issue of prolactin's effect on human copulatory behavior has become clouded because of lack of precision in summarizing studies such as this. Many bibliographies include this as a study showing that impotence is induced by hyperprolactinemia. Yet a review of the actual data shows that the majority of patients with hyperprolactinemia had plasma testosterone levels below normal and that all but one patient had significant elevations in plasma testosterone associated with pharmacological reduction of serum prolactin levels. One should also be conscious of the large increase in prolactin in these patients before treatment. This is quite different from studies which attempt to persuade one that a 30% or 50% increase in prolactin without alterations in plasma testosterone levels is sufficient explanation for impotence and is sufficient cause for unblinded treatment with bromocriptine. In our experience, only men with dramatic elevations in prolactin associated with low testosterone levels characteristically respond to bromocriptine treatment. In fact, the prolactin itself is probably of no consequence. Rather, the induced Leydig cell deficiency is critical.

the second. The stage is now set for review of a parsimonious endocrine evaluation.

ENDOCRINE EVALUATION OF MEN WITH ERECTILE DYSFUNCTION

The actual endocrine evaluation of the man with a chief complaint of impotence without evidence of other illness is straightforward and rather modest. Clues for Leydig cell failure can be gleaned from the history. A patient who complains about loss of libido in addition to erectile dysfunction is more likely to have low testosterone levels. The patient who notes onset of gynecomastia or reduced shaving frequency has an even greater chance of being found hypogonadal.

Physical examination concentrates on whether or not the patient has regression of male hair pattern, gynecomastia, or small, soft testes. In the absence of any of these historical symptoms or physical signs, testosterone levels in men under the age of 50 are almost inevitably in the normal range.

The key endocrine test is a plasma testosterone level. Some authors might persuasively argue that the free testosterone is the more sensitive test, but the total testosterone level is probably sufficient. A low testosterone level should be followed up by basal LH and FSH levels. If either is high, testing with GnRH is not indicated. If the basal LH and FSH levels are not high, GnRH responsiveness should be assessed. A useful test involves the intravenous administration of 100 mg of GnRH in a bolus with LH levels measured at 30 min. One can also measure FSH levels at 45 min, but this does not add useful information.[135] Failure to demonstrate gonadotropin responsiveness should be followed by a thorough anatomical and functional evaluation of the anterior pituitary gland. It is not approriate to review that evaluation at this time.

Despite my stand that prolactin levels are not useful unless there is evidence of Leydig cell hypofunction, one could argue that plasma prolactin levels should be obtained in all men with erectile dysfunction. Certainly I would favor drawing prolactin levels in all men with decreased testosterone levels. When a high prolactin level is found, anatomical study of the sella turcica is indicated (by computerized tomography, if possible). I shall not discuss the further evaluation of space-occupying lesion of the sella turcica at this time.

I have no faith that any other hormonal evaluations are appropriate in otherwise asymptomatic patients with erectile dysfunction. Suggestions that erectile dysfunction can be the sole presenting complaint for patients with adrenocortical dysfunction or thyroid disease in the absence of any physical stigmata of endocrine disease are frankly frivolous.

Hormonal Therapies for Demonstrable Endocrinopathies

Adherence to the parsimonious evaluation outlined here results in only a few rational therapeutic approaches. In the man with demonstrably low plasma testosterone levels which are not shown to be due to pituitary or hypothalamic disease (this clinical setting is more likely to be encountered in the patient over the age of 50), replacement with testosterone cypionate (or a similar long-acting compound) in a dose of 200 mg intramuscularly every other week reliably induces normal levels of circulating testosterone. It is probably good therapy for both the patient and the physician to remeasure the plasma testosterone during treatment and confirm that a change has taken place. Oral androgens interfere with the proper measurement of plasma testosterone and may not be as biologically effective.[136]

Patients with demonstrable pituitary disease may still require replacement therapy after the tumor has been appropriately treated. If the patient with pituitary destruction wishes to restore fertility, combined gonadotropin therapy is employed.[137,138] A workable regimen uses 1500–2000 IU of human chorionic gonadotropin intramuscularly twice weekly until plasma testosterone levels are in the normal range. Then one ampule of human menopausal gonadotropin is given additionally every other day for at least 6 months (and, in most cases, a great deal longer) until spermatogenesis is restored.

Patients with hyperprolactinemia and low plasma testosterone levels without demonstrable pituitary tumors may profit from treatment with bromocriptine.[129] Generally, it is prudent to initiate therapy with 1.25 mg daily and build up to 2.5 mg twice daily if the patient does not develop significant side effects. Larger doses are rarely used. There is some reason to believe that androgen therapy alone will not be useful in these patients.[127] In most cases, patients with high prolactin levels who have demonstrable pituitary tumors will have to undergo surgical resection of the tumor as well as undergoing treatment with bromocriptine.[129]

Other endocrine studies such as thyroid hormone levels, cortisol levels, glucose-tolerance tests, or tests of pituitary function are unwarranted in men whose sole presenting complaint is erectile dysfunction and who do not have evidence of systemic disease on physical examination.

ENDOCRINE CONSIDERATIONS FOR FUTURE RESEARCH: SPECULATIONS DERIVED FROM STUDIES OF MAMMALS

In light of all that is known about copulatory behavior in mammals, it is surprising how little attention has been paid to the possible importance of exteroceptive stimuli in humans. The hormonal status of a man's sexual partner is not considered to be of importance, and yet the more frequent occurrence of erectile dysfunction in older patients also means that the partners of such patients are more likely to be postmenopausal. Future studies of erectile dysfunction in humans might well attempt to assess the hormonal status of the partners. It is possible, for instance, that erectile dysfunction is less frequently encountered in men whose postmenopausal partners are on standard combined estrogen–progesterone therapy than in men whose partners are no longer estrogenized.

I think it is particularly important that investigators be stimulated to consider broader areas of study because of the rather dismal record thus far. Detailed endocrine evaluations of men with erectile dysfunction have usually failed to uncover clinically useful data. When one realizes that countless mammalian studies demonstrate that one must induce dramatic changes in androgen levels before reduction in copulatory behavior can be attributed to an endocrine etiology, the failure to find differences in androgens accounting for sexual dysfunction in the absence of frank hypogonadism ought to have been predicted.

REFERENCES

1. Beach FA: Cerebral and hormonal control of reflexive mechanisms involved in copulatory behavior. *Physiol Rev* 47:289–316, 1967
2. Davidson JM, Levine S: Endocrine regulation of behavior. *Ann Rev Physiol* 34:375–408, 1972
3. Pfaff DW: *Estrogens and Brain Function*, New York, Springer-Verlag, 1980
4. Goebelsmann U, Mishell DR:The menstural cycle, in Mishell DR, Davajan V (eds): *Reproductive Endocrinology, Infertility and Contraception*. Philadelphia, F. A. Davis, 1979, pp 67–90
5. Donovan BT: The regulation of the secretion of follicle-stimulatory hormone, in Harris GW, Donovan BT (eds): *The Pituitary Gland*, Volume 11. Berkeley, University of California Press, 1966, pp 49–99
6. Harris GW, Campbell HJ: The regulation of the secretion of luteinizing hormone and ovulation, in Harris GW, Donovan BT (eds): *The Pituitary Gland*, Volume 11. Berkeley, University of California Press, 1966, pp 99–166
7. Martini L: Hypothalamic control of gonadotropin secretion in the male, in Rosenberg E, Paulsen CA (eds): *The Human Testis*. New York, Plenum Press, 1970, pp 187–206
8. Vigersky RA: Pituitary–Testicular axis, in Lipschultz LI, Howards SS (eds): *Male Infertility*. New York, Churchill Livingstone, 1983, pp 19–41

9. Gorski RA: Localization and sexual differentiation of the nervous structures which regulate ovulation. *J Reprod Fertil* 1(suppl 1):67–88, 1966

10. Pfeiffer CA: Sexual differences of the hypophyses and their determination by the gonads. *Am J Anat* 58:195–226, 1936

11. Wagner JW, Erwin W, CritchlowV: Androgen sterilization produced by intracerebral implants of testosterone in neonatal female rats. *Endocrinology* 79:1135–1142, 1966

12. Arai Y, Gorski RA: Protection against the neural organizing effect of exogenous androgen in the neonatal female rat. *Endocrinology* 82:1005–1009, 1968

13. Arai Y, Gorski RA: Critical exposure time for androgenization of the developing hypothalamus in the female rat. *Endocrinology* 82:1010–1014, 1966

14. Morley JE: The endocrinology of the opiates and opioid peptides. *Metabolism* 30:195–209, 1981

15. McEwen BS, Davis PG, Parsons B, et al: The brain as a target for steroid hormone action. *Ann Rev Neurosci* 2:65–112, 1979

16. Davidson JM: Effect of estrogen on the sexual behavior of male rats. *Endocrinology* 84:1365–1372, 1969

17. Dewsbury DA: Patterns of copulatory behavior in male mammals. *Qu Rev Biol* 47:1–33, 1972

18. Diamond M: Intromission pattern and species vaginal code in relation to induction of psuedopregnancy. *Science* 169:995–997, 1970

19. Malsbury C, Pfaff DW, Neural and hormonal determinants of mating behavior in adult male rats, in Caria LD (ed): *Limbic and Autonomic Nervous Systems Research.* New York, Plenum Press, 1974, pp 85–136

20. Harris GW, Levine S: Sexual differentiation of the brain and its experimental control. *J Physiol* 181:379–400, 1965

21. Pfaff DW: Morphological changes in the brains of adult male rats after neonatal castration. *J Endocrinol* 36:415–416, 1966

22. Garcia JA, Ferreira AC: Cytometry of the hypothalamus after large doses of estrogen. *Acta Neuroveg* 8:283–286, 1955

23. Pfaff DW: Autoradiographic activity in rat brain after injection of tritiated sex hormones. *Science* 161:1355–1356, 1968

24. Kang HK, Singh B, Anand BK, et al: Effect of gonadal hormones on electrical activity of brain in adult monkeys. *J Reprod Fertil* 27:298–299, 1971

25. Donoso AG, Stefano FJE, Biscardi AM, et al: Effects of castration on hypothalamic catecholamines. *Am J Physiol* 212:737–739, 1967

26. Lisk RD: Neural localization for androgen activation of copulatory behavior in the male rat. *Endocrinology* 80:754–761, 1967

27. Heimer L, Larsson K: Impairment of mating behavior in male rats following lesions in the preoptic–anterior hypothalamus continuum. *Brain Res* 3:248–263, 1967

28. Malsbury CW: Facilitation of male rat copulatory behavior by electrical stimulation of the medial preoptic area. *Physiol Behav* 7:797–805, 1971

29. VanDis H, Larsson K: Induction of sexual arousal in the castrated male rat by intracranial stimulation. *Physiol Behav* 6:85–86, 1971

30. Davidson JM: Neurohormonal bases of male sexual behavior. *Int Rev Physiol* 13:225–254, 1977

31. F eder HH: The comparative actions of testosterone propionate and 5 -androstan-17-ol-3-one propionate on the reproductive behavior, physiology and morphology of male rats. *J Endocrinol* 51:241–252, 1971

32. Bramley PS: Territoriality and reproductive behavior of roe deer. *J Reprod Fertil* 11(suppl):43–70, 1970

33. Donne TE: *The Game Animals of New Zealand.* London, John Murray, 1924
34. Neaves WB: Changes in testicular Leydig cells and in plasma testosterone levels among seasonally breeding rock hyrax. *Biol Reprod* 8:451–466, 1973
35. Skinner JD: The effect of season on spermatogenesis in some ungulates. *J Reprod Fertil* 13(suppl):29–37, 1971
36. Marshall FHA: On the change-over in the oestrous cycle in aminals after transferance across the equator with further. observations on the evidence of the breeding seasons and the factors controlling sexual periodicity. *Proc Roy Soc London* B122:413–428, 1937
37. Millar RP, Glover TD: Seasonal changes in the reproductive tract of the male rock hyrax, Procavia capensis. *J Repro Fertil* 23:497–499, 1970
38. Reiter RJ: Pineal control of a seasonal reproductive rhythm in male golden hamsters exposed to natural daylight and temperature. *Endocrinology* 92:423–430, 1973
39. Yeates NTM: The breeding season of the sheep with particular reference to its modification by artifical means using light. *J Agric Sci* 39:1–43, 1949
40. Reiter RJ, Hester RJ: Interrelationships of the pineal gland, the superior cervical ganglia and the photoperiod in the regulation of the endocrine systems of hamsters. *Endocrinology* 79:1168–1170, 1966
41. Romero JA; Influence of diurnal cycles on biochemical parameters of drug sensitivity: The pineal gland as a model. *Fed Proc* 35:1157–1161, 1976
42. Lincoln GA, Youngson RW, Short RV: The social and sexual behavior of the red deer stag. *J Reprod Fertil* 71 (suppl 11):103, 1970
43. Jainudeen MR, Katongole CB, Short RV: Plasma testosterone levels in relation to musth and sexual activity in the male asiatic elephant, Elephas maximus. *J Reprod Fertil* 29:99–103, 1972
44. Lincoln GA: Seasonal changes in the pineal gland related to the reproductive cycle in the male hare, Lepus europaeus. *J Reprod Fertil* 46:489–491, 1971
45. McMillin JM, Seal US, Keenlyne KD, et al: Annual testosterone rhythum in the adult white-tailed deer. *Endocrinology* 94:1034–1040, 1974
46. Lincoln GA, Guinness F, Short RV: The way in which testosterone controls the social and sexual behavior of the red deer stag. *Hormones Behav* 3:375–396, 1972
47. Smals AGH, Kloppenborg PWC, Bernard TJ: Circannual cycle in plasma testosterone levels in man. *J Clin Endocrinol Metab* 42:979–982, 1976
48. Timoneu SO, Lokki O, Wichmann K, et al: Seasonal changes in obstetrical phenomena. *Acta Obstet Gynecol Scand* 44:507–533, 1965
49. Timoneu S, Carpen E: Multiple pregnancies and photoperiodicity. *Ann Chir Gynaecol Fenniae* 57:135–138, 1968
50. Doering CH, Kraemer HC, Brodie KH, et al: A cycle of plasma testosterone in the human male. *J Clin Endocrinol Metab* 40:492–500, 1975
51. Young WC: The hormones and mating behavior, in Young WC (ed): *Sex and Internal Secretions.* Baltimore, Williams & Wilkins, 1961, pp 1173–1239
52. Clegg MT, Beamer W, Bermant G: Copulatory behavior of the ram, Ovis aries, III: Effects of pre- and postpubertal castration and androgen replacement. *Animal Behav* 17:712–717, 1969
53. Mattner PE, Braden A, George JM: Incidence and duration of sexual inhibition in young rams. *J Reprod Fertil* 149–150, 1971
54. Hard E, Larsson K: Effects of precoital exposure of male rats to copulating animals upon subsequent mating performance. *Animal Behav* 17:540–541, 1969
55. Carlsson SG, Larsson K: Mating in male rats after local anesthetization of the gland penis. *Z Tierpsychol* 21:854–856, 1964

56. Saginor M, Horton R: Reflex release of gonadotropin and increased plasma testosterone concentration in male rabbits during cpoulation. *Endocrinology* 82:627–630, 1968
57. Rowe FA, Edwards DA: Olfactory bulb removal: Influences on the mating behavior of male mice. *Physiol Behav* 8:37–41, 1972
58. Bermant G, Taylor L: Interactive effects of experience and olfactory bulb lesions in male rat copulation. *Physiol Behav* 4:13–17, 1969
59. Doty R, Carter CS, Clemens LG: Olfactory control of sexual behavior in the male and early-androgenized female hamster. *Hormones Behav* 2:325–335, 1971
60. Heimer L, Larsson K: Mating behavior of male rats after olfactory bulb lesions. *Physiol Behav* 2:207–209, 1967
61. Klein LL: Observations on copulation and seasonal reproduction in two species of spider monkeys, Ateles belzebuth and A. geoffroy. *Folia Primatol* 15:233–248, 1971
62. Michael RP, Zumpe D: Aggression and gonadal hormones in captive rhesus monkeys (Macaca mulatta). *Animal Behav* 18:1–10, 1970
63. Michael RP, Keverne EB: Primate sex pheromones of vaginal origin. *Nature* 225:84–85, 1970
64. Herbert J: Hormones and reproductive behavior in rhesus and talapoin monkeys. *J Reprod Fertil* 11(suppl):119–140, 1970
65. Carr WJ, Loeb LS, Wyle NR: Responses to feminine odors in normal and castrated male rats. *Compar Physiol Psychol* 62:336–338, 1967
66. Vandenbergh JG: Endocrine coordination in monkeys: Male sexual responses to the female. *Physiol Behav* 4:261–264, 1969
67. Vandenbergh JG: The influence of the social environment on sexual maturation in male mice. *J Reprod Fertil* 24:383–390, 1971
68. Koverne EB, Michael RP: Sex-attractant properties of ether extracts of vaginal secretions from rhesus monkeys. *J Endocrinol* 51:313–322, 1971
69. Cheal ML, Sprott RL: Social Olfaction: A review of the role of olfaction in a variety of animal behaviors. *Psychol Reports* 29:195–243, 1971
70. Gleason K, Reynierse JH: The behavioral significance of pheromones in vertebrates. *Psychol Bull* 71:58–73, 1969
71. Ralls K: Mammalian scent marking. *Science* 171:445–449, 1971
72. McClintock MK: Menstrual synchrony and suppression. *Nature* 229:244–245, 1971
73. Comfort A: Likelihood of human pheromones. *Nature* 230:432–433, 1971
74. Koranyi L, Endroczi E, Tarnok F: Sexual behavior in the course of avoidance conditioning in male rabbits. *Neuroendocrinology* 1:144–157, 1966
75. Le Boeuf BJ, Peterson RS: Social status and mating activity in elephant seals. *Science* 163:91–93, 1969
76. Sade DS: Determinants of dominance in a group of free-ranging rhesus monkeys, in Altmann S (ed): *Social Communication Among Primates,* Chicago, University of Chicago Press, 1967, pp 99–1146
77. Calhoun JB: A behavioral sink, in Bliss EL (ed): *Roots of Behavior.* New York, Harper & Row, 1967, pp 295–315
78. Hanby JP, Robertson LT, Phoenix CH: The sexual behavior of a confined troop of Japanese macaques. *Folia Primatol* 16:123–143, 1971
79. Marsden HM, Holler NR: Social behavior in confined populations of the cottontail and the swamp rabbit. *Wildlife Monographs* #13, 1964
80. Mech LD: *The Wolf.* Garden City, New York, The American Museum of Natural History, 1970
81. Vessey S: Effects of chlorpromazine on aggression in laboratory populations of wild house mice. *Ecology* 48:367–376, 1967

82. von Holst D: Sozial Stress bei Tupajas *Z Vergleich Physiol* 63:1–58, 1969

83. Rose RM, Gordon TP, Bernstein IS: Plasma testosterone levels in the male rhesus: Influences of sexual and social stimuli. *Science* 178:643–645, 1972

84. Baldwin JD: Reproductive synchronization in squirrel monkeys (Saimiri). *Primates* 11:317–326, 1970

85. Christian JJ: Fighting maturity and population density in Microtus pennsylvanicus. *J Mammalogy* 52:556–567, 1971

86. MacLennan RR, Bailey ED: Seasonal changes in aggression hunger and curiosity in ranch mink. *Can J Zool* 47:1395–1401, 1969

87. Clark G, Birch HS: Hormonal modifications of social behavior: I. The effect of sex-hormone administration on the social status of a male-castrate chimpanzee. *Psychosom Med* 7:321–329, 1945

88. Tollman J, King JA: The effects of testosterone propionate on aggression in male and female (57 BL/10) mice. *Br J Animal Behav* 4:147–149, 1956

89. Rose, RM, Holaday JW, Berstein IS: Plasma testosterone, dominance rank and aggressive behavior in male rhesus monkeys. *Nature* 231:366–368, 1971

90. Romaniuk, A. Representation of aggression and flight reactions in the hypothalamus of the cat. *Acta Biol Exp* 25:177–186, 1965

91. Rothballer, AB: Aggression defense and neurohumors, in Clement CD, Lindsey DB (eds): *Aggression and Defense.* Berkeley, University of California Press, 1967, pp 135–170

92. Delgado JMR: Social rank and radio-stimulated aggressiveness in monkeys. *J Ner Ment Dis* 144:383–390, 1967

93. Bailey ED: Social interaction as a population-regulating mechanism in mice. *Can J Zool* 44:1007–1012, 1966

94. Christian, JJ: Endocrine adaptive mechanisms and the physiologic regulations of population growth, in Mayer WV, Van Gelder RG (eds): *Physiological Mammalogy,* Volume 1. New York, Academic Press, 1963, pp 153–189

95. Myers K, Poole WE: A study of the biology of the wild rabbit, Oryctolagus cuniculus, in confined populations. *CSIRO Wildlife Res* 6:1–41, 1961

96. Petrusewicz K, Wilska T: Investigation of the influence of inter-population relations on the result of fights between male mice. *Ekol Polska* (series A) 7:357–390, 1959

97. Rowe FD, Redfern R: Aggressive behavior in related and unrelated wild house mice (Mus musculus). *Ann Appl Biol* 64:425–431, 1969

98. Yeaton RI: Social behavior and social organization in Richardson's ground squirrel (Spermophilus Richardson ii) in Saskatchewan. *J Mammal* 53:139–147, 1972

99. Eisenberg JF: Studies on the behavior of Peromyscus maniculatus gambelli and Peromyscus californicus parasiticus. *Behavior* 19:177–207, 1962

100. Michael RP, Zumpe D: Rhythmic changes in the copulatory frequency of rhesus monkeys (Macaca mulatta) in relation to the menstrual cycle and a comparison with the human cycle. *J Reprod Fertil* 21:199–201, 1970

101. Dixon AJ, MacKintosh JH: Effects of female urine upon the social behavior of adult male mice. *Animal Behav* 19:138–140, 1971

102. Lee CT, Brake SC: Reactions of male fighters to male and female mice untreated or deodorized. *Psychonom Sci* 24:209–211, 1971

103. Mugford RA, Nowell NW: Pheromones and their effect on aggression in mice. *Nature* 226:967–968, 1970

104. Mugford RA, Nowell NW: The preputial glands as a source of aggression-promoting odors in mice. *Physiol Behav* 6:247–249, 1971

105. Mugford RA, Nowell NW: The relationship between endocrine status of female opponents and aggressive behavior of male mice. *Animal Behav* 19:153–155, 1971

106. Baumgarten HG, Owman C, Sjoberg NO: Neural mechanisms in male fertility, in Sciarra JJ, Markland C, Speidel JJ (eds): *Control of Male Fertility*. Hagerstown, Maryland, Harper & Row, 1975, pp 26–40

107. Benson GS, McConnell J: Erection, emission and ejaculation: Physiological mechanism, in Lipshultz LI, Howards SS (eds): *Male Fertility*. New York, Churchill Livingston, 1983, pp 165–186

108. Kedia K, Markland C: Effect of sympathectomy and drugs on ejaculation, in Sciarra JJ, Markland C, Speidel JJ (eds): *Control of Male Fertility*. Hagerstown, Maryland, Harper & Row, 1975, pp 240–248

109. Brown-Séquard CE: The effects produced on man by subcutaneous injections of a liquid obtained from the testicles of animals. *Lancet* 2:105–107, 1889

110. Pirke KM, Doerr P: Age related changes and interrelationships between plasma testosterone, oestradiol and testosterone-binding globulin in normal adult males. *Acta Endocrinol* 74:792–800, 1973

111. Ver Meulen A, Rubens R, Verdonck L: Testosterone secretion and metabolism in male senescence. *J Clin Endocrinol Metab* 34:730–735, 1972

112. Stearns EL, MacDonnell JA, Kaufman BJ, et al: Declining testicular function with age. *Am J Med* 57:761–766, 1974

113. Rubens R, Dhont M, Vermeulen A: Further studies on Leydig cell function in old age. *J Clin Endocrinol Metab* 39:40–45, 1974

114. Slag MF, Morley JE, Elson MK, et al: Impotence in medical clinic outpatients. *JAMA* 249:1736–1740, 1983

115. Ismail AAA, Davidson DW, Loraine JA, et al: Assessment of gonadal function in impotent men, in Irvine WJ (ed): *Reproductive Endocrinology*. Edinburgh, E.P.S. Livingstone, 1970, pp 138–147

116. Legros JJ, Palem M, Servais J, et al: Basal pituitary–gonadal function in impotency evaluated by blood testosterone and LH assays, in Lissak K (ed): *Hormones and Brain Function*. New York, Plenum Press, 1973, pp 527–529

117. Lawrence DM, Swyer GIM: Plasma testosterone and testosterone binding affinites in men with impotence, oligospermia, azoospermia and hypogonadism. *Br Med J* 1:349–351, 1974

118. Kolodny C, Kahn CB, Goldstein HH, et al: Sexual dysfunction in diabetic men. *Diabetes* 23:306–309, 1974

119. Faerman I, Vilar O, Rivarola MA, et al: Impotence and diabetes. *Diabetes* 21:23–30, 1972

120. Ellenberg M: Impotence in diabetes: The neurologic factor. *Ann Intern Med* 75:213–219, 1971

121. Benkert O: Studies on pituitary hormones and releasing hormones in depression and sexual impotence. *Progr Brain Res* 42:25–36, 1975

122. Cooper AJ, Ismail AAA, Harding T, et al: The effects of clomiphene in impotence. *Br J Psychiatry* 120:327–330, 1972

123. Jones M, Fang VS, Rosenfield RL, et al: Parameter of response to clomiphene citrate in oligospermic men. *J Urol* 124:53–61, 1980

124. Lange JD, Brown WA, Wincze JP, Zwick W: Serum testosterone concentration and penile tumescence changes in men. *Horm Behav* 14:267–270, 1980

125. Bancroft J, Wu FCW: Changes in erectile responsiveness during androgen replacement therapy. *Arch Sexual Behav* 2:59–66, 1983

126. Besser GM, Parke L, Edwards CRW, et al: Galactorrhea: Successful treatment with medication of plasma prolactin levels by brom-ergocryptine. *Br Med J* 3:669–672, 1972

127. Carter JN, Tyson JE, Tolis G, et al: Prolactin-secreting tumours and hypogonadism in 22 men. *N Engl J Med* 229:847–852, 1978

128. Franks S, Jacobs HS, Martin N, et al: Hyperprolactinemia and impotence. *Clin Endocrinol* 8:277–287, 1978

129. Prescott RWG, Kendall-Taylor P, Hall K, et al: Hyperprolactinaemia in men: Response to bromocriptine therapy. *Lancet* 1:245–249, 1982

130. Thomas MO, McNeilly AS, Hergan G, et al: Long-term treatment of galactorhoea and hypogonadism with bromocriptine. *Br Med J* 2:419–422, 1974

131. Besser GM, Thorner MO: Bromocriptine in the treatment of the hyperprolactinemia–hypogonadism syndromes. *Postgrad Med J* 52(suppl 1):64–70, 1976

132. Fonzo D, Faglia G, Ambrosi B, et al: The role of prolactin in the regulation of male sexual functions, in Frajese G, Hafez ESE, Conti C, et al (eds): *Oligospermia: Recent Progress in Andrology.* New York, Raven Press, 1981, pp 147–153

133. Zarate A, Canales ES, Soria J, et al: Ovarian refractoriness during lactation in women: Effect of gonadotropic stimulation. *Am J Obstet Gynecol* 112:1130–1132, 1972

134. Wong TW, Jones TM: Hyperprolactinemia and male infertility. *Arch Pathol Med* 108:35–39, 1984

135. Wollesen F, Swerdloff RS, Odell WD: LH and FSH responses to luteinizing-releasing hormones in normal adult, human males. *Metabolism* 25:845–864, 1976

136. Jones TM, Fang VS, Landau RL, et al: The effects of fluoxymesterone administration on testicular function. *J Clin Endocrinol Metab* 44:121–128, 1977

137. MacLeod J: The effects of urinary gonadotropins following hypophysectomy and in hypogondotropic eunnchoidism, in Rosenberg E, Paulsen CA (eds): *The Human Testis.* New York, Plenum Press, 1970, pp 577–588

138. Vermeulen A: Hormonal treatment of male infertility, in Frajese G, Hafez ESE, Conti C, et al: *Oligospermia: Recent Progress in Andrology.* New York, Raven Press, 1981

7

Other Causes of Erectile Impotence

HARRY W. SCHOENBERG

Erectile impotence may result from a miscellaneous group of problems that are neither vasculogenic, endocrine, nor neurogenic in origin. This group includes impotence which is (1) drug-induced; (2) secondary to renal failure and transplantation; (3) secondary to priapism; (4) secondary to pelvic surgery; and (5) secondary to trauma.

DRUGS

A large number of drugs interfere with normal erections.

Chronic alcohol abuse is associated with impotence, probably because of liver involvement and failure to detoxify estrogen.

Estrogen therapy for carcinoma of the prostate even at low doses causes a high degree of impotence by suppression of androgen secretion and loss of libido.

Many agents used in the management of arterial hypertension are associated with erectile impotence. Beta blockers, some diuretics (aldactone), centrally acting agents and vasodilators, and ganglionic blockers all produce impotence in some hypertensive patients.

HARRY W. SCHOENBERG • Department of Surgery, Section of Urology, University of Chicago, Chicago, Illinois 60637.

Alpha-blocking agents such as phenoxybenzamine are associated with retrograde ejaculation.

Many other drugs, including barbiturates, hypnotics, antihistamines, and tranquilizers are sporadically associated with erectile impotence.

RENAL FAILURE AND TRANSPLANTATION

Patients with uremia from chronic renal failure frequently (about 50%) suffer from erectile impotence. A number of factors may be related to impotence in this situation. Testicular atrophy with loss of Leydig cells and decreased testosterone levels play some part. In uremia, serum testosterone is decreased, follicle-stimulating hormone is normal, and luteinizing hormone is generally increased. Disturbances in the hypothalamic–pituitary–gonadal axis with elevated prolactin levels have been noted in patients with chronic renal failure and may be associated with impotence.[1] Patients on a chronic dialysis program have accelerated atherosclerosis, and this may in some instances contribute to impotence on a vasculogenic basis. A uremic neuropathy demonstrated by delayed conduction times may also be implicated.[2] Renal transplantation may have a beneficial effect on impotence, but when a second transplant is required, it is associated with a high degree of impotence (65%), probably because both internal iliac vessels have been sacrificed.[3] In potent male patients undergoing a second renal transplant, it has been suggested that an end-to-side anastomosis be made between the renal artery and the external iliac artery, thus sparing the remaining hypogastric vessel.

PRIAPISM

Although most cases of priapism are ultimately classified as idiopathic, there are a larger number of specific causes or frequently associated disease states.[4] The idiopathic group includes priapism associated with prolonged sexual stimulation or continuous masturbation. The more specific group includes a long list of causes such as sickle cell anemia, leukemia, glucose phosphate isomerase deficiency, prostatitis, urethritis, urethral trauma, multiple sclerosis, infectious myelitis, traumatic lesions of the spinal cord, and tumors of the prostate and kidney. A significant number of patients will be impotent following priapism. Impotence in this situation is secondary to the fibrosis and destruction of the corpora cavernosa. Because no large randomly treated series is available for review, it is difficult to assess the efficacy of early relief of priapism on the subsequent development of impotence. A number of active methods are available for the treatment of priapism, including irrigation of the corpora, vascular shunts between the saphenous vein and corpora cavernosa, or shunts between the corpora cavernosa and corpus spongiosum. Until more data are available, there are theoretical reasons why prolonged priapism is more likely to damage the corpora than is a brief episode. Therefore, most urologists suggest active surgical therapy of idiopathic priapism rather than allowing priapism to run its natural course. Aggressive treatment of the primary disorder in secondary priapism is appropriate.[5]

PELVIC SURGERY

Major cancer surgery in the male pelvis is today a frequent cause of erectile impotence. The most common procedures in this category are abdominal peritoneal resection for carcinoma of the rectum; radical prostatectomy, either retropubic or perineal for carcinoma of the prostate; and cystoprostatectomy for carcinoma of the bladder. Walsh and Donker are currently experimenting with methods of preserving potency while carrying out radical prostatectomy.[6] Some younger men undergoing total proctocolectomy for ulcerative colitis will be rendered impotent even though the scope of this operation is somewhat less than the one performed for a malignant lesion. Simple enucleation of the prostate for benign disease or transurethral prostatectomy rarely produces organic impotence. Retroperitoneal lymphadenectomy as performed for carcinoma of the testes is frequently associated with disturbances of ejaculation, and Donahue and co-workers noted ejaculatory impotence in all patients undergoing bilateral suprahilar (renal hilus) lymphadenectomies. Erectile potency, however, was maintained.[7]

TRAUMATIC LESIONS

Traumatic rupture of the membranous urethra in association with severe pelvic fractures has in the past been associated with a high incidence of urethral stricture formation and erectile impotence. In the past, it was general practice to align the urethra over a catheter, working both through the penile urethra and through the bladder, or, if necessary, through the perineum. More recently, Morehouse and MacKinnon[8] have recommended that no urethral instrumentation be carried out, but that a simple suprapubic cystostomy be done at the time of injury. This technique, originally proposed by Johanson,[9] avoids infection of the large pelvic hematoma that always forms in this type of injury, and in their hands this therapy has resulted in a far lower incidence of both urethral stricture and impotence.[8] This is an important concept since most of the men suffering impotence in this fashion are young.

Radiation therapy is a form of trauma to the pelvic structures. One of the reasons for its popularity in the management of carcinoma of the prostate utilizing both interstitial and external-beam modalities is a decrease in the incidence of erectile impotence as compared to radical prostatectomy. Interstitial radiation usually accompanied by pelvic lymphadenectomy is generally reported to have a low incidence of associated impotence in the range of 1–5%. External-beam radiation carries a considerably higher incidence of impotence ranging up to 45% in various reports. However, the effect of chronic illness, debilitation, and psychic depression associated with progressive malignant disease makes it difficult to identify an etiology for impotence in this situation.[10]

DIAGNOSIS

The diagnosis of the varieties of impotence in this miscellaneous group is often obvious if one is careful not to forget that any of these lesions may produce a psychic trauma from which impotence may also result. We therefore feel it essential that, in the evaluation of impotence resulting from any of these factors, the psychiatric evaluation not be overlooked because of the presence of some obvious organic cause. From the standpoint of treatment, frequently drug-related impotence can be managed by withdrawal of the drug where feasible or substitution of another equivalent agent particularly in patients with hypertension. When the organic nature of the lesion has been established, prosthetic surgery may be offered to the patient. Of course, if a partner is present, her attitude toward this surgery should be considered, and the presence of any emotional contraindication to this form of therapy should be ruled out.[11]

REFERENCES

1. Waltzer WC: Sexual and reproductive function in men treated with hemodialysis and renal transplantation. *J Urol* 121:713–716, 1981
2. Bottaccini MR, Gleason DM: Krane RJ, Siroky MB (eds): in *Clinical Neurourology*. Fluid mechanics of micturition. Boston, Little, Brown, 1979, Chapter 2, p 52
3. Gilles RF, Waters WB: Sexual impotence: The overlooked complication of a second renal transplant. *J Urol* 121:719–720, 1979
4. Schoenberg HW, Banno JJ: Corporal shunts for priapism, in Lipshultz LI, Corriere JN

Jr, Hafez ESE (eds): *Clinics in Andrology*, Volume 2. *Surgery of the Male Reproductive Tract*. The Hague/Boston/London, Martinus Nijhoff, 1980, Chapter 12, pp 135–142

5. Wasmer JM, Carrion HM, Mekras G: Evaluation and treatment of priapism. *J Urol* 125:204–207, 1981

6. Walsh PC, Donker PJ: Impotence following radical prostatectomy: Insight into etiology and prevention. *J Urol* 128:492–497, 1982

7. Donahue JP, Perez JM, Sinhorn LH: Improved management of nonseminomatous testis tumors. *J Urol* 121:425–428, 1979

8. Morehouse DD, MacKinnon KJ: Management of prostatomembranous urethral disruption: 13-year experience. *J Urol* 123:173–174, 1980

9. Johanson B: Reconstruction of the male urethra in strictures. *Acta Chir Scand* Suppl 176, 1953

10. Cupps RE, Utz DC, Fleming TR, et al: Definitive radiation therapy for prostatic carcinoma: Mayo Clinic experience. *J Urol* 124:855–859, 1980

11. Schoenberg HW, Zarins CK, Segraves RT: Analysis of 122 unselected impotent males subjected to multidisciplinary evaluation. *J Urol* 127:445–447, 1982

8

Evaluation of the Etiology of Erectile Failure

R. TAYLOR SEGRAVES, HARRY W. SCHOENBERG, and
KATHLEEN A. B. SEGRAVES

Although patients complaining of erectile problems have pestered, perplexed, and intrigued physicians for centuries, the differentiation of organic from psychological causes of impotence has assumed greater significance in the minds of most physicians within the past 5–10 years. Part of this reawakening of interest on the part of physicians is the development of genuine treatment alternatives. In the recent past, therapeutic alternatives were extremely limited. In the vast majority of cases, specific etiologies could rarely be established, yet the patient still demanded a remedy to his difficulty. Exogenous testosterone was frequently utilized although the majority of evidence suggests that it was rarely useful in men with normal gonadal function.[1] If testosterone supplementation did not have a placebo effect, the physician was left with a choice of psychiatric referral or consideration of a penile prosthetic device. Twelve years ago, neither of these alternatives was completely acceptable. Prosthetic devices consisted mainly of semirigid silicone rods which usually had less than normal length and girth and which left the patient with permanent erectile state, making concealment a problem.[2] Similarly, the predominant psychiatric treatment

R. TAYLOR SEGRAVES and KATHLEEN A. B. SEGRAVES • Department of Psychiatry, Tulane University Medical Center, New Orleans, Louisiana 70112. HARRY W. SCHOENBERG • Department of Surgery, Section of Urology, University of Chicago, Chicago, Illinois 60637.

for erectile problems was long-term insight-oriented psychotherapy, a treatment of questionable success.[3] In 1970, the medical profession became aware of new brief symptom-oriented counseling methods for the treatment of sexual difficulties.[4] In contrast to earlier treatment methods, the behavioral approaches had respectable outcome data and a brief treatment duration. Most physicians could feel comfortable referring a patient for such a service. In 1973,[5] Scott and associates reported the first implantation of an inflatable silicone rubber penile prosthesis. With subsequent improvement of the prosthesis, this device enables an impotent patient to stimulate normal erection and flaccidity. Similarly, normal length and girth are appropriated. Thus, the contemporary physician is faced with at least two major treatment alternatives, making differential diagnosis more important than in previous years. The possibility of correctable vascular and endocrine abnormalities also highlights the current importance of differential diagnosis.

In the recent past, it was routinely assumed that the preponderance of cases of erectile dysfunction were psychologically based.[6-8] By implication, the physician had minimal motivation for an extensive evaluation as he anticipated significant findings to be infrequent. However, recent research has suggested that organogenic causes of impotence may be more common than previously realized.[9,10] Spark and associates[11] reported that 35% of a series of 105 impotent men were found to have abnormalities of the hypothalamic–pituitary–gonadal axis. Correction of the problem was usually associated with restoration of potency. This report was particularly disturbing in that many of these men had been reassured by their private physicians that the problem was psychologically based. Thirteen percent of Spark's patients were in psychotherapy at the time of referral. Similarly, Karacan and his co-workers[12] at Baylor University have found that approximately one half of all patients screened for noturnal penile tumescence are found to have records suggestive of organogenic impotence. Other clinical series[13-16] have suggested that at least 30% of impotent men will be found to have organic etiologies to their problems.

DIFFERENTIATION OF ORGANIC FROM PSYCHOGENIC IMPOTENCE

In a minority of cases of erectile insufficiency, the history and clinical presentation will essentially establish the diagnosis. Obvious examples would include the hypertensive patient whose erectile problem began after a change in hypotensive medication or the healthy recently married man who experienced erectile failure for the first time on his wedding night.

Unfortunately, a sizable majority of patients will present with histories that do not allow an easy diagnostic differentiation. In such cases, the physican faces a choice between extensive laboratory testing or missing possibly treatable organic pathology. A reasonable evaluation of impotence might include several nights of noctural penile tumescence (NPT) testing in a neurophysiology laboratory, an endocrine evaluation including evaluation of thyroid, adrenal, and androgen function, assessment of pelvic blood flow, and physical examination.[17] Psychological testing[18] and sacral nerve conduction[19] studies might also be included at certain centers. If a multidisciplinary team approach is utilized, the medical bill may include visits by urological and vascular surgeons, by an endocrinologist, and by a psychiatrist. The resulting bill could easily be several thousand dollars. Some of the specialized laboratories are unavailable in certain communities. Clearly, most physicians would consider routine inclusion of such laboratory investigations of impotence as a disservice to patients.[20]

USE OF HISTORICAL DATA

Many physicians would assume that the presence of frequent strong erections under any circumstances[21,22] indicates that the vascular, endocrine, and neurological systems are probably intact and that the erectile difficulty is predominantly psychogenic. Thus these physicians would question the patient closely about the presence and quality of masturbatory[23-25] and early-morning erections,[27] and erections with alternative partners.[25,26] Certain other characteristics, such as abrupt onset and loss of erection after vaginal intromission,[16,23] are considered by some investigators as more reflective of psychogenic erectile problems.

Magee,[28] in a review of the literature on psychogenic impotence, emphasized the necessity of precise standards of erectile quality and frequency in investigations of impotent patients. For example, he noted that certain authors considered semifirm erections or erections sufficient for coitus once a year to indicate normal function. Segraves, Schoenberg, and co-workers[13] attempted to define historical data more precisely as meeting the criteria for psychogenic and organic impotence. For example, a provisional diagnosis of psychogenic impotence was made only if one of the five following criteria based on historical data were met: (1) full erections upon awakening occurring 2 or more times per week for the past 3 months and lasting until micturition, (2) normal masturbatory erections as judged by the patient, (3) normal erections with an alternative partner as judged by the patient and sufficient for intercourse, (4) normal erections after trial of behavioral sex therapy, and (5) frequent full, lasting erections during noncoital activity. The diagnosis of organogenic impotence rested on a history of inadequate erectile function in multiple contexts plus the presence of an organic condition known to cause impotence. Utilizing these criteria, 12% of a series of 93 impotent men could not be assigned to probable etiological groups. The percentage of men with impotence of unknown etiology would probably have been much larger if a trial of behavioral sex therapy had not been frequently employed as a diagnostic aid.

At least three investigations have assessed historical data in men with organic or psychogenic impotence. Kockett and co-workers[29] compared answers to 88 questions in a semistandardized interview in 16 men with psychogenic impotence (average age 33.8, no detectable physical disease) and ten diabetics with erectile problems. All patients received a standardized physical and neurological examination as well as the repeated determination of testosterone and luteinizing hormone. Diabetics with impotence were significantly different from men with psychogenic impotence on four historical variables. Diabetics reported decreased erectile turgidity during foreplay, during masturbation, and with spontaneous erections. Similarly, diabetics significantly more often than men with psychogenic impotence reported that erectile behavior during masturbation was as bad as or worse than during coital activities. Abel and his colleagues[30] at Columbia University reported that certain items in the sexual history can distinguish between impotence of psychogenic or organic etiology. Sixty diabetic males complaining of impotence were administered a structured interview including questions regarding 18 specific sexual symptoms and also completed nocturnal penile tumescence testing. Nocturnal penile tumescence measures were used to assign men to psychogenic and organic categories. Seven symptoms were extremely effective in differentiating organic from psychogenic impotence. Four of these symptoms referred to erectile capacity: (1) "Every time I try to get an erection it is less than a 100% full erection," (2) "I never wake up in the morning or during the night with a 100% full erection," (3) "during oral sex or masturbation I always get less than a 100% full erection," and (4) "I frequently or always fail to get a 100% full erection." Three of the symptoms referred to the ejaculatory reflex: (1) "It frequently or always takes me longer to reach ejaculation than it used to," (2) "The amount I ejaculate is frequently or always less than it used to be," and (3) "I rarely or never ejaculate prematurely." Abel and co-workers concluded that by relying on the sexual history alone (the seven questions cited above), 38% of impotent diabetics could be spared the expense of further diagnostic workup. In a study of the relationship between serum testosterone, prolactin, and sexual behavior, Segraves, Schoenberg, and Ivanoff[31] compared answers to eight questions concerning sexual function in 52 men with complaints of impotence. The absence of early-morning erections (upon awakening) and a complaint of decreased libido were significantly related to abnormal serum testosterone levels. The complaint of decreased libido was a particularly strong predictor of decreased serum testosterone levels. Seven of nine men with low serum testosterone had complaints of low libido. One half of the men complaining of low libido were found to have abnormally depressed serum testosterone levels. The presence of masturbatory erections, a pattern of obtaining and losing erections, a complaint of semiturgid erections during coitus, a complaint of total absence of erectile activity, a fluctuating course, or sudden onset of the problem was not related to etiology. In an unpublished report, the authors of this chapter studied the effectiveness of 18 sexual history questions in predicting the etiology of erectile complaints. All patients were subjected to extensive biomedical evaluation including nocturnal penile tumescene testing, doppler determination of penile blood flow, and serum testosterone and prolactin monitoring. Only two sexual history questions appropriately assigned etiology: firm lasting erections upon awakening and turgid noncoital erections predicted a psychogenic etiology to the problem. Condra and associates[32] also reported that firm early morning erections were the best discriminator between men with biogenic and psychogenic impotence.

The available evidence suggests that the clinician can use historical data with a certain degree of reliability to make a differential diagnosis of the etiology of impotence. Historical data indicating the presence of decreased erectile turgidity in noncoital activities is highly suggestive of an organic etiology to the problem. The finding that prolonged ejaculatory latency may also be predictive of organic impotence in diabetics probably is reflective of a peripheral neuropathy affecting nerve pathways influencing ejaculation as well as those controlling erections in many diabetics. The complaints of decreased libido in the sexual history appears to warrant an endocrine workup.

There are several disadvantages to relying on sexual history alone to make a differential diagnosis between psychogenic or organogenic impotence. One of the major problems is that certain sexual behaviors may occur so infrequently in certain subgroups that large numbers of patients cannot be diagnosed by history alone.[33] The discrepancy between coital and noncoital sexual activity can be quite useful in diagnosing psychogenic impotence. However, many men with psychogenic impotence report total absence of erections during noncoital activity. Many older married men, particularly of lower socioeconomic backgrounds, totally deny masturbatory activity after marriage. Similarly, many men in their sixties and seventies may report absent or infrequent erections upon awakening yet remain coitally potent. In other words, these historical items can be useful when present. However, in certain subgroups of impotent men, one has to rely on different sources of information. Another difficulty is that there is frequently a discrepancy between subjective and objective measures of rigidity. Most men tend to underrate their degree of penile tumescence.[34] This phenomenon may be even more common in men with psychogenic erectile problems.

It is of note that obtaining and then losing an erection and obtaining erections with alternate sex partners did not prove especially useful in distinguishing organic from psychogenic erectile problems in diabetics. A history of obtaining turgid erections, maintaining them for prolonged periods of foreplay, and losing erections only when coitus is attempted has often been considered as indicative of psychogenic impotence. On occasion a patient with pelvic vascular problems may report normal erectile function in the supine position which is lost after thrusting is initiated. In patients with unilateral occlusion of the external iliac artery and contralateral stenosis of the internal iliac, the ipsilateral internal iliac artery may serve as the main blood supply to the leg. Thus, shunting of blood away from the pelvis (pelvic steal syndrome)[35] during active thrusting might explain the loss of erection after penetration. The finding by Abel and associates that performance with alternative partners was not always an effective discriminator of psychogenic and organogenic problems fits with observation of other investigators that men with hyperprolactinemia or decreased serum testosterone may report erectile failure with the spouse but success with an alternative partner.[11,33,36,37] These observations suggest an interaction between biological and psychological factors. In many cases, it appears that partial organic suppression of function may be overridden by unusual and powerful environmental events (e.g., the novel stimulus of an extramarital affair).

USE OF PERSONALITY QUESTIONNAIRES

Clearly, the use of sexual history to differentiate the etiology of sexual complaints has certain disadvantages. The value of the information obtained is partially dependent on the skill and patience of the interviewer. Also, a proper sexual history may require an inordinate amount of the physician's time in reserved patients. For these and other reasons, many professionals have hoped that various self-administered personality questionnaires would be useful in the differential diagnosis of sexual problems.

The literature in this area of inquiry includes many failures to find consistent psychological patterns in psychologically impotent men or failures to replicate findings of previous investigators. Before reviewing these studies, it is worth emphasizing the absolute necessity of including a control group of men with organic impotence in an attempt to define a relationship between personality and psychogenic impotence. In other words, finding significant personality differences between psychologically impotent men and potent normals may provide little information other than that the experience of impotence often has devastating psychological effects.

Cooper[38] in 1969 investigated 43 men with erectile problems by psychiatric interview and the neuroticism scale questionnaire.[39] Although a control group was not utilized, elevated scores on the questionnaire were uncommon. Cooper also felt that the diagnosis of neurotic disorder was infrequent in this population. Cooper[40] in 1968 also administered the Foulds Hostility scale[41] to 64 patients with either erectile or ejaculatory complaints. A control group was not utilized. The patients with sexual dysfunction did demonstrate higher hostility levels as compared to norms for the scale. The absence of a control group of men with organic causes of impotence seriously limits the usefulness of this finding. The male impotence test[42] has been reported to discriminate between psychogenic and organic impotence. This particular instrument has been criticized for methodological shortcomings.[43] The original findings were not replicated by other investigators,[44] and thus that particular instrument is seldom utilized today.

The Minnesota Multiphasic Personality Inventory (MMPI) is the instrument used most frequently in the assessment of men with erectile problems.[16,45,46] Surprisingly, there is minimal evidence that the MMPI reliably differentiates between psychological and organic impotence. Beutler and co-workers[44] examined MMPI scores in relationship to nocturnal penile tumescence evaluations in 32 men with erectile disturbances. No significant differences were noted on any of the MMPI scales. Beutler and associates used a criterion group of ten patients representing the extremes of nocturnal penile tumescene to derive a decision rule to differentiate organic from psychogenic impotence. The presence of an MMPI masculinity—feminity score greater than 60 combined with a standard score greater than 70 on another scale was reported to indicate a greater probability that the problem was psychogenic. However, subsequent investigators have not been able to replicate the Beutler finding. Staples and co-workers[47] investigated the relationship between MMPI scores and nocturnal penile tumescence recording in 18 impotent patients. The decision rule advocated by Beutler and associates was not found to differentiate psychogenic from biogenic impotence. Similarly, Marshall and co-workers[48] administered the MMPI in organogenic and ten psychogenic cases of erectile failure. The decision rules advocated by Beutler were again found to misclassify most patients. Using a discriminant function analysis, the authors found provisional evidence in support of a decision rule contrary to that reported previously. They concluded "that the MMPI cannot yet be included as part of the process of determining the etiology of impotence" (p. 408). More recently, Martin and associates[48] reported that the MMPI and California Psychological Inventory were both ineffective in the differential diagnosis of impotence.

The other instrument most frequently employed in the evaluation of erectile problems is the Derogatis Sexual Functioning Inventory (DSFI).[50,51] In contrast to the MMPI, the DSFI was specifically designed to be a multidimensional measure of human sexual functioning. This questionnaire takes approximately 45–60 min to complete and consists of ten subscales. Two of the subscales were modified from previous questionnaires. The psychological-symptoms subscale is comprised of the brief symptom inventory, which is a brief form of the symptom checklist (the SCL-90),[52] and the affects subscale is taken from the affects balance scales.[53] The other eight scales were specifically developed to measure sexual attitudes and behavior. The sexual-information subscale consists of 26 true–false items that measure accuracy of sexual information. The sexual-attitude subscale is designed to measure sexual attitudes along the liberalism–conservatism dimension. Typical items of this scale include "Premarital intercourse is beneficial to later marital adjustment" and "Homosexuality is perverse and unhealthy." Patients are required to indicate their degree of agreement or disagreement with such statements. The gender-role-definition subscale consists of 30 gender-stereotyped adjectives; subjects are asked to indicate the degree to which such adjectives apply to themselves. Typical adjectives include whimsical, compassionate, vigorous, and decisive. The measure utilized is a difference score obtained by subtracting feminity from masculinity scores. The sexual-fantasy subscale consists of 20 sexual themes that might have appeared in the subjects' dreams or daydreams. The higher the score, the greater the number of daydreams. The sexual-drive and -experience subscales essentially consist of lists of sexual activities. For the sexual-experience scales, the total number of experiences checked is the final score. For the sexual-drive scale, the frequency of various sexual activites is summed to give a total score. Sexual satisfaction is scored by the answer to ten true–false questions. A typical question is "I am not very interested in sex." Most questionnaires also include a rating scale of satisfaction.

Derogatis and co-workers[54] reported a study of 28 patients with a complaint of erectile disturbance. Fifty percent of these patients were diagnosed as having organogenic impotence, and 50% were felt to have psychogenic problems. Diagnostic decisions were reached in multidisciplinary conferences. The report unfortunately omitted information concerning the type and extent of medical evaluation. Each of these patients completed the DSFI. Two subtests differentiated psychogenic from organogenic cases. Psychogenic males reported significantly more sexual experiences (p < 0.05) and a hyperpolarized masculine role definition (p < 0.001). A cutting-score analysis[55] suggested that individuals with gender-role-definition scores of −5 should be assigned a psychogenic diagnosis. This decision role produced an efficiency of 89.2% in correct etiological assignment. Examination of individual symptom dimensions on the symptoms subscale suggested that biogenic cases were more symptomatic on most scales, although these differences were rarely statistically In summary, men with psychogenic impotence appeared to be characterized by increased sexual experience and a hyperpolarized masculine gender role. The authors[54] stated that these findings suggested that psychogenic impotence may be characterized by a counterphobic attitude toward sex in men with rigid masculine-role patterns.

> The evidence strongly suggests that the evolution of a polarized or sex-typed role definition renders the individual who adopts it disproportionately vulnerable to sexual disorders. Sexual relationships become limited to a relatively inflexible set of stylized behaviors, often compulsively executed, that are highly resistant to alteration or adaptation to new circumstances. [p. 239]

Melman and Redfield[56] administered the DSFI to 39 patients with erectile problems. The diagnostic evaluation of these patients always included physical examination and a complete neurological evaluation. Fasting blood glucose, plasma testosterone and prolactin, pudental nerve conduction velocities, and nocturnal penile tumescence studies were frequently employed as diagnostic facilitations. The DSFI scores of a subsample of 16 men with organic impotence were compared with those of ten men with psychogenic impotence. They failed to replicate the finding of Derogatis et al.[54] that cutting scores on the gender-role subscale could be used to differentiate organic from psychogenic impotence. Patients with organic complaints tended to have greater sexual satisfaction (p < 0.02) than men with psychogenic complaints. It is of note that this finding is contrary to the previously mentioned Derogatis study.

Similarly, Segraves, Schoenberg, and co-investigators[57] examined DSFI scores in 12 men with impotence of organic etiology and 51 men with psychogenic impotence. Diagnostic criteria for psychogenic and organogenic impotence were clearly specified. Repeated comparisons of the impotent men on DSFI subscales failed to differentiate organic from psychogenic etiology. A number of the DSFI scales were found to be significantly associated with demographic variables such as age, race, marital status, social class, and duration of problem. For example, age was significantly and negatively associated with various measures of sexual drive. However, older age was positively related to sexual satisfaction. Similarly, being married was highly negatively related to sexual drive. For these reasons, the authors formed a psychogenic cohort, trying to match each organic case with a psychogenic case of the same race and similar age, marital status, duration of complaint, and social class. A comparison of the organic group with the newly formed psychogenic cohort failed to identify significant differences. The significant differences noted by Melman and Redfield[56] were not confirmed in this study. The psychological distress scale of the DSFI is equivalent to the SCL-90. Therefore, the nine subscales—somatization, obsessive–compulsive, interpersonal sensitivity, depression, anxiety, hostility, phobic anxiety, paranoid ideation, and psychoticism—were individually scored. Again, no signficant differences were noted between the two groups of patients.

Clearly, the research to date does not provide convincing evidence that psychological testing is useful in the differentiation of psychogenic from organogenic impotence. The failure to find differences of psychological test scores may be due to methodological difficulties in the studies conducted or to an actual absence of such differences. The obvious source of methodological error would be the incorrect assignment of cases to criterion groups. Although none of the studies reported routinely employed nocturnal penile tumescence testing or measurement of pudendal nerve latencies, all studies made considerable effort to fully investigate possible cases of organogenic impotence. The study by Segraves and co-workers[57] strictly followed objective criteria in assignment of cases. Although it appears unlikely that incorrect diagnostic assignment is responsible for the failures to replicate, this remains a possibility until a future investigator repeats these studies using stricter diagnostic criteria, requiring nocturnal penile tumescence testing and pudendal nerve conduction studies in all subjects at a minimum. Similarly, it is possible that psychological differences exist which the current instruments did not detect. Probably, the most sophisticated sexual attitude questionnaire to date was developed by Eysenck.[58] Unfortunately, this instrument has received minimal use in the United States to date.

Possibly, this or other questionnaires might detect a difference between men with organogenic and psychogenic impotence. However, it is also possible that such differences do not exist, when one considers the heterogeneity of the groups being compared.

> Inability to achieve erections in marital coitus is an observable end result of many possible psychologic etiologies....Even cases of chronic psychogenic impotence constitute an extremely heterogeneous group. Within this sample, the appearance of psychological erectile dysfunction appeared related to a myriad of causes ranging from individual psychopathology to chronic marital dysfunction in otherwise healthy individuals. In other cases, the onset of impotence appeared clearly related to a significant psychological stress such as widowhood, becoming divorced, or the death of a child or parent.[57]

The very hetereogenity of the population may explain the pattern of irreproducible results in this field of inquiry. It is, of course, entirely possible that a definable subgroup of men with psychogenic impotence may have demonstrable personality differences from men with organic impotence and that these personality differences may reflect some of the psychological factors influencing the etiology.

NOCTURNAL PENILE TUMESCENCE TESTING

Originally, it was hoped that NPT testing would prove to be the ultimate discriminating procedure in determining the etiology of erectile problems. The existence of NPT has been known since the work of Ohlmeyer and co-workers[59] and of Halverson.[60] The association between NPT and rapid eye movement (REM) sleep was noted by Serinsky and Kreitman,[61] and Karachan[62] was one of the first investigators to suggest that measurement of NPT could be used to ascertain prognosis in erectile dysfunction. Subsequent studies by Karachan's group[63-68] and by Fisher and co-workers[69-72] have elucidated the relationship between NPT and REM sleep. Karachan and co-workers[73-77] have suggested that the presence of full sustained erections during sleep is indicative of psychogenic impotence whereas the absence of turgid erections during REM sleep is indicative of organogenic impotence. NPT testing has been incorporated into the routine evaluation of erectile problems at many treatment centers.[78-85]

More recently, investigators have become aware of the limitations of NPT testing in the differential diagnosis of erectile problems. These limitations include both technical difficulties and serious questions concerning the basic assumptions underlying NPT testing.

Initially, changes in penile circumference were used as the sole measure of nocturnal erectile capacity.[84] However, it soon became apparent that there are tremendous interindividual differences in circumference changes with erections and that the relationship between circumference change and turgidity is not always direct. In other words, some men may be observed to have large circumference change and still have an erection too flaccid to permit vaginal penetration.[86-88] Because of these interindividual differences in the relationship between circumference change and penile rigidity, most centers have relied on subjective ratings or direct tests of penile rigidity during sleep.[89] In many centers, the patient may be awakened during an NPT episode, and the patient and investigator may estimate the percentage of full erection obtained. Clearly, such a procedure is quite crude and introduces an element of subjectivity into the procedure.[90] The timing of the rigidity estimate may also present a problem. In other words, the technician may sample an inadequate erection whereas adequate erections were present during other periods of the sleep cycle. Some clinicians have attempted to use artificially produced erections (infusion of saline into the corpus cavernosum) as a standard by which to assess NPT.[91,92] For example, an adequate or full erection could be defined as an erection equaling or exceeding 85% of the maximum corporeal infusion circumference. The complication rate and overall patient acceptability of such a procedure are unknown. Similarly, the definition of adequate tumescence remains arbitrary, and this procedure does not solve the problem of the unclear relationship between tumescence and rigidity.[90–94] Another approach to this problem has been direct measurement of buckling pressure.[95] A pressure device is pressed against the glans of the penis toward the base, and the pressure required for buckling the penis is recorded in millimeters of mercury. Pilot data suggests that a penis too soft for vaginal penetration will buckle at pressures of 60 mm Hg or less. A penis that does not buckle until it encounters a pressure of 100 mm Hg is regarded as sufficiently turgid to enter most vaginas. Values between 60 and 100 mm Hg are indeterminate. Clearly, the direct measurement of buckling pressure is a major advance. Again, timing of the measurement sample may present a problem, and the decision regarding adequate "buckling pressures" is somewhat arbitrary. Another technical problem with NPT testing is the decision regarding the minimal number of nights of recording required. Various medical centers range from 1 to 3 nights of recording as the standard procedure, and the minimal number of required nights in the laboratory is unclear. This is far from an academic question as some neurophysiology laboratories charge more than $700 for 1 night of NPT testing.

Perhaps more troublesome to the validity of NPT testing are recent questions regarding the basic assumptions underlying this test procedure. This test rests on the assumption that the absence of sufficient nocturnal erections, given the presence of normal sleep architecture, indicates that the problem is organic in etiology. This assumes that psychological events during sleep are incapable of suppressing end-organ function. This assumption remains unproven, and certain evidence raises the probability that it may be false. Karacan and associates[96] reported that dreams with a high anxiety content were associated with no or irregular erections during dream sleep. It is important to note that normal volunteers were used in this study. If psychologically impotent males had been used, one might have expected this relationship to be much stronger. Similarly, Fisher and co-workers[97,98] reported anecdotal evidence that dream content and nocturnal erectile capacity might be highly correlated. Rapid detumescence and absent erections were often associated with dreams with anxiety, homosexual, or incestuous themes. Again normal volunteers were studied. There is some evidence in the literature that at least a small number of men with psychogenic impotence may not have nocturnal erections, and thus the problem could be erroneously diagnosed as biogenic if NPT measures were used as the sole criterion. Kahn and Fisher[99] reported an investigation of 21 aged male volunteers. The average age of these patients was 80.5 years. All patients were studied for a minimum of 3 nights' sleep. Of particular note is that two of the elderly men in the sample did not demonstrate full erections during sleep although they reported normal coital activities outside the laboratory. Fisher, Schiavi, and co-workers[70] investigated 30 patients with erectile problems. These patients had an average age of 48 years. Two men among the patients with a diagnosis of psychogenic impotence are especially interesting. One man obtained only semiflaccid sleep erections yet upon follow-up was found to have had full erections during masturbation and intercourse. Another patient had essentially no NPT during 4 nights of recording. However, he obtained full erections during self-stimulation, suggesting that the erectile mechanism was intact. The author is personally aware of at least three men who demonstrated minimal or no nocturnal penile erectile activity at the University of Chicago neurophysiology laboratory who subsequently reported erections sufficient for coitus. One insulin-dependent diabetic was observed to have a virtually flat nocturnal tumescence record. However, with the excitement involved in extramarital situations, he was able to obtain erections sufficient for vaginal penetration. It is of note that this man had documented peripheral neuropathy and erections of decreased, yet sufficient turgidity. The other two men had similar histories in that coital erections were decreased in turgidity but significantly more functional than the nocturnal penile tumescence record would have indicated. These cases are a potent reminder that we have minimal information concerning the general physiological activation responsible for nocturnal erections and have no evidence that this arousal mechanism is equivalent in intensity to environmental stimuli. It is also of note that the magnitude and frequency of nocturnal erections in various psychiatric conditions has not been studied. One immediately wonders whether affective syndromes with so-called vegetative signs (sleep and appetite suppression) may not also be associated with disturbance of the erectile mechanism during sleep.

On the other side of the picture, there is reason to suspect that certain organic conditions might be misdiagnosed as psychogenic if one relied on NPT testing alone. For example, certain patients with a pelvic steal syndrome may report normal erections which are lost only during active coital thrusting.[100,101] The loss of erection is due to a shunting of blood from the pelvis to ischemic extremities during active coital thrusting. Presumably, such men could have normal NPT records as the sleeping state would make minimal requirements for collateral blood flow. In hyperprolactinemia, a situational or episodic erectile impairment may be observed clinically (M.F. Schwartz et al., personal communication). In certain men, erectile function may persist during masturbation or with alternative partners. The NPT pattern in such men is unknown. Wasserman and associates[90] reported a patient with hyperprolactinemia whose erectile circumference was only marginally influenced. However, erectile turgidity was abnormal.

There is some evidence indicating the existence of two separate erectile pathways in man, one elicited by psychogenic and the other by relfexogenic stimuli.[101] This evidence comes mainly from studies of sexual function in spinal-cord-injured patients. Bors and co-workers[103,104] have attempted to correlate the location of spinal injury with the preservation or interruption of sexual function. This work suggests the presence of reflexogenic erections elicited by stroking the penis or by a full bladder or rectum. The afferent branches of this reflex arc are the pudendal and pelvic nerves. The efferent pathway is a parasympathetic outflow (nervi erigentes) from the sacral cord, S2–S4. Psychogenic erections are mediated by a sympathetic nervous system thoracolumbar outflow from the T12 to the L1 region of the cord. The eliciting stimuli for this reflex are predominantly auditory, visual, and imaginative stimuli which arouse erotic centers in the brain. The evidence for the existence of both reflexogenic and psychogenic erectile pathways is not definitive. However, if two such pathways exist, NPT recordings are presumably measuring only one of the two pathways and perhaps underestimating erectile function in certain cases.

In conclusion, the presence of firm nocturnal erections suggests that a patient's problem is probably not organically based. Two possible exceptions to this statement include hyperprolactinemia and the pelvic steal syndrome. However, the significance of decreased or absent nocturnal penile tumescence is unclear. Although it probably portends an organic etiology in most cases, the possibility exists that some men with psychogenic impotence may not have nocturnal erections.

Other Laboratory Procedures

Because of their low cost relative to NPT recording and greater specificity as to etiology, pudendal nerve velocity studies[105-110] and penile blood pressure are frequently employed as screening procedures. Each of these procedures obviously indicates the presence or absence of an abnormality in a given system and cannot be used to rule out organicity in general (e.g., the presence of normal pudendal nerve conduction studies does not rule out other organic etiologies). In each of these procedures, normal values are known. However, the degree of deviance from normality sufficient to cause erectile failure is not known for either procedure. For this reason, these procedures are best utilized for cases of erectile failure where a probable organic basis has already been established. At this point, penile blood pressure and pudendal nerve conduction studies can be effectively utilized to investigate neurological and vascular contributions to the problem. Their relative low cost indicates that they probably should be included in a screening battery.

Endocrinological causes of erectile failure are reviewed in Chapter 6. As idiopathic hypogonadism and hyperprolactinemia may present as episodic or situational erectile failure, historical data alone may not identify such cases. Similarly, it is unclear whether NPT is disturbed in such patients. Although the exact role of testosterone and prolactin in erectile potency is unclear, some minimal screening of androgen function is probably indicated in almost all cases of erectile incapacity.

SCREENING PROTOCOL FOR ESTABLISHING ETIOLOGY OF IMPOTENCE

BACKGROUND

Much of the information concerning the diagnostic evaluation of erectile complaints has evolved in the last 5–10 years or is in the process of being established. Accordingly, there is considerable variation from practitioner to practitioner and from center to center in screening procedures. However, there appears to be uniformity in that most centers stress multisystem and multidisciplinary evaluations of such patients. Such an evaluation usually involves endocrinological, neurological, vascular, and psychological examinations of the complaints. Most of the variation between medical centers involves different procedures for evaluating each of the different systems serving erectile functions. For example, some centers utilize psychological testing whereas others require psychiatric evaluation. Similarly, some centers use NPT testing for all patients; others use this screening device in selected cases. Because of the lack of firmly established guidelines, diagnostic evaluation of this complaint still requires clinical artistry as well as clinicial science.

Montague[23] describes the screening procedures utilized at the Cleveland Clinic. He stresses the importance of the original medical and sexual history. At this time, the clinician can establish certain provisional hypotheses regarding etiology. The medical history should, of course, concern the presence of chronic diseases (e.g., diabetes mellitus, alcoholism, renal failure), prior surgical procedures (e.g., radical perineal prostatectomy, abdominoperineal resection of the rectum), and use of pharmacological agents (e.g., anticholinergics, antihypertensives). The sexual history should document the specific circumstances of the dysfunction, the state of libido, and adequacy of genital sensation. Montague also recommends that the physician specifically enquire about the sexual and marital history. The physical examination should include assessment of the penis for plaques, size and consistency of the testicles, sphincter tone, bulbocavernosus reflex, saddle sensation, sensation and reflexes in the lower extremities, and lower-extremity pulses. The clinician should also examine for the presence of gynecomastia and masculine hair distribution. Routine laboratory screening should include serum testosterone, glucose tolerance, and a general survey such as the SMA-12 or -18 (e.g., for liver or renal disease). If the serum testosterone is abnormal, prolactin, follicle-stimulating hormone, and luteinizing hormone should be assessed to determine if the hypogonadism is primary, secondary to testicular abnormality or secondary to pituitary disease. Montague recommends that vascular etiologies be further investigated with the Doppler ultrasound probe comparing penile to brachial pressures and looking for abnormalities in the wave form of the pulse volume. If abnormalities are found in this screening procedure, arteriography of the aortic bifuration, each internal iliac, and the internal pudendal circulation should follow. Corporeal cavernosography is recommended for cases of suspected venous outflow problems (i.e., chordee). Psychiatric assessment of all patients and their partners is recommended if the urologist knows a suitable psychiatrist. Montague appropriately emphasizes that not all psychiatrists are interested or experienced in the area of sexual dysfunction. He also recommends routine administration of the MMPI and the California Psychological Inventory and feels that these instruments are useful in the diagnostic evaluation of depression. He mentions the use of NPT testing but does not indicate whether it should be routinely or selectively employed. It is also unclear whether penile blood flow measures are routinely employed.

Nath and the colleagues[17] at the Boston University School of Medicine recently described a multidisciplinary approach to the evaluation of impotence which resembles that described by Montague. In their approach, patients are seen by urological, psychiatric, neurological, endocrine, and vascular specialists. Each patient routinely undergoes psychiatric evaluation, a full medical and sexual history, physical examination, NPT testing, Doppler evaluation of penile blood flow, and endocrine screening. Their approach differs from the approach described by Montague in several ways: (1) psychological testing is not employed, (2) penile blood flow is assessed before and after leg exercise (the pelvic steal test), (3) serum testosterone, luteinizing hormone, and prolactin levels are routinely assessed in all patients, and (4) all patients undergo a neurological evaluation. In patients with suspected neurological lesions, cystometrography and pudendal nerve velocity (sacral latency testing) are employed. NPT testing is employed as part of the complete assessment battery and is regarded as primarily useful when the NPT results are inconsistent with the patient's history.

Karachan and co-workers[73-77] at Baylor have had some of the most extensive experience evaluating erectile complaints. They employ a multidisciplinary evaluation involving urologists, neurologists, psychiatrists, and psychologists. Their evaluation approach differs somewhat from that of other centers in terms of the primacy attached to the NPT record. Patients undergo 3 nights of NPT recording routinely, accompanied by measures of penile rigidity, recording of activity in the bulbocavernosus and ischiocavernosus muscles, and measurement of penile pulse volume during nocturnal erections. Each patient is also seen by a psychiatrist, and testosterone and prolactin levels are routinely obtained. It is of note that this center also employs one of the most extensive psychological questionnaire assessments. Patients are routinely administered the following tests: the MMPI, the profile of mood states, the state-trait anxiety inventory, the Institute of Living scale, the fundamental interpersonal relations orientation–behavior questionnaire, the Rotter locus of control questionnaire, and the draw-a-person test.

Numerous other investigators have reported their screening protocols.[14,26,27,30,92,111-114] These reports differ mainly in their special emphasis of selected parts of the evaluation. For example, Abel and associates[30] specifically emphasize the importance of the sexual history, and Barry and Hodges[27] emphasize the importance of psychological testing.

A RECOMMENDED PROTOCOL

In this section, a recommended protocol for the evaluation of erectile complaints will be described (Figure 1). The basis for this recommended diagnostic approach is an attempt to balance costs of various procedures against their relative yield. In other words, the approach advocated will emphasize the selective employment of investigative procedures rather than the exhaustive exclusion of all possible etiologies.

Sexual History

The initial physician–patient interaction for any disorder usually begins with a detailed history of the presenting complaint followed by a careful past medical history and a review of symptoms.[115,116] During this time the physician establishes rapport and credibility with the patient and begins to form provisional hypotheses concerning etiology. These hy-

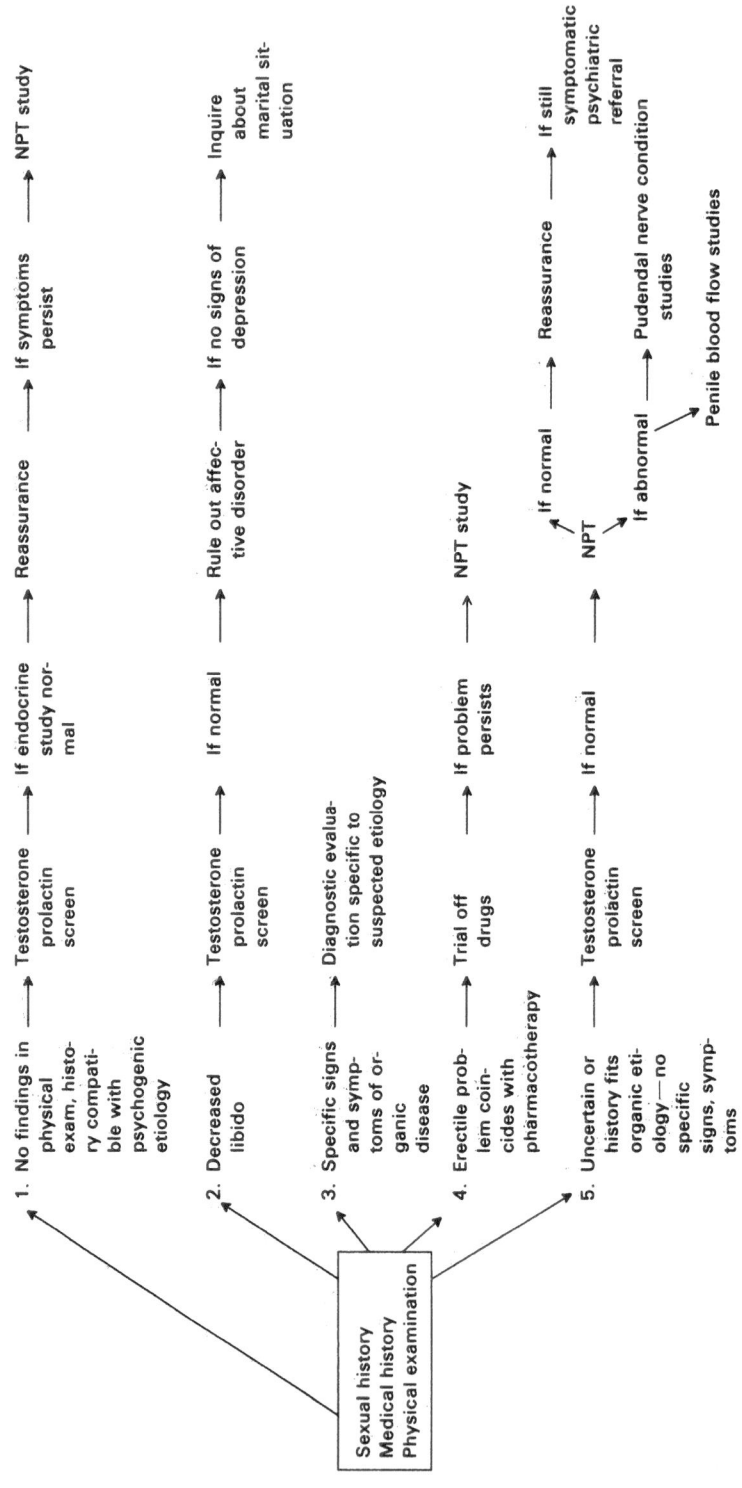

Figure 1. Protocol for evaluation of impotence.

potheses are further investigated during the physical examination and by ordering appropriate diagnostic tests and procedures. The physician's investigation of sexual complaints follows the same general format. Because of patient embarrassment concerning sexual matters, the history taking may require considerable skills in putting the patient at ease such that specific details of the complaint can be elicited.

If the patient presents with an erectile problem as his chief complaint, this should be explored in a straightforward way. As with most medical complaints, the physician should ask the patient to describe his problem, document the time and manner of onset, the nature of its progression, its current status, and concurrent medical–psychological events. Although the physician should first encourage the patient to describe his problem in his own words, many patients require considerable assistance in providing specific details regarding the dysfunction. For certain patients who are remarkably poor medical historians, the physician can occasionally help the patient to provide a more coherent history by asking certain questions. For example, it may help to first ask the patient to describe his last sexual experience. The physician can then ask the patient specific details about that experience. Subsequently, the physician can direct the patient to the time when he first noticed a problem. Sometimes, this attempt at time orientation can help a confused patient to orient his presentation in a manner helpful to the physician.

One of the first goals of the differential diagnostic process during the history taking is to ascertain whether the problem is truly an erectile problem. It is not uncommon to be referred patients by other physicians who have received exogenous testosterone and other interventions and who do not really have erectile problems. For example, these men may complain that they are impotent, whereas a detailed sexual history may reveal something quite different. It is not unusual for a man to complain that he is impotent but during a detailed sexual history to discover that his real problem is that he ejaculates rapidly and then experiences difficulty in reobtaining an erection.

A provisional differential diagnosis as to psychogenic or organogenic impotence can often be made during the sexual history. The presence of full sustained erections occurring frequently in any situation is strong evidence that the problem is probably psychogenic. For example, it is important to know whether the problem is difficulty obtaining or maintaining erections and whether the patient has erections under any circumstances. The physician needs to specifically inquire about erections during foreplay, during phantasy, upon awakening, during masturbation, and with alternative partners. If the patient reports that he has only partial erections in all circumstances, there is strong reason to suspect that his problem is organic. If the patient reports that he continues to have intercourse by stuffing a semifirm erection into his wife's vagina, the physician's suspicion of an organic basis should be heightened. This suggests that the erectile failure is not precluding sexual intimacy and thus is less likely to serve a psychological function. Table 1 lists some of the questions during the sexual history which may be especially useful in establishing a preliminary differential diagnosis. As previously mentioned, a situational pattern of erectile failure can occasionally occur in men with hyperprolactinemia. Similarly, a report of firm sustained erections during foreplay which are lost after intromission might suggest either psychogenic impotence or a pelvic steal syndrome.

At the same time that the physician is documenting the erectile problem, he will also wish to inquire about the ejaculatory reflex and libido. A history of delayed ejaculation or of retrograde ejaculation is suggestive evidence of an autonomic neuropathy which may also be responsible for the erectile problem. The presence of premature ejaculation is compatible with the diagnosis of psychogenic impotence.

A complaint of decreased libido is not diagnostic, but it should alert the physician to three probable causes: endocrinopathy, affective disorder, or relationship discord.

Medical History

The medical history should be complete and cover at least the following areas: (1) general physical health and chronic diseases, (2) diseases known to specifically influence erectile function, (3) past surgery, and (4) a review of all current pharmacotherapy.

It is becoming clear that the presence of chronic debilitating disease may interfere with sexual functioning although the erectile mechanism per se is intact. For example, men with cardiac failure or advanced emphysema may experience fatigue or shortness of breath during sexual activity.[116] Many men experience erectile problems after myocardial infarctions. In these men, a careful sexual history may reveal considerable anxiety about a "coital coronary" or even the presence of severe angina during foreplay.[118-124] Two patients seen by the authors clearly illustrate the role of poor general health in sexual failure. A 50-year-old man with terminal chronic lymphocytic leukemia complained of coital erectile failure. This man received monthly blood transfusions after which he reported firm erections upon awakening and firm masturbatory erections. Later in the month, as his hematocrit began to fall, he reported the absence of early-morning and masturbatory erections. Another man with metastatic carcinoma of the colon reported total suppression of both libido and sexual

Table 1. Sexual History Data Useful in Differential Diagnosis

A. Items possibly suggestive of psychogenic etiology[a]
   1. Abrupt onset unassociated with any medical event of note (e.g., starting antihypertensive medication, spinal trauma)
   2. Adequate erections during foreplay lost before intromission
   3. Significant psychosexual stress preceding or accompanying onset (e.g., divorce, affair)
B. Items possibly suggestive of an organic etiology[b]
   1. Concurrent report of delayed ejaculation
   2. Concurrent report of retrograde or absent ejaculation
   3. Report of decreased genital sensation
   4. Report of adequate erections during foreplay or in passive male sexual position which are lost if active thrusting is begun
C. Items highly suggestive of a psychogenic etiology[c]
   1. Full erections during foreplay
   2. Full erections during masturbation
   3. Full spontaneous erections
   4. Masturbatory erections firmer than coital erections
D. Items highly suggestive of an organic etiology[d]
   1. Coital erections always less than 100%
   2. Early-morning erections never completely firm
   3. Masturbatory erections less than 100%
   4. Always fails to obtain full erections

[a] These items have not been empirically validated as discriminators between psychogenic and organogenic impotence.
[b] Items 1 and 2 provide presumptive evidence of an autonomic peripheral neuropathy also affecting the ejaculatory reflex. Item 3 is suggestive of a peripheral neuropathy. Item 4 is possibly suggestive of a pelvic steal syndrome.
[c] From Kockett et al.[29]
[d] From Abel et al.[30]

function during periods of active chemotherapy. During periods off chemotherapy, libido and noncoital erections returned. Both men were aided by a simple explanation of the process involved and instructions to limit sexual activities to those periods when general well-being was present. The point we are attempting to establish is that the physician needs to consider nonspecific debilitating effects of a variety of physical conditions and medical interventions in his assessment of medical factors possibly contributing to erectile failure. In a minority of cases, advice to the patient to restrict sex activities to periods of good physical stamina or correction of the underlying medical disorder will restore good erectile function. In such cases, a careful history and good clinical judgement may lead to the appropriate intervention and preclude the necessity for an expensive diagnostic assessment.

A large number of disease processes are known to directly impair erectile function. The presence of such diseases does not prove that the disease caused the erectile problem. For example, psychogenic impotence

can occur in diabetic men[125] and behavioral sex therapy has been reported
to reverse erectile dysfunction in men with diabetes mellitus.[126] However,
the presence of a possible etiology suggested by the history may point the
way to an abbreviated workup. If a patient has a documented history of
peripheral vascular disease, one should proceed to check femoral and ankle
pulses during the physical examination. Monitoring of penile blood flow
might be the logical next step. In such cases, a full endocrine workup is
obviously unnecessary. Similarly, a diabetic with erectile failure and other
evidence of peripheral neuropathy would be immediately suspected to have
neurogenic impotence. In such cases, the physical examination should include a careful neurological examination including checking the bulbocavernosus reflex. One then might proceed directly to pudendal nerve
conduction studies. A summary of pertinent physical findings is listed in
Table 2. In many cases, a careful history will establish probable etiologies.
A reasoned approach to the use of laboratory facilities can thus spare the
patient unnecessary medical costs. The number of medical conditions reported to be possibly related to erectile problems is extensive. A partial
listing is given in Table 3.

The review of the past medical history should include a careful review
of previous surgical procedures to document whether the onset of the
erectile problem coincided with such a procedure. A variety of surgical
procedures may produce impotence. These include radical perineal prostatectomy, abdominoperineal resection of the rectum, retroperitoneal
lymphadenectomy, and surgery of the abdominoaorticoiliac arteries.

Table 2. Physical Examination of Impotent Men

System	Physical signs
Endocrine	Change in hair or skin texture
	Absence of secondary sex characteristics
	Gynecomastia
	Abnormal size or consistency of testes
Neurological	Decreased sensation
	Motor deficits
	Changes in deep tendon reflexes
	Decreased sphincter tone
	Abnormal bulbocavernosus reflex
Vascular	Change in hair or skin in lower extremities
	Decreased femoral, ankle, penile pulses
Local	Plaques or fibrosis in corpora cavernosa

Table 3. Medical Conditions Associated with Impotence

Neurogenic
  Diabetes mellitus
  Alcoholic neuropathy
  Spinal cord injury
  Temporal lobe lesions
  Postpelvic radiation
  Neurotoxicity associated with cancer chemotherapy
Endocrine
  Hypothyroidism
  Cushing's disease
  Addison's disease
  Hypogonadism
  Pituitary adenomas
Vascular
  Peripheral vascular disease
  Leukemic infiltration of corpora cavernosa
  Thrombosis associated with sickle cell disease
Other
  Renal failure
  Peyronie's disease

Pharmacological agents influencing erectile function are reviewed in Chapter 2. Clearly, a careful pharmacological history is required. In particular, the physician needs to document whether the onset of an erectile problem coincided with the initiation of a given drug or with a change in dosage. Almost any pharmacological agent should be suspected as responsible. Several factors preclude the listing of drugs known to cause erectile problems. First, there has been minimal systematic investigation in this area. The bulk of evidence consists of case reports of varying merit. Second, there is still considerable uncertainty regarding the neurotransmitters involved in both the central and peripheral sexual pathways. Thus, one cannot predict which agents might be expected to inhibit sexual function. In addition, many drugs may indirectly influence sexual function by their side effects on endocrine activity. From a practical viewpoint, a history of concurrence of a sexual problem and the initiation of any pharmacological agent should be taken seriously. If possible, the agent should be discontinued for a trial period while assessing for the return of potency. If discontinuance of the drug is medically contraindicated, an alternative agent should be tried. In rare cases, one will encounter men with severe essential hypertension which can be controlled only by hypotensive agents that also render the man impotent. In most cases, the appropriate first step is drug discontinuance. If this intervention suffices, a full diagnostic workup including NPT, an endocrine battery, and other procedures would clearly be both unnecessary and a disservice to the patient.

Physical Examination

In most patients, the history should be followed by a thorough physical examination. The physical examination serves various purposes providing an opportunity for the physician to (1) follow up on presumptive
diagnostic possibilities uncovered during the history, (2) look for physical
signs of other diseases which might influence potency, and (3) reassure
the patient that his problem is being taken seriously. If the history reveals
a gradual diminution of libido in the absence of symptoms of a depressive
disorder and there is no evidence of marital discord, the physician might
suspect an endocrinological aspect to the complaint. During the physical
examination, special attention should be paid to changes in skin and hair
texture, the presence of secondary sex characteristics, gynecomastia, and
testicular size and consistency. In diabetic patients, the physical examination should search for evidence of peripheral neuropathy and focus on
sensation, motor deficits, and deep tender reflexes especially in the lower
extremities. This examination should be followed by an examination of
sphincter tone and the bulbocavernosus reflex. In patients suspected of
having peripheral vascular disease, the physical examination should include
assessment of skin and hair changes in the lower extremities as well as
examination of ankle, femoral, and penile pulses. In all patients, the physical examination should include careful palpation of the penis for evidence
of plaques and fibrosis. During the physical examination, evidence may
be found suggesting the presence of other conditions affecting sexual function such as thyroid disease, Cushing's disease, Addison's disease, or renal
failure. Many men with obvious psychogenic impotence may require a
careful physical examination plus a variety of other diagnostic procedures
before they are willing to consider the possibility of an interpersonal etiology to their complaint. In such cases, diagnostic tests may be more useful
for their psychological impact than for their aid in medical evaluation.

Chemical Laboratory Tests

There is minimal evidence concerning which chemical laboratory tests
should be included in a routine evaluation of erectile complaints. Serum
testosterone levels probably should be part of the routine evaluation, especially if there is any sign of a disturbance in libido. As previously mentioned, it is unclear whether androgen levels are directly related to erectile
capacity independent of libido. It is possible that erectile complaints in
hypogonadal men are secondary to decreased libido and consequent performance anxiety. It is also unclear how often exogenous androgen administration restores erectile potency in hypogonodal men.[126] Hyerprolactine-

mia can mimic psychogenic impotence.[128] (M. F. Schwartz et al., personal communication). In a small number of cases, situational impotence may be the first sign of a pituitary adenoma.[129,130] Although hyperprolactinemia is usually associated with low serum testosterone, this is not a consistent relationship.[131] Thus, it appears that serum prolactin levels should be part of the routine evaluation of all complaints of erectile dysfunction. A finding of an abnormally low testosterone should, of course, be further evaluated measuring follicle-stimulating hormone and luteinizing hormone.

Montague[23] recommends that a general survey (complete blood count plus an SMA-12 or SMA-18) be included as part of the routine evaluation. Such a screen would presumably detect significant liver or renal disease as well as elevated glucose levels. There is no evidence to date to indicate whether this should be part of the routine assessment of impotent men. In view of its minimal cost, this probably deserves to be included in the routine assessment. Although diabetes is associated with erectile problems, it is unclear whether a glucose tolerance test merits being included in the routine assessment.

Some investigators[132] have reported thyroid disease in impotent patients. However, there is insufficient evidence to date to state that thyroid function tests should be routinely ordered. Similarly, it is unclear whether routine assessment of adrenal function is warranted.

Other Diagnostic Procedures

Unfortunately, a careful history, medical examination, and routine chemical laboratory work will not reveal a probable etiology in many patients. Unless the physician has a strong suspicion of a psychogenic basis (in which case a trial of behavioral sex therapy might be indicated), NPT testing should be considered. As previously mentioned, this testing should include monitoring of sleep stages and some direct test of penile rigidity. The presence of a normal nocturnal erection pattern can safely be presumed to establish the diagnosis of psychogenic impotence. The absence of nocturnal erections provides suggestive but inconclusive evidence of an organic etiology. The search for an organic etiology can be further pursued by neurological and vascular studies. If a peripheral neuropathy is suspected, the next logical step is to proceed to pudendal nerve conduction studies. An abnormal conduction time provides evidence of peripheral neuropathy in the pudendal nerve. Unfortunately, a normal pudendal nerve conduction velocity does not rule out a peripheral autonomic neuropathy as responsible for the erectile complaint. It is possible for a neuropathy to selectively damage the pelvic autonomic nerves without affecting the pudendal nerve. If facilities for monitoring pudendal nerve conduction are unavailable, a cystometrogram can be utilized to provide evidence of pelvic neuropathy. The pelvic parasympathetic nerves involved in erectile function also innervate the bladder. Thus, an abnormal cystometrogram and cystogram provide evidence of a pelvic autonomic neuropathy.[133]

In the presence of an abnormal nocturnal tumescence test and a normal pudendal nerve conduction velocity, penile flow studies should be performed. The presence of pulses in the penis and the penile systolic blood pressure can be determined with a Doppler ultrasound probe. It is unclear whether this study should be routinely included in the assessment of all men with erectile problems. In our experience, clinically significant reductions in penile blood flow are rarely encountered in men without other evidence of peripheral vascular disease. The outcome of surgical correction of identifiable lesions is still unclear.[134] In other words, it is uncertain how often such a procedure will render information that allows the physician to restore normal function. However, the procedure is relatively inexpensive in most centers and thus probably merits inclusion as a general screening device. Identification of a lesion would, of course, be followed up by appropriate vascular studies. To date, there is minimal evidence to suggest that pelvic and internal pudendal arteriography, phalloarteriography, and corporal cavernosography should be routinely performed in impotent men with normal penile blood pressure. There is some evidence that penile blood pressure should be assessed before and after minor exertion to check for the pelvic steal syndrome.

In our experience, approximately 15% of men with erectile complaints who are subjected to multidisciplinary evaluation will have impotence of unknown etiology. The history will be suggestive of an organic problem. Nocturnal penile tumescence testing will be compatible with an organic diagnosis. Yet, a complete evaluation by urology, psychiatry, neurology, endocrinology, and vascular surgery will fail to reveal any disease process. These patients are a constant reminder of how little we know about the physiology of erectile function and of the infancy of the field of medical sexology.

REFERENCES

1. Bancroft J: Hormones and human sexual behavior. *Br Med Bull* 37:153–158, 1981
2. Scott FB, Fishman IJ, Light JK: An inflatable penile prosthesis for treatment of diabetic impotence. *Ann Intern Medic* 92:340–342, 1980
3. Segraves RT: Treatment of sexual dysfunction. *Compr Ther* 4:38–43, 1978
4. Masters WH, Johnson VG: *Human Sexual Inadequacy*. Boston, Little, Brown, 1970
5. Scott FB, Bradley WB, Timm GW: Management of erectile impotence. *Urology* 2:80–86, 1973

6. Tyler EA: Sexual-incapacity therapy, in Freedman DX, Dyrud JE (eds): *American Handbook of Psychiatry Treatment*. New York, Basic Books, 1975
7. Kaplan HS: *The New Sex Therapy*. New York, Brunner/Mazel, 1974
8. Wagner G, Green R: *Impotence, Physiological, Psychological, Surgical Diagnosis and Treatment*. New York, Plenum Press, 1981
9. Strauss EB: Impotence from a psychiatric standpoint. *Br Med J* 1:697–699, 1950
10. Martin, LM: Erectile impotence — It can be highly treatable. *Geriatrics* 35:79–83, 1980
11. Spark RF, White RA, Connolly PB: Impotence is not always psychogenic. *JAMA* 243:750–755, 1980
12. Karacan I, Salis PJ, Williams RL: The role of the sleep laboratory in diagnosis and treatment of impotence, in Williams RL, Karacan I (eds): *Sleep Disorders, Diagnosis and Treatment*. New York, John Wiley, 1982
13. Segraves RT, Schoenberg HW, Zarins CK, et al: Characteristics of erectile dysfunction as a function of medical care system entry point. *Psychosom Med*, 43:227–234, 1981
14. Kaplan D, Melman A: An analysis of the first seventy patients in a center for male sexual dysfunction. Paper read at Society for Sex Therapy and Research, Charleston, South Carolina, 1982
15. Goldman A, Fishkin RE, Cohen S, et al: Multidisciplinary approach to the evaluation and treatment of male sexual dysfunction. Paper read at Society for Sex Therapy and Research, Charleston, South Carolina, 1982
16. Shrom SH, Lief HI, Wein AJ: Clinical profile of experience with 130 consecutive cases of impotent men. *Urology*, 13:511–515, 1979
17. Nath RL, Menzolan JO, Kaplan KH, et al: The multidisciplinary approach to vasculogenic impotence. *Surgery* 89:124–144, 1981
18. Furlow WL: Surgical treatment of erectile impotence using the inflatable penile prosthesis. *Sexual Disabil* 1:299–306, 1978
19. Khan Z, Melman A: Use of the evoked scaral potential in the diagnosis of male impotence. *Sexual Disabil* 4:105–107, 1981
20. Tyler EA: Sexual-incapacity therapy, in Freedman DX, Dyrud JE (eds): *American Handbook of Psychiatry*, Volume V, *Treatment*. New York, Basic Books, 1975
21. Ellis A: Treatment of erectile dysfunction, in Leiblum SR, Pervin LA (eds): *Principles and Practice of Sex Therapy*. New York, Guilford, 1980
22. Ellis A: Treatment of erectile dysfunction, in Leiblum SR, Pervin LA (eds): *Principles and Practice of Sex Therapy*. New York, Guilford, 1980
23. Montague DK: Clinical evaluation of impotence. *Urol Clin North Am* 8:103, 1981
24. Mills LC: Sexual disorders in the diabetic patient, in Oaks, WW, Melchiode GA, Ficher I (eds): *Sex and the Life Cycle*. New York, Grune & Stratton, 1976
25. Schiavi RC: Psychological treatment of erectile disorders in diabetic patients. *Ann Intern Med* 92:337–339, 1980
26. Martin LM: Impotence in diabetes: An overview. *Psychosomatics* 22:1–5, 1981
27. Barry JM, Hodges CV: Impotence: A diagnostic approach. *J Urol* 119:575–578, 1978
28. Magee MC: Psychogenic impotence: A critical review. *Urology* 15:435–442, 1980
29. Kockett G, Feil W, Revenstorf D, et al: Symptomatology and psychological aspects of male sexual inadequacy: Results of an experimental study. *Arch Sex Behav* 9:457–475, 1980
30. Abel GG, Becker JV, Cunningham-Rathner J, et al: Differential diagnosis of impotence in diabetics: The validity of sexual symptomatology. *Neurol Urodynamics* 1:57–69, 1982
31. Segraves RT, Schoenberg HW, Ivanoff J: Serum testosterone and prolactin levels in erectile dysfunction. *Sex Marital Ther* 9:19–26, 1983
32. Condra M, Morales A, Surridge P, Fenemore J: Evaluation of the urological assessment in impotence: Findings with a new diagnostic rating scale. *J Urol* 13:486–490, 1984

33. Segraves RT: Male sexual dysfunction. Paper read at annual meeting of Society for Sex Therapy and Research, Charleston, South Carolina, June, 1982
34. Schaefer HH, Tregerthan GJ, Colgan AH: Measured and self-estimated penile erection. *Behav Ther* 7:1–7, 1976
35. Kedia KR: Vascular disorders and male erectile dysfunction. *Urol Clin North Am* 8:153–168, 1981
36. Schwartz MF, Bauman J, Kolodny RC: Prolactin levels in men presenting with sexual dysfunction. Paper read at Society for Sex Therapy and Research, New York, 1981
37. Schumacher S: The physiological basis of sexology and sex therapy. Paper read at Society of Sex Therapy and Research, New York, 1981
38. Cooper AJ: Disorder of sexual potency in the male: A clinical and statistical study of some factors related to short-term prognosis. *Br J Psychiatry* 115:709–719, 1969
39. Scheier IH, Cattell RA: *Handbook for the Neuroticism-Scale Questionnaire.* The NSQ, Champaign, Ill.: Institute for Personality and Ability Testing, 1961
40. Cooper AJ: Hostility and male potency disorders. *Compr Psychiatry* 9:621–626, 1968
41. Foulds GA: *Personality and Personal Illness* London, Tavistock, 1965
42. Senoussi AI: *The Male Impotence Test* Los Angeles, Western Psychological Services, 1964
43. Ellis A: The male impotence test, in Buros OK (ed): *The Seventh Mental Measurement Yearbook.* Highland Park, New Jersy, Gryphon Press, 1972
44. Beutler LE, Karacan I, Anch AM, et al: MMPI and MIT discriminators of biogenic and psychogenic impotence. *J Consul Clin Psychol* 43:899–903, 1975
45. Osborne D: Psychological evaluation of impotent men. *Mayo Clin Pro* 51:363–366,1976
46. Beutler LE, Scott FB, Karacan I: Psychological screening of impotent men. *J Urol* 116:193–197, 1976
47. Staples RB, Ficher IV, Shapiro M, et al: A re-evaluation of MMPI discriminators of biogenic and psychogenic impotence. *J Consult Clin Psychol* 48:543–545, 1980
48. Marshall P, Surridge D, Delva N: Differentiation of organic and psychogenic impotence on the basis of MMPI decision rules. *J Consult Clin. Psychol* 48:407–408, 1980
49. Martin LM, Rodgers DA, Montague DK: Psychogenic differentiation of biogenic and psychogenic impotence. *Arch Sex Behav* 12:475–485, 1983
50. Derogatis LR, Melisaratos N: The DSFI: A multidimensional measure of sexual functioning. *J Sex Marital Ther* 5:244–281, 1979
51. Derogatis LR, Meyer JK: A psychological profile of the sexual dysfunctions. *Arch Sex Behav* 8:201–223, 1979
52. Deogatis LR, Rickels K, Rock AF: The SCL-90 and the MMPI. A step in the validation of a new self-report scale. *Br J Psychiatry* 128:280–289, 1976
53. Derogatis LR: *The Affect Balance Scale.* Baltimore, Clinical Psychometrics, 1975
54. Derogatis LR, Meyer JK, Dupkin CN: Discrimination of organic versus psychogenic impotence with the DSFI. *J Sex Marital Ther* 2:229–240, 1976
55. Rorer JG, Hoffman PJ, LaForge GE, et al: Optimum cutting scores to discriminate groups of unequal size and variance. *J App Psychol* 50:153–158, 1966
56. Melman A. Redfield J: Evaluation of the DSFI as a test of organic impotence. *Sexual Disabil* 4:108–114, 1981
57. Segraves RT, Schoenberg HW, Zarins CK, et al: Discrimination of organic versus psychological impotence with the DSFI: A failure to replicate. *J Sex Marital Ther* 7:230–238, 1981
58. Eysenck HJ: *Sex and Personality.* Austin: University of Texas Press, 1976
59. Ohlmeyer P, Brilmayer H, Hüllstrung H: Periodische Norgänge im Schat. *Pflevegers Arch* 248:559–560, 1944
60. Halverson HM: Genital and sphincter behavior of the male infant. *J Genet Psychol* 56:95–136, 1940

61. Serinsky A, Kreitman N: Two types of ocular motility occurring in sleep. *J Appl Physiol* 8:1–10, 1955
62. Karachan I: Clinical value of nocturnal erection in the prognosis and diagnosis of impotence. *Med Aspects Hum Sexuality* 4:27–34, 1970
63. Karachan I, Hursch CJ, Williams RL: Some characteristics of nocturnal penile tumescence during puberty. *Pediatr Res* 6:529–537, 1972
64. Karachan I, Murch CJ, Williams RL, et al: Some characteristics of nocturnal penile tumescence in young adults. *Arch Gen Psychiatry* 26:351–356, 1972
65. Hursch CJ, Karachan I, Williams RL: Some characteristics of nocturnal penile tumescence in early middle-aged males. *Compr Psychiatry* 13:539–548, 1972
66. Karachan I, Hursch CJ, Williams RL: Some characteristics of nocturnal penile tumescence in elderly males. *J Gerontol* 27:39–45, 1972
67. Karachan I, Williams RL, Thonby IJ: Sleep-related tumescence as a function of age. *Am J Psychiatry* 132:932–937, 1975
68. Karachan I, Salis PJ, Ware PC, et al: Nocturnal penile tumescence and diagnosis in diabetic impotence. *Am J Psychiatry* 135:191–197, 1978
69. Fisher C, Schiavi R, Edwards A: Quantitative differences in nocturnal penile tumescence (NPT) between impotence of psychogenic and organic origin. *Sleep Res* 6:49, 1977
70. Fisher C, Schiavi R, Edwards A: Evaluation of nocturnal penile tumescence in the differential diagnosis of sexual impotence: A quantitative study. *Arch Gen Psychiatry* 36:431–437, 1979
71. Fisher C, Gross J, Zuch J: Cycle of penile erection synchronous with dreaming (REM) sleep. *Arch Gen Psychiatry* 12:29–45, 1965
72. Fisher C, Shiavi R, Lear H, et al: The assessment of nocturnal REM erection in the differential diagnosis of sexual impotence. *J Sex Marital Thera* 1:277–289, 1975
73. Karachan I: Diagnosis of erectile impotence in diabetes mellitus. *Ann Intern Med* 92:334–337, 1980
74. Karachan I, Ilaria RL: Nocturnal penile tumescence (NPT): The phenomenon and its role in the diagnosis of impotence.*Sexual Disabil* 1:260–267, 1978
75. Karachan I: Advances in the diagnosis of erectile impotence. *Med Aspects Hum Sexuality* 2:85–94, 1978
76. Karachan I, Scott FB, Salis PJ, et al: Nocturnal erections, differential diagnosis of impotence, and diabetes. *Biol Psychiatry* 12:373–380, 1977
77. Karachan I, Salis PJ: Diagnosis and treatment of erectile impotence. *Psychiatr Clin North Am* 3:97–lll, 1980
78. Rosen RC: Genital blood flow measurement: feedback application in sexual therapy. *J Sex Marital Ther* 2:184–196, 1976
79. Bohlen JG: Sleep erection monitoring in the evaluation of male erectile failure. *Urol Clin North Am* 8:119–134, 1981
80. Hatch JP: Psychophysiological aspects of sexual dysfunction. *Arch Sex Behav* 10:49–64, 1981
81. Martin LM: Erectile impotence — It can be highly treatable. *Geriatrics* 35:79–83, 1980
82. Wabrek AJ: Nocturnal penile tumescence (NPT). *Connecticut Med* 45:559–562, 1981
83. Tordjman G: Male erectile impotence, in Gemme R, Wheeler CC (eds): *Progress in Sexology* New York, Plenum Press, 1976
84. Marshall P, Surridge D, Delva N: The role of nocturnal penile tumescence in differentiating between organic and psychoogenic impotence: The first stage of validation. *Arch Sex Behav* 10:1–10, 1981
85. Vliet LW, Meyer JK: Erectile dysfunction: Progress in evaluation and teatment. *Johns Hopkins Med J* 151:246–258, 1982
86. Abel GG: Sexual psychophysiology. Paper read at Society for Sex Therapy and Research,

Charleston, South Carolina, 1982

87. Marshall P, Morales A, Surridge D: Unreliability of nocturnal penile tumescence recording and MMPI profiles in assessment of impotence. *Urology* 17:136–139, 1981

88. Wein AJ, Fishkin R, Carpiniello VL, et al: Expansion without significant rigidity during nocturnal penile tumescence testing: A potential source of misinterpretation. *J Urol* 126:343–344, 1981

89. Wasserman MD, Pollak CP, Speilman AJ, et al: The differential diagnosis of impotence. *JAMA* 243:2038–2042, 1980

90. Wasserman MD, Pollak CP, Spielman AJ, et al: Theoretical and technical problems in the measurement of nocturnal penile tumescence for the differential diagnosis of impotence. *Psychosom Med* 42:575–585, 1980

91. Morales A, Marshall PG, Surridge DH, et al: Corporeal calibration: A discriminatory test for impotence. *J Urol* 128:41–44, 1982

92. Godec CJ, Cass AS: Quantification of erection. *J Urol* 126:345–347, 1981

93. Allen RP: Editorial comment. *J Urol* 128:43, 1982

94. Allen RP: Erectile impotence: Objective diagnosis from sleep-related erections (nocturnal penile tumescence). *J Urol* 126:353, 1981

95. Karacan I, Salis PJ, Williams RL: The role of the sleep laboratory in diagnosis and treatment of impotence, in Williams RL, Karacan I (eds): *Sleep disorders: Diagnosis and Treatment.* New York, John Wiley, 1982

96. Karacan I, Goodenough DR, Shapiro A, et al: Erection cycle during sleep in relation to dream anxiety. *Arch Gen Psychiatry* 15:183–189, 1966

97. Fisher C, Gross J, Zuch J: Cycle of penile erection synchronous with dreaming (REM) sleep. *Arch Gen Psychiatry* 12:29–45, 1965

98. Fisher C: Dreaming and sexuality, in Loewensten RM, Newman LM, Schur M, Solnit AJ (eds): *Pschoanalysis: A General Psychology.* New York, International Universities Press, 1966

99. Kahn E, Fisher C: REM sleep and sexuality in the aged. *J Geriatr Psychiatry* 11:181–189, 1969

100. Kedia KR: Vascular disorders and male erectile dysfunction. *Urol Clin North Am* 8:153–168, 1981

101. Nath RL, Menzoian JO, Kaplan KH, et al: The multidisciplinary approach to vasculogenic impotence. *Surgery* 89:124–133, 1981

102. Weiss HD: The psysiology of human penile erection. *Ann Inter Med* 76:793–799, 1972

103. Bors E, Commar AE: Neurological disturbances of sexual function with special reference to 529 patients with spinal cord injury. *Urol Rev* 10:191–222, 1960

104. Bors E, Turner RD: Neurologic urology, in Kaufman JJ (ed): *Advances in Diagnostic Urology.* Boston, Little, Brown, 1964

105. Bors E, Blinn KA: Bulbocavernosus reflex. *J Urol* 82:128–130, 1959

106. Pierce JM, Roberge JT, Newman MM: Electromyographic demonstration of bulbocavernosus reflex. *J Urol* 83:319, 1960

107. Ertekin C, Reel F: Bublocavernosus reflex in normal men and in patients with neurogenic bladder and/or impotence. *J Neurol Sci* 28:1–15, 1976

108. Siroky MB, Sax DS, Krane RJ: Sacral signal tracing: The electrophysiology of the bulbocavernosus reflex. *J Urol* 122:661–664, 1979

109. Blaiva JG, Zayed AH, Labib KB: The bulbocavernosus reflex in urology: A prospective study of 299 patients. *J Urol* 126:197–199, 1981

110. Haldeman S, Bradley WE, Bhatia NN, et al: Pudendal evoked responses. *Arch Neurol* 39:280–283, 1982

111. Morgan RJ, Pryor JR: The investigation of organic impotence. *Br J Urol* 52:571–574, 1980

112. Smith AD: Causes and classification of impotence. *Urol Clin North Am* 8:79–89, 1981
113. Beutler LE, Gleason DM: Integrating the advances in the diagnosis and treatment of male potency disturbance. *J Urol* 126:338–342, 1981
114. Wincze JP: Assessment of sexual disorders. *Behavi Assessment* 4:257–271, 1982
115. Tumulty PA: Conversing with patients and obtaining a history, in Harvey AM, Cluff LE, Johns RJ, et al (eds): *The Principles and Practice of Medicine*. New York, Appleton-Century-Crofts, 1968
116. Green R: Taking a sexual history, in Green R. (ed): *Human Sexuality: A Health Practitioner's Text*. Baltimore, Williams & Wilkins, 1979
117. Schumacher S, Lloyd CW: Physiological and psychological factors in impotence. *J Sex Res* 17:40–53, 1981
118. Cole CM, Levin EM, Whitley JO, et al: Brief sexual counseling during cardiac rehabilitation. *Heart Lung* 8:124–129, 1979
119. Cole CM: A treatment strategy for postmyocardial sexual dysfunction. *Sexual Disabil* 2:122–129, 1979
120. Waxberg JD: Sexual counseling techniques for coronary bypass patients. *Behav Med* 6:30–33, 1979
121. Masur FT: Resumption of sexual activity following myocardial infarcation. *Sexual Disabil* 2:98–114, 1979
122. McLane M, Krop H, Mehta J: Psychosexual adjustment and counseling after myocradial infarction. *Ann Intern Med* 92:514–519, 1980
123. Kushnir B, Fox KM, Tomlinson IW, et al: Primary ventricular fibillation and resumption of work, sexual activity, and driving after first acute myocardial infarction. *Br Med J* 4:609–611, 1975
124. Sanders JD, Sprenkle DH: Sexual therapy for the post coronary patient. *J Sex Marital Ther* 6:174–186, 1980
125. Schiavi RC: Psychological treatment of erectile disorders in diabetic patients. *Ann Intern Med* 92:337–339, 1980
126. Renshaw DC: Sexual function and diabetes. *Psychosomatics* 20:54–60, 1979
127. Bancroft J: Changes in erectile responsiveness during androgen replacement therapy. *Arch Sex Behav* 12:59–66, 1983
128. Spark RF, White RA, Connolly PB: Impotence is not always psychogenic: Newer insights into hypothalamic–pituitary–gonadal dysfunction. *JAMA* 243:750–754, 1980
129. Carter JN, Tyson JE, Tolis G, et al: Prolactin-secreting tumors and hypoganadism in 22 men. *N Engl J Med* 29:847–852, 1978
130. Franks S, Jacobs HS, Martin N, et al: Hyperprolactinaemia and impotence. *Clin Endocrinol* 8:277–287, 1978
131. Nagulesparen M, Ang V, Jenkins JS: Bromocriptine treatment of males with pituitary tumors, hyperprolactinaemia, and hypogonadis. *Clin Endocrinol* 9:73–78, 1978
132. Moutjoy CQ, Davies TF: Erectile impotence. *Br Med J* 1:176–177, 1970
133. Ellenberg M: Sexual function in diabetic patients. *Ann Intern Med* 92:331–333, 1980
134. Kedia KR: Vascular disorders and male erectile dysfunction. *Urol Clin of North Am* 8:153–168, 1981

9

Psychiatric Evaluation of Penile Prosthesis Candidates

LARRY GOLDMAN and R. TAYLOR SEGRAVES

Technical advances in genitourinary surgery have led to an increased frequency of penile prosthesis placements to correct male erectile problems. A recent report estimated that more than 20,000 rigid and more than 1500 inflatable prostheses had been placed, mainly in the last 5–10 years.[1] The surgical literature is extensive, and much has been written about technique, complications, and surgical outcome. On the other hand, relatively little besides "clinical impressions" has appeared in the literature about psychosocial outcome. In a thorough review of surgical outcomes, Sotile[2] emphasized that almost all the published outcome data concerned objective function of the prosthetic device, and that considerably less attention had been paid to the subjective effects of surgery on the patient and his partner.

Many urologists and almost all psychiatrists would agree that some psychological screening of implant candidates is good clinical practice. There is, however, no uniformly agreed upon protocol for such screening. For example, some centers require an assessment not only of the patient but of his partner as well, whereas others evaluate only the patient. In addition, there is considerable diversity between centers in their views toward implant surgery when the patient's impotence is known to be psychogenic.

LARRY GOLDMAN • Department of Psychiatry, University of Illinois, Chicago, Illinois 60680.   R. TAYLOR SEGRAVES • Department of Psychiatry, Tulane University Medical Center, New Orleans, Louisiana 70112.

The primary obstacle to the development of an acceptable standardized screening protocol is the conspicuous absence of a well-established data base. Little is known about psychosocial outcome after implant surgery and even less is established about predictors of such outcome. Thus there is much uncertainty as to the major variables to be assessed in psychiatric screening of implant candidates. Given the absence of well-designed follow-up studies of psychosexual adjustment after surgery, attitudinal differences along professional lines have arisen and are presently difficult to resolve. Psychiatrists and psychologists are highly cognizant (sometimes overly so) of the symbolic meaning of the penis, and many tend to regard the prospect of genitourinary surgery with a certain degree of apprehension or abhorrence. This is particularly so given that most of these professionals have had little exposure to the recipients of penile prosthetic devices, and that they have encountered (or treated) many men whose erectile function has been improved by psychological therapies. The philosophical orientation of many mental health professionals was expressed by Bullard and his colleagues:

> As a group, we believe that a surgical approach to the treatment of erectile dysfunction should be used only after its suitability for the individual client has been assessed by extensive counseling. We are concerned lest enthusiastic representations about the procedure mislead a person into seeking a pat surgical solution for a problem that may have deep intrapsychic and interpersonal ramifications. The surgical procedure may result in a penis capable of being inserted into a vagina, but the client's distress about relationship problems or his concern with personal adequacy may remain unchanged.[3]

Some urologists tend to see things somewhat differently, stressing that the etiology of the impotence should not be a major concern, and that adverse psychological sequelae to surgery are infrequent. These surgeons remember the joy of many men upon surgical restoration of potency and know of men impotent after years of psychological therapy. The difference in perspective between urologists and mental health professionals can be appreciated by considering differences in practice: urologists tend to see patients for a briefer period of time, focus on surgical recovery and mechanical function rather than psychological material, seldom see sexual partners, and infrequently find out about long-term follow-up. Thus it is hardly surprising that they tend to downplay the significance of emotional and interpersonal factors in their selection of surgical candidates. Gerow, a urologist, puts it plainly:

> The surgeon merely serves as a technician who implants the prosthesis so that the patient is able to use his penis for satisfying coital function . . . . Psychoneurotic functional overlay disappears in large part when the patient receives a penile implant.[4]

Given the current uncertainties regarding evluation for penile prosthesis surgery, prudent patient care at this time requires a multidisciplinary team approach with representation from urology, vascular surgery, endocrinology, and psychiatry at a minimum. Other specialty consultation (e.g., neurology) should be available for certain cases. Effective screening of surgical candidates requires a particular alliance between the psychiatrist and the urologist, an alliance which not only involves mutual appreciation of the other discipline's strengths and limitations, but which requires a lengthy reciprocal educational effort.

Goin and Goin[5] discuss the process of finding and "taming" (teaching) a psychiatrist to do psychological screening of candidates for plastic surgery procedures. They emphasize the need to select a psychiatrist with the interest and skills to do such screening as not all psychiatrists are capable of doing so. They use the analogy of not referring a patient for rhinoplasty to a master hand surgeon. Psychiatrists appropriate for screening candidates for penile prosthesis surgery would have experience in sexual and marital treatments as well as in evaluating surgical patients more generally. Similarly, a psychiatrist needs to convey to the surgeon the types of questions he can actually answer and the services he can provide a patient.

The authors believe that a productive alliance can be achieved between physicians from different specialities which is not only mutually helpful and educational, but more important, contributes to good patient care.

The major goals of this chapter are to discuss what the psychiatrist can offer the urologist in screening potential implant candidates and to describe a rational system for screening such patients given the present limitations of knowledge in the field. We shall begin by discussing goals for screening, establishing outcome variables, and reviewing what is actually known about psychosocial outcome following penile prosthesis surgery. The chapter will conclude with specific recommendations about screening and a discussion of the needed clinical research in this area.

GOALS FOR SCREENING

There is a suprisingly small literature on the psychiatric assessment of candidates for surgical treatment of impotence, and the existing literature tends to mirror the main themes involved in screening candidates for any surgical procedure. For example, Osborne,[6] in discussing screening goals at the Mayo clinic, stressed that the evaluation should assist in determing the etiology of the erectile dysfunction, identifying patients who require nonsurgical intervention, and identifying patients for whom surgery might precipitate emotional problems. Maddock[7] described similar goals in use at the University of Minnesota, adding that such screening may be useful in cases where the balance between organic and psychological causes of the dysfunction is uncertain. The major screening objectives are determination of etiology, identification of contraindications, identification of patients for whom alternative treatment is indicated, and assessment of patients in need of associated psychiatric treatment.

DETERMINATION OF ETIOLOGY

Although a number of investigators[6-12] feel that a careful psychiatric examination can help establish the etiology of erectile dysfunction, the evidence for such a claim is far from convincing. Such an examination may indeed identify psychopathological or interpersonal factors associated with the erectile dysfunction; however, this does not necessarily establish a causal relationship.[13-15] Certain psychodynamic assumptions about the etiology of erectile dysfunction are based on uncontrolled observations of selected patient groups and have not been empirically substantiated.[16] Abel and co-workers recently reported low correlations between clinical judgements of etiology and subsequent assessment by nocturnal penile tumescence study.[17]

On the other hand, a detailed sexological interview establishing current levels of erectile function can help in establishing the etiology of the dysfunction. For example, a sexual history indicative of episodic erectile failure is highly suggestive of a psychogenic etiology. It is becoming clear that psychological factors frequently interact with organic pathology in the development of erectile dysfunction.[16] Thus one can view impotence as a disorder with psychogenic and organic components each of which occurs along a continuum. Even in men with unequivocal organic illness, there may be psychological factors contributing as well to the impotence.

For further information on etiologies, see Chapter 1.

IDENTIFICATION OF CONTRAINDICATIONS

Situations in which an absolute psychiatric contraindication to surgery exist are uncommon. Serious sequelae to surgery, such as psychosis, major affective illness, or other conditions that might necessitate psychiatric hospitalization, are far easier to diagnose than to predict. Similarly, claims that neurotic and unstable personality types react poorly to surgery are not well substantiated.[18]

Nonetheless, there are clearly a number of conditions that might make surgery a risky proposition. Examples include significant depression (particularly if suicidal ideation is present); psychosis (particularly if there are delusions about the surgeon or the surgery); marked hostility and suspiciousness, which often make postoperative satisfaction unlikely (and litigation too likely); and surgery-seeking behavior, where unconscious wishes for punishment or mutilation motivate the request for surgery.

In addition, there are numerous situations in which no contraindication exists, but where there is reason to believe that surgery will not be a complete success. Some of these situations may present unexpected ethical considerations. Not infrequently a patient requests implant surgery with the (conscious or unconscious) expectation that it will solve a nonsexual problem as well, such as improving personal relationships or saving a troubled marriage. Such patients may strenuously resist accepting that these expectations may be (or are) quite unrealistic. Proceeding with surgery may not lead to grave consequences, but there might be a higher likelihood of patient (or partner) dissatisfaction or of nonuse of the prosthesis.

Perhaps a more serious problem arises if the patient's dysfunction plays a crucial role in stabilizing a marriage or in maintaining the wife's psychological stability. Surgical restoration of potency may seriously compromise the marriage or the wife's mental health. Such a situation raises the question of the physician's responsibility to an institution (marriage) or a person other than the patient alone.

IDENTIFICATION OF ALTERNATIVE TREATMENT

If a psychiatric disorder is causing the patient's impotence or would contraindicate surgery, it is clear that treatment must first be directed at the disorder, much as one would bring diabetic ketoacidosis under control before proceeding with elective surgery.

Behaviorally oriented sex therapy is a treatment which is now generally available, of proven efficacy, of short duration, and of modest expense, and which has minimal complications.[19] These features suggest that it ought to be regarded as a first-line treatment for impotence of psychogenic etiology or perhaps even in cases where the etiology is equivocal. It is also an appropriate treatment for cases of impotence with a small organic basis and further psychological overlay exacerbating the organic deficit: sex therapy may improve the clinical situation sufficiently to obviate or postpone the need for surgery.[3,20–22] A common example would be a diabetic whose anxiety about a marginal decrement in turgidity renders him completely impotent. Alleviation of the performance anxiety by sex therapy may restore potency. Patients with these indications for sex therapy could, of course, be considered for surgery if sex therapy was unacceptable or unsuccessful.

Finally, sex counseling might be an appropriate treatment in cases of organic impotence if the patient either refuses or has a medical contraindication to surgery. Therapy would be directed at development of an increased repertoire of noncoital sexual activities.

ASSESSMENT FOR ASSOCIATED PSYCHIATRIC TREATMENT

There are three types of situations in which psychiatric treatment concomitant with implant surgery might be warranted. The first would be for patients with concurrent psychiatric condictions who need ongoing treatment, such as lithium and psychotherapy for patients with bipolar (manic–depressive) disorder. Second, patients (or couples) with significant unease discussing sexual matters or with severely constricted sexual activity might well benefit from counseling to facilitate communication and use of the new prothesis. Finally, psychiatric treatment might be useful in cases where the surgery or restored potency may introduce disequilibrium in the patient or the relationship might need follow-up to help adaptation.[23] Even in cases in which such problems cannot be predicted, an alliance formed during the assessment may make treatment of unanticipated complications easier. An example of this would be the resolution by brief therapy by the assessing psychiatrist of postsurgical ejaculatory inhibition in a passive–aggressive man who had used his vasculogenic impotence as a weapon in struggles with his wife.

GOALS FOR SURGERY

Clearly the narrowest goals for an acceptable surgical outcome are the strictly technical ones: good wound healing, acceptable cosmetic results, minimal pain, absence of mechanical problems (e.g., kinking of tubing), and a phallus long and hard enough to effect penetration of a vagina. These goals can be readily assessed by the surgeon.

The situation is more complicated in considering the "softer" psychosocial or more subjective goals. In the first place, the goals are more difficult to define. Regular use of the prosthesis may be defined as the coital frequency just prior to impotence, but this level itself might have been near zero or the duration of the impotence might have been very long and the patient thus considerably older. Use of a statistical norm instead presents its own problem if the patient's preimpotence activity was significantly above or below the norm.

Second, apparently reasonable goals might contradict one another. A patient delighted with the prosthesis who only uses it in extramarital affairs may score high on a patient satisfaction measure but poorly on a marital improvement rating. Similar situations exist if the patient is pleased with the prosthesis but the partner refuses sex or if the partner loves the prosthesis but the patient is unhappy.

Finally, it may not be possible to causally link a change in a patient's psychological status or marital relationship with the surgery itself. A patient's dramatic rise in self-esteem may indeed be because of surgically restored potency, but if other life events such as a job promotion or a parent's recovery from a serious illness occur about the same time, such a connection may not be so warranted.

Such difficulties complicate interpretation of outcome data, and they speak to a need for particular clarity in research designs evaluating surgical outcomes. For the purpose of reviewing outcome studies thus far, five goals have been selected. Unfortunately there is no neat mapping between these goals and data report in most studies, and there is certainly no one-to-one mapping between these and the screening goals described previously. The goals are

1. The patient is satisfied with the outcome,
2. The patient's partner is satisfied with the outcome,
3. The patient uses the prosthesis regularly,
4. The patient experiences an improvement or at least maintenance of psychological well-being, and
5. The patient and his partner's relationship improves or at least remains the same.

OUTCOME STUDIES

Thirty-one studies[1,24-53] reporting outcomes of penile prosthesis surgery were reviewed by the authors to try to draw some conclusions that would be useful in screening candidates for the surgery. These reports span 22 years and represent a total of 2173 subjects, about 70% receiving rigid prostheses and 30% inflatable. Twenty-five of these studies (which will be referred to as Type 1) are concerned primarily with surgical technique and results, and they contain varying amounts of psychosocial outcome data. Six studies (Type 2) specifically address psychosocial outcome and complications.

It will become obvious that almost all the studies are far from optimal for this purpose of this section. Some of the case reports or small studies provide considerable data about the subjects but leave the reader wondering about how representative the results were. Many of the larger studies are flawed by omission of data, failure to describe how they were obtained, and absence of follow-up past the immediate postoperative period. Questionnaire studies are clear about methodology but are invariably plagued by incomplete returns and thus a possibly biased sample population. Results based on patient interviews may be hampered by patient dissimulation (e.g., overreporting positive results so as not to displease the surgeon) or by lack of interviewer sophistication. As Kaufman (a urologist himself) states: ". . . for most urologists . . . [no] complaint from the patient is tantamount to an excellent result."[1]

Keeping all the limitations in mind, each of the five outcome goals listed in the previous section will be reviewed in the light of the existing outcome data. For each goal an attempt will be made not only to reach some overall conclusions, but also to reach some for difficult patient subgroups (e.g., by age, etiology of impotence, type of prosthesis) as well.

PATIENT SATISFACTION

Table 1 presents information from studies in which patient satisfaction with the prosthesis was reported. The inquiry to the patient generally took the form of "Are you satisfied?" or "Would you repeat the surgery if you had to do it all over again?" Not included are studies without quantification (e.g., Kaufman and Raz's[31] report that "patients are almost uniformly happy . . ."). Note that n, the number of subjects listed in column 2, is the number of patients asked rather than the total number reported in the article: patients with poor surgical results or lost to follow-up are thus usually not included.

For all studies included, the overall satisfaction with the prosthesis is 86%. The satisfaction varies from a low of 60% in the small group of Gee et al.[46] to 100% in four studies. The Type 1 studies yield a higher rate of satisfaction (88%) than the Type 2(78%).

Although range of duration of follow-up is given in most studies, it is unclear even in these at which point in the range patients were evaluated. Gerstenberger et al.[53] reported an increase of 10% in satisfaction among their patients following their evaluations (at 6 months postoperation or later) when previously unrecognized complications were recognized and corrected. On the other hand, it is impossible to be sure that patients evaluated relatively soon postoperatively might not later become dissatisfied after the novelty of the "honeymoon period" wore off.

The studies seem to have little to say about patient age and its relation to outcome. Although patients undergoing surgery have ranged in age from 20 to 85, there were only two impressions relating age to satisfaction. Loeffler and Iverson[48] denied that there was a correlation in their group

Table 1. Patient Satisfaction

Source	N	N satisfied (%)	R/I[a]
Type 1			
Loeffler and Sayegh[24]	2	2 (100)	R
Loeffler et al.[25]	5	5 (100)	R
Gee et al.[30]	15	10 (67)	R
Mallory and Voneschenbach[34]	39	35 (90)	I
Gottesman et al.[38]	56	56 (100)	R
Merrill and Swanson[42]	15	14 (93)	R
Gee et al.[46]	15	9 (60)	R
Loeffler and Iverson[48]	72	46 (64)	R
Scott et al.[49]	174	169 (97)	I
Total	393	346 (88)	
Type 2			
Kaufman et al.[1]	90	70 (78)	R
Segraves et al.[44]	15	15 (100)	R and I
Gerstenberger et al.[53]	61	45 (74)	I
Total	166	130 (80)	

[a] R, rigid; I, inflatable.

of 72 patients, as did Gerstenberger et al.[53] in theirs. It may be that there is no particular link.

Nine studies reported on subjects who had received rigid prostheses. Of 236 subjects, 187 or 79% were satisfied. Of the 282 subjects (four studies) receiving inflatable prostheses, 257 or 91% were satisfied. Sotile[2] reported a 16.7% complication rate with the rigid devices versus 31.2% for the inflatable with 65% of the hydraulic device complications requiring additional surgery. The inflatable prosthesis is considerably more expensive, requires a longer operation, and necessitates a longer postoperative hospital stay.[54] Thus it seems likely that the increased satisfaction with inflatable prostheses is due to factors that override economic, surgical, and postoperative considerations. Mainly cited is the simulation of a more natural erection only when desired.

The relationship between the etiology of the impotence and the patient's satisfaction with the prosthesis remains poorly described. Beheri[26] was the first to report on surgical treatment for psychogenic impotence. He claimed that more than 95% of his 700 patients were functionally impotent. He provided no outcome figures but gave a strong impression of highly favorable results. His only caveat was cryptic. "Patients who should not be accepted for the operation include highly neurotic patients. . . .They do improve after their operation but they never cease to complain."

Lash[28] reported on 13 psychologically impotent patients, all of whom had "gratifying results" following insertion of a rigid prosthesis. Apfelberg et al.[32] reported a patient who requested removal of his silicone implant because of "renewed sexual confidence." Small's[35] 260 patients included 40 with psychogenic impotence; all results in this group were reported as excellent, although one patient had prolonged discomfort in the glans. One of Merrill and Swanson's[42] patients with impotence secondary to alcoholism (whether this represented psychological, neurological, endocrinological, or other sequelae is not stated) was dissatisfied (as was his wife), and he did not use his rigid implant. Scott et al.[49] stated that of their ten patients with psychogenic impotence (by sleep study diagnosis), nine were satisfied with their inflatable prostheses and one was lost to follow-up. In their follow-up study, Kaufman et al.[1] noted that 84% of their patients operated on for psychogenic impotence were completely or somewhat satisfied as compared to 76% (author's calculation) of the group with an organic etiology. It should be noted that their data resulted from a mail-in questionnaire returned by 49 of the 90 subjects to whom it was sent; the findings, as they warn, are subject to an unknown bias. Both subjects of Segraves et al.[44] with psychogenic impotence were satisfied with their implants, but as discussed later, there were other complications. Finally, Gerstenberger et al.[53] denied a correlation between etiology and satisfaction in their 11 patients. These data, though scanty, suggest that from the perspective of patient satisfaction alone, psychogenic impotence may not be a contraindication for penile prosthetic surgery.

PARTNER SATISFACTION

Although the data in the previous section were presented with more than a little reservation and skepticism, one should be even less sanguine about reports of partner satisfaction with prostheses. Twelve of the thirty-one studies made no mention at all of patient satisfaction, and 16 neglected partner satisfaction. Of the remaining 15, half offered some quantitative data, but only five involved direct inquiry of the partner. Thus only 42 direct partners responses have been reported upon in this literature. The figures in Table 2 summarize the reports in which there was some quantitation of partner satisfaction. The first group of studies relied exclusively on patient reports; the second group, consisting of only two reports, presented partner responses (not included is the report of Krauss et al.[52] which, although it included partner reporting, provided no sample size).

Besides the overall paucity of data, the discrepancy between patient and partner reports is the striking feature of the tables. The first report of partner satisfaction was in 1964 by Loeffler et al. in which a patient re-

Table 2. Partner Satisfaction

Source	N	N satisfied (%)	R/I[a]
Type 1			
Gee et al.[30]	15	10 (67)	R
Finney[33]	20	20 (100)	R
Gottesman et al.[38]	56	56 (100)	R
Merrill and Swanson[42]	15	14 (93)	R
Gee et al.[46]	15	9 (60)	R
Gerstenberger et al.[53]	61	44 (72)	I
Total	182	153 (84)	
Type 2			
Segraves et al.[42]	6	5 (83)	R and I
Kramarsky-Binkhorst[45]	31	13 (42)	I
Total	37	18 (48)	

[a] R, rigid; I, inflatable.

ceiving an acrylic rod claimed to have "the happiest wife in Santa Clara county."[25] The tendency to ask only the patient and to accept even the hyperbolic responses as accurate* continued until the 1978 report by Kramarsky-Binkhorst.[45] Her study merits a closer look.

She contacted 60 recipients of penile implants to request permission to interview their partners. Twenty-nine, just under half, refused. Of the 31 women interviewed, there were a number of difficulties: five experienced initial dyspareunia (three cases of which remitted), five had trouble coping with their partner's "hypersexuality," and seven complained that the prosthesis was too short, too thin, or likely to buckle. Finally, she noted that four women had been unaware of the surgery until her interviews, in spite of having had sex using the prosthesis.

Other reports have been only descriptions of individual cases. Gee et al.[46] described a patient whose wife, initially unaware of the operation, subsequently refused intercourse. Krauss et al.[52] discussed two cases of partner dissatisfaction: one was a wife, "under strict orders" by her husband not to express reservations preoperatively, who had persistent postoperative complaints about the adequacy of the erection. The second case was a wife whose preoperation support and encouragement did a rapid turnaround following surgical restoration of her husband's potency. Segraves et al. also reported a case of partner dissatisfaction in a man with psychogenic impotence. Despite preoperative agreement by both husband and

* The authors certainly would not suggest that all enthusiastic responses represent an exaggeration. Segraves et al.[44] quote the wife of a prosthetic recipient: "I have a bionic husband. All women should be so lucky."

wife, the wife became extremely unhappy about the rigid prothesis after hospitalization. She insisted on a second surgery for an inflatable prosthesis, which was done, but her complaints continued.[44]

Besides the obvious conclusion that more research is needed in this area, it seems that partner satisfaction is not what implant recipients (or their doctors) claim it to be. As an additional point of confusion, Kaufman et al. reported that 67% of their patients would have undergone the operation even though there might be partner dissatisfaction.[1]

REGULAR USE

Five reports[1,40,42,44,53] specifically provide data on coital frequency following implantation. Several caveats are in order. First, apart from the married patients in the group of Segraves et al.,[44] frequency of intercourse is provided solely by patient report. Second, only two reports[42,53] compared frequency of intercourse before and after surgery, although both of these examined the frequency before the onset of impotence. Finally, specific follow-up time was not always provided.

Merrill and Swanson[42] in 1976 were the first to report some systematic data on this variable. Of their 15 patients only one (see p. 206) reported no use. Ten patients reported coitus once per week and four twice to three times per week. In the same issue of the same journal Nellans et al.[40] reported their series of 23 patients receiving Small–Carrion implants. Two patients did not have coitus after surgery, two obese patients had difficulty in penetration, and two patients had coitus only once.

At a minimum of 6 months after implantation of an inflatable prosthesis, Gerstenberger et al. sent questionnaires to 96 patients to evaluate their own and their partners' satisfaction with the implant.[53] Sixty-one patients responded. No patients reported no use of the prosthesis at all, although 27 reported no coitus during the 6 months preceding surgery (hardly surprising since they were presumably impotent), and three patients reported no coitus prior to the onset of the impotence. Taking their figures (and using 1 for patients reporting intercourse 1 time or less per month and 5 for those reporting 5 times or more) one can calculate averages of 3.03, 0.97, and 2.75 episodes of intercourse per month for the group prior to impotence, during the 6 months before surgery, and postoperatively, respectively. Taking into account the increment in patient age between the onset of impotence and surgery and the likely difficulties in the interpersonal relationship owing to the impotence, these figures suggest a rather close postoperative return to preimpotence sexual activity. It was also noted in this study that there was a statistically significant difference in coital frequency between the patients satisfied and those dissatisfied with the prostheses (as one might guess, the satisfied patients had more sex).

Kaufman et al. used a similar method "to assess the social, sexual, and psychological status of patients one year after implantation of Small–Carrion prosthesis."[1] They sent questionnaires to 90 randomly selected patients; 49 were returned. Fourteen percent of the respondents denied intercourse postoperatively as compared to only 4% prior to the onset of impotence. The group *mode* increased from once to 2–3 times per week. Using different calculations, (figuring <1/month = 0, 1/week = 4, 2–5/week = 10, 4–5/week = 18, >5/week = 20), one comes up with a group mean for intercourse per month of 6.8 and 5.3 prior to impotence and postoperatively, respectively. The decrement in this group (which appeared to be about twice as sexually active as Gerstenberger's) again seems fairly small. Noteworthy also in this study was the finding that 57% of the respondents felt the quantity of sexual intercourse was better postoperatively than before the onset of impotence.

Segraves et al. recently reported on 15 men who had received either Scott or Small–Carrion implants.[44] Of the seven unmarried men, three had not used the prosthesis at all (at least 8 months after surgery) and one had used it only three times in 2½ years. Two of the remaining men reported intercourse 1–2 times per week, one 1–2 times per month. The married group of eight fared somewhat better; none had no use, one man had intercourse 10 times in 2 years (all in extramarital affairs), and the remainder (and their spouses) reported intercourse once or once to twice a week. The one patient in this married group with psychogenic impotence was discussed in the previous section.

Renshaw,[55] in an editorial arguing for better pre- and postoperative evaluation of patients and their partners, quoted Kramarsky-Binkhorst's informal poll of Veterans Administration (VA) Hospital house staff to the effect that "most of these damn things (implants) never get used anyway."[45] The one hundred sixty-three patients discussed in this section are a small and (in the reports using questionnaires) selective group, but the VA residents' impression is not wholly borne out by them. A sizable proportion (perhaps up to one quarter) of recipients of implants either do not or rarely engage in coitus postoperatively and the remainder seem to return to their approximate frequency of intercourse prior to the onset of impotence. Although rare use or nonuse of the implant may not always be a bad outcome,* this subset needs better description to minimize its ranks.

---

* Consider, for example, the report by Segraves et al. of a single man who did not use the prosthesis at all during the 6 months after surgery, but who experienced increased self-esteem and productivity because "now I'm free to flirt with women and to feel competent competing with other men."[44]

PSYCHOLOGICAL STATUS

As discussed earlier, this is perhaps the most difficult outcome measure to assess. Both enhancement of self-image as well as emotional distress following implant surgery may be missed by a cursory interview or may be impossible at times to link up with the surgery. These ambiguities are reflected in the paucity of attention to this measure in the literature.

Gee et al.[46] reported a probable psychiatric complication in 1974. A 31-year-old man preoperatively diagnosed as "a paranoid schizophrenic with severe sexual maladjustment" had an excellent surgical result but required implant removal 3 months later because of an infection caused by a bite. It is not far-fetched to suppose that the patient's preexisting illness was affected by the surgery and that his infection stemmed from this (he may, for example, have requested or induced the bite to "undo" the surgery). Two patients of Mallory and Voneschenbach similarly required reoperation following a bite to the prosthesis; regrettably, further details were not provided. Another of their patients "continued to have problems with interpersonal relationships" and did not have regular intercourse.[34]

One concern of psychoanalytically oriented psychiatrists has been that psychogenic impotence represents a defense, and that surgical correction would lead to symptom substitution or other decompensation. Such an example was reported by Krauss et al.[52]: 6 months after implantation for psychogenic impotence, their patient developed testicular pain without evident organic etiology which interfered with use of his prosthesis.

There are several cases indicating felicitous results. Two patients of Segraves et al.[44] told of enhanced confidence around women in spite of not actually using their prosthesis; already mentioned was the patient of Apfelberg et al. with psychogenic impotence who had his prosthesis removed because of renewed confidence.[32]

The only study to specifically ask about emotional adjustment was that of Kaufman et al.[1] Eighty percent of their sample of 49 patients reported general emotional adjustment postoperatively as adequate to excellent. Nevertheless, 58% of the patients attributed some emotional adjustment problems to the implant. Patient self-image changed following surgery: the percent describing themselves as quite happy rose from 18 to 49 between pre- and postoperative assessment, and the percent describing themselves as somewhat unhappy dropped from 47 to 16. Two percent postoperatively described disliking themselves versus 4 percent before surgery.

Any conclusions here are highly tentative at best, but individual complications may be unlikely, and there is a general trend toward improved adjustment and self-esteem for most implant recipients. It is necessary again to caution that problems are likely to be underrepresented in the literature compared to successes. For example, many complaints about the prosthesis (particularly prolonged pain, but also site or slight deviations) may represent either physiological problems or latent psychological complications.

RELATIONSHIP STATUS

As with individual psychological status, this outcome may be difficult to assess although some of the markers (e.g., dissolution of the relationship, refusal of sex) may be clearer. There is also a certain abitrariness about including some results here rather than in the section on partner satisfaction.

Aside from the patient of Gee et al.[46] whose wife refused intercourse after implantation (p. 207), the first report of relationship discord following implant surgery was the case described by Stewart and Gerson.[27] This long case report described a man who became paraplegic (and impotent) following an automobile accident and who married 3 years later. After 2 years of marriage the patient had a Scott prosthesis placed, and his wife left him within 3 days of his return home from the hospital. It is of considerable note that both the patient and his wife were interviewed preoperatively by two psychiatrists. The wife later reported that she had played down her misgivings in these interviews, and the authors concluded that her fears of intimacy (noted but understandably not viewed as a contraindication preoperatively) may have been augmented by the possibility of intercourse. They expressed reservations about prosthetic surgery for patients married after the onset of the impotence.

A similar dynamic may have been operative in the case of Segraves et al. of a psychogenically impotent man whose girl friend of 3 years refused intercourse on the grounds that coitus would symbolize commitment.[44]

Respondents to the questionnaire of Gerstenberger et al.[53] reported considerable improvement in the nonsexual aspects of their relationships: 61% reported an improvement (42 much, 19 slight) whereas only 7% reported a worsening. Ninety-three percent reported either no change in marital status or a new marriage. The remaining four patients (who were separated, divorced, or widowed) denied a relationship between the change and the implant.

Similar positive effects were noted by Kaufman et al.[1] Fifty-one percent of their respondents reported increased closeness in their relationships, and 57% rated their marital adjustment very good or excellent after implantation compared to 30% preoperatively. On the other hand, 18% reported more distance after surgery and an additional 8% reported total avoidance.

It seems that most relationships are improved or remain unchanged following prosthetic surgery. Once again, however, there seems to be a sizable subset of the recipient population whose relationship deteriorates in the face of renewed potency. This subset too is poorly characterized (is it, for example, the same subset that does not use the prosthesis?). Nonetheless, patients or partners with particular difficulties in intimacy (which may be reduced by impotence) or a compelling need for absent potency may be at particular risk.

CONCLUSIONS

From the data presented here, the following conclusions are advanced:

1. There is a strong need for more research into outcomes of penile prosthetic surgery. Studies thus far are marred by inadequate duration of follow-up, bias introduced by use of mail-in questionnaires, failure to contact partners, limited reporting of presurgical variables (e.g., duration of impotence, sexual activity levels, psychiatric findings) and other shortcomings. A large study, perhaps from several centers, using a design like Maddock's,[7] might answer a lot of questions.

2. A large percentage of men (80–90%) are pleased with the outcome regardless of their age, type of prosthesis received, or specific organic etiology.

3. Too few patients with psychogenic impotence have received implants and been reported to draw firm conclusions, but most of those reported seem to be as satisfied as the organically impotent patients.

4. A high percentage of implant recipients report partner satisfaction but perhaps one third or more of the partners reported as satisfied do not agree if asked directly.

5. Following implant surgery, a small group of patients (a) will not use or will rarely use the implant, (b) will have a deterioration in their relationships with their sexual partner, or (c) will experience some decrement in psychological well-being. It is unclear whether these three categories represent separate subgroups or the same patients. It is also not clear yet how to identify these patients preoperatively.

6. Most implant recipients and their partners return to a coital frequency about that of the period prior to impotence.
7. Most recipients and their partners experience increased closeness in their relationship after surgery.
8. There is a period of adjustment for both patient and partner following surgery, which requires ability to adapt to increased intimacy, a change in sexual partners, possible dyspareunia, and in some cases transient patient hypersexuality.

AN APPROACH TO SCREENING

The previous section makes it obvious that many questions about screening remain unanswered, and it underscores the point that screening, no matter how conscientious, may be as much an art as a science. For example, the couple reported by Stewart and Gerson[27] had a scrupulous preoperative evaluation with a nonetheless disappointing outcome, whereas two patients of Segraves and colleagues[44] had reasonable results in spite of moderate preoperative reservations. The dilemma at present, with so much unknown, is that overrigorous screening may result in few bad outcomes but deprive many men of the opportunity for a prosthesis, whereas too-lax screening may produce too many unhappy patients and partners.

Figure 1 shows a decision tree (flow chart) for psychiatrically evaluating candidates for implant surgery, based on the material discussed throughout this chapter. The tree does not contain steps involved in reaching a diagnosis based on organic etiology, such as physical examination, endocrine studies, and vascular workup, as these procedures are reviewed in detail in other chapters.

The first step consists of a thorough interview of the patient. In addition to a review of the presenting complaint, a detailed sexological history should be obtained. The patient should be asked about present and past psychopathological states, particularly looking for depressive symptomatology, psychosis, pronounced suspiciousness, or substance abuse. Questioning about the patient's expectations after implantation is mandatory, and this must include an assessment not only of conscious, reasonable hopes, but also of hints of (or obvious) unrealistic ones as well. The interviewer must secure an adequate data base, but must also appreciate the patient's sensitivities and the need for a possible therapeutic alliance as well.

The first decision in this tree regards the presence or absence of a

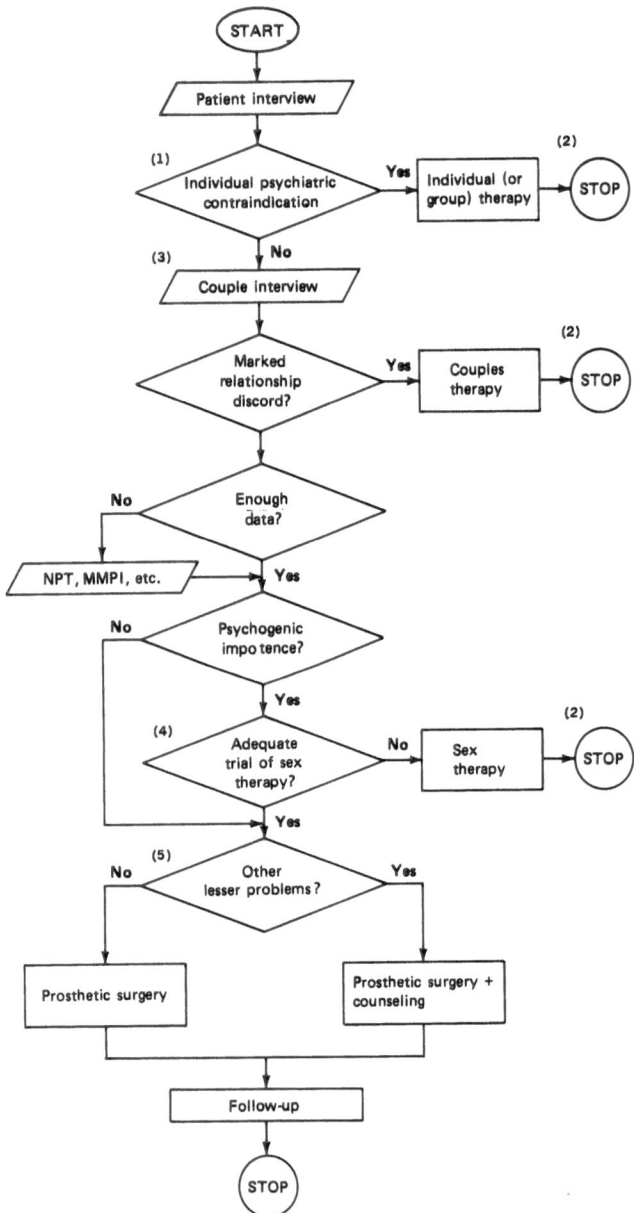

Figure 1. Screening decision tree.

psychiatric contraindication much as discussed in the section on screening goals. The patient with a contraindication could then be referred for appropriate treatment and, of course, later be reevaluated if necessary.

The second step in this scheme consists of an interview with the patient and his partner. Here too, a sexological history, an assessment of expectations, and a probe for psychopathology should be made, but in addition some evaluation of the couple's relationship can also be obtained. Not all centers secure such a joint interview, and of course not all patients have regular partners or will grant permission to see the partner. Nonetheless, this seems a critical step in evaluation and should probably be included whenever possible. If sufficient pathology is observed in the partner or the relationship to mitigate against surgery, marital or other therapy should be offered, and consideration of surgery taken up later if desired.

Under most circumstances this would provide an adequate data base on which to base treatment recommendations. Additional tests, such as the nocturnal penile tumescence study or the Minnesota multiphasic personality inventory, may be indicated in some situations or as part of a research protocol.[6,7,13,56]

In cases of psychogenic impotence, mixed organic and psychogenic impotence, or perhaps even equivocal cases (i.e., where etiology remains unclear), a trial of behaviorally oriented sex therapy is probably the next best step if the patient and his partner are amenable. If the couple refuses or have already failed to respond to an adequate trial of sex therapy (how adequate needs to be ascertained as part of the screening process), then the patient may be cleared for surgery. It is worth understanding that the entire risk-versus-benefit accounting of prosthetic surgery for men with clear-cut psychogenic impotence is not yet known, and surgery on such patients, particularly without a trial of sex therapy, may almost be considered experimental.

The screening process should clarify which patients may be approved for surgery without further psychiatric intervention and which may need simultaneous surgical and psychiatric treatments. See the discussion of assessment for associated psychiatric treatment for further discussion.

Finally, adequate follow-up should address not only technical outcome but also some estimation of whether the five screening goals of this chapter were met. This requires direct inquiry of both the patient and his partner (if possible about satisfaction, utilization, and personal and relationship well-being). Such follow-up not only is critical to optimal patient care, but would also contribute to the much-needed professional fund of knowledge about the effects of this surgery on our patients and on their lives.

REFERENCES

1. Kaufman JJ, Boxer RJ, Boxer B, et al: Physical and Psychological results of penile prosthesis: A statistical survey. *J Urol*, 126:173–175, 1981
2. Sotile WM: The penile prosthesis: A review. *J Sex Marital Ther* 5(2):90–102, 1979
3. Bullard DG, Mann J, Caplan H, et al: Sex counseling and the penile prosthesis. *Sexual Disabil* 1(3):184–189, 1978
4. Treatment of impotence by penile implants (medical news). *JAMA* 241(1):16–17, 1979
5. Goin JM, Goin MK: *Changing the body: Psychological effects of plastic surgery*. Baltimore, Williams & Wilkins, 1981
6. Osborne D: Psychologic evaluation of impotent men, *Mayo Clin Proc* 51:363–366, 1976
7. Maddock JW: Assessment and evaluation protocol for surgical treatment of impotence. *Sexual Disabil* 3(1):39–49, 1980
8. Rosenheim E, Neumann M: Personality characteristics of sexually dysfunctioning males and their wives. *J Sex Res*, 17:124–138, 1981
9. O'Connor JF, Stern LO: Developmental factors in functional sexual disorders. *NY State J Med*, 42:1838, 1972
10. Meyer JK, Schmidt CW, Lucas MJ, et al: Short-term treatment of sexual disabilites: Interim report. *Am J Psychiatry* 132:172, 1975
11. El-Senoussi JA, Coleman DR, Tauber AS: Factors in male impotence. *J Psychol* 48:3–46, 1959
12. Noy P, Wollstein S, Kaplan-DeNour A: Clinical observations on the psychogenesis of impotence. *Br J Med Psychol*, 39:43–53, 1966
13. Beutler LE, Karacan I, Anch AM, et al: MMPI and MIT discriminators of biogenic and psychogenic impotence. *J Consul Clin Psychol* 43:899–903, 1975
14. Beutler LE, Scott FB, Karacan I: Psychological screening of impotent men. *J Urology* 116:193–197, 1976
15. Cooper AJ: Factors in male sexual inadequacy: A review. *J Nerv Ment Dis* 149:337–359, 1969
16. Schiavi RC: Psychological determinants of erectile disorders. *Sexual Disabil* 4:86–92, 1981
17. Abel GG, Becker JV, Cunningham-Rather J, et al: Differential diagnosis of impotence in diabetics: The validity of sexual symptomatology. *Neurourol Urodynamics* 1:57–69, 1982
18. Abram, HS: Therapeutic consultation with the surgical patient, in Wittkower ED, Warners H (eds): *Psychosomatic Medicine. Its Clinical Applications*. Hagerstown, Maryland, Harper & Row, 1977
19. Kaplan HS: *The New Sex Therapy*. New York, Brunner/Mazel, 1974
20. Schiatri RC: Psychological treatment of erectile disorders in diabetic patients. *Ann Intern Med* 92(2):337–339, 1980
21. Renshaw DC: Impotence in diabetics. *Dis Nerv System* 36:369–371,
22. Renshaw DC: Impotence in diabetics, in LoPiccolo J, LoPiccolo L (eds): *Handbook of Sex Therapy*. New York, Plenum Press, 1978
23. Segraves RT: *Marital Therapy: A combined Psychodynamic–Behavior Approach*. New York, Plenum Press, 1982
24. Loeffler RA, Sayegh ES: Perforated acrific implants in management of organic impotence. *J Urol* 84(4):559–561, 1960
25. Loeffler RA, Sayegh ES, Lash H: The artificial os penis. *Plast Reconstruct Surg* 34(1):71–74, 1964

26. Beheri GE: Surgical treatment of impotence. *Plast Reconstruc Surg* 38(2)92–97, 1966
27. Stewart TD, Gerson SN: Penile prosthesis: Psychologic factors. *Urology* 7(4):400–402, 1976
28. Lash H: Silicone implant for impotence. *J Urol* 100:709–710, 1968
29. Pearman RO: Insertion of a silastic penile prosthesis for the treatment of organic sexual impotence. *J Urol* 107:802–806, 1972
30. Gee WF, McRoberts JW, Ansell JS: Penile prosthetic implant for the treatment of organic impotence. *Am J Surg* 126:698–700, 1973
31. Kaufman JJ, Raz S: Use of implantable prosthesis for the treatment of urinary incontinence and impotence. *A J Surg* 130:244–250, 1975
32. Apfelberg DB, Maser MR, Lash H: Surgical management of impotence. *AM J Surg* 132:336–337, 1976
33. Finney RP: New hinged silicone penile implant. J Urol 117:585–587, 1977
34. Mallory TR, Voneschenbach AC: Surgical treatment of erectile impotence with inflatable penile prosthesis. *J Urol* 118:49–51, 1977
35. Small MP: The Small–Carrion penile prosthesis. *Urol Clin North Am* 5(3):549–561, 1978
36. Brown JS: Surgical treatment of impotence. *NY State Med* 42:1897–1900, 1978
37. Small MP: Small–Carrion penile prosthesis. *Mayo Clin Proc* 51:336–338, 1976
38. Gottesman JE, Kosterb S, Das S, et al: The Small–Carrion Prosthesis of male impotency. *J Urol* 117:289–290, 1977
39. Morales PA, Scavez JB, Delgado, J, et al: Penile implant for erectile impotence. *J Urol* 109:641–645, 1973
40. Nellans RE, Naftel W, Stein J, et al: Experience with Small–Carrion penile prosthesis in the treatment of organic impotence. *J Urol* 115:280–283, 1976
41. Furlow WL: The current status of the inflatable penile prosthesis in the management of impotence: Mayo Clinic experience updated. *J Urol* 119:363–364, 1978
42. Merrill DC, Swanson DA: Experience with the Small–Carrion penile prosthesis. *J Urol* 115:277–279, 1976
43. Small MD: Small–Carrion penile prosthesis: A report on 160 cases and review of the literature. *J Urol* 119:365–368, 1978
44. Segraves RT, Schoenberg HW, Zarines CK: Psychosexual adjustment after penile prosthesis surgery. *Sexual Disabil* 5:222–229, 1982
45. Kramarsky-Binkhorst S: Female partner perception of Small–Carrion implant. *Urology* 12(5): 545–548, 1978
46. Gee WF, McRoberts JW, Raney JO, et al: The impotent patient: Surgical treatment with penile prosthesis and psychiatric evaluation. *J Urol* 114:41–43, 1974
47. Melman A: Experience with implantation of the Small–Carrion penile implant for organic impotence. *J Urol* 116:49–50, 1976
48. Loeffler RA, Iverson RE: Surgical treatment of impotence in the male. *Plast Reconstruct Surg* 58(3):293–297, 1976
49. Scott FB, Byrd GJ, Karacan I, et al: Erectile impotence treated with an implantable, inflatable prosthesis. *JAMA* 241(24):2609–2612, 1979
50. Furlow WL: Surgical management of impotence using the inflatable penile prosthesis. *Mayo Clin Proc* 51:325–328, 1976
51. Furlow WL: Surgical treatment of impotence using the inflatable penile prosthesis. *Sexual Disabil* 1(4):299–306, 1978
52. Krauss DJ, Bogin D, Culebras A: The failed penile prosthetic implantation despite technical success. *J Urol* 129:969–973, 1983

53. Gerstenberger DL, Osborne D, Furlow WL: Inflatable penile prosthesis. *Urology* 14(6):583–587, 1979

54. Controversy over penile implants for impotence. *Medical World News* pp 25–27, January 10, 1977

55. Renshaw DC: Inflatable penile prosthesis (editorial). *JAMA* 241(24):2637–2638, 1979

56. Karacan I, Salis PJ, Ware JC, et al: Nocturnal penile tumescence and diagnosis and diabetic impotence. *Am J Psychiatry* 135:191–197, 1978

10

Penile Prosthesis
Implantation

DAVID M. BARRETT and WILLIAM L. FURLOW

Numerous causes for failure of the penis to achieve adequate rigidity for vaginal penetration have become apparent, and sophisticated methods have been developed for determining more accurately the particular cause in a given case. The therapeutic options remain limited, however, especially in patients with true organic disease. Fortunately, the surgically implantable penile prosthesis has evolved into an effective, reliable means of establishing penile rigidity suitable for intromission. This chapter will deal with such prostheses from the standpoint of historical significance, patient selection, device selection, surgical technique, and future considerations.

HISTORY OF PENILE IMPLANTS

The first reported attempts at reconstructing the penis for the purpose of providing rigidity for intercourse were made by Bogoras[1] in 1936 and by Frumkin[2] in 1943, when they created an os penis by implanting resected rib into the dorsal aspect of the penis. In 1948 Bergman and associates[3] reported on plastic reconstruction of an amputated penis, which included placement of a rib graft for rigidity. Although intercourse was accomplished, the grafted rib was totally absorbed in a few years.

DAVID M. BARRETT and WILLIAM L. FURLOW • Department of Urology, Mayo Clinic and Mayo Foundation, and The Mayo Medical School, Rochester, Minnesota 55905.

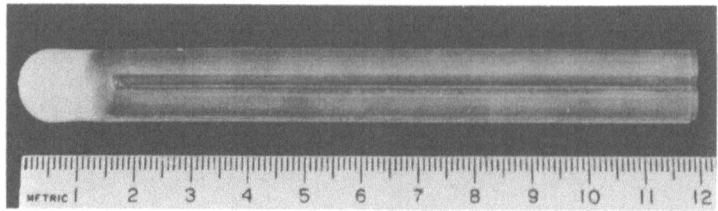

Figure 1. Pearman prosthesis. (From Furlow.[10] By permission of the J.B. Lippincott Company.)

Placement of acrylic penile splints was reported by Scardino[4] in 1950 and Goodwin and Scott[5] in 1952. In the five cases, two prostheses were tolerated for more than 5 years, but three were removed—two because of patient intolerance and one because of infection.

In 1960 Beheri incised the tunica albuginea and used dilators to create tunnels into the corpus cavernosum, into which he placed paired polyethylene rods. He later reported a series of 700 cases of varying categories of erectile dysfunction treated successfully with his prosthesis.[6]

Concurrently, Loeffler and Sayegh[7] began using perforated acrylic implants between the corpora cavernosa. Later, with Lash and associates,[8] they used a similar prosthesis in the surgical treatment of Peyronie's disease.

Pearman was one of the first to use silicone; in 1967[9] he reported placing a single-rod prosthesis between Buck's fascia and the tunica albuginea on the dorsal aspect of the penis (Figure 1).[10] This technique proved to be unsatisfactory, as many of the patients complained of pain. Eventually he placed the prosthesis beneath the tunica albuginea in the created central tunnel, using Hegar dilators.[11] The Lash–Maser[12] silicone rod prosthesis also was designed to be implanted centrally within the corpora, but the

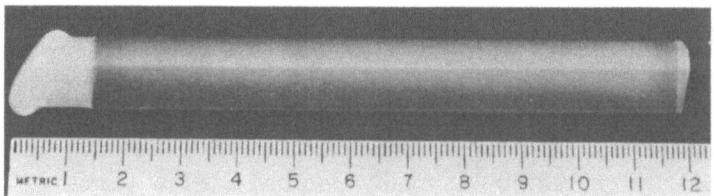

Figure 2. Lash prosthesis. (From Furlow.[13] By permission of the American Diabetes Association.)

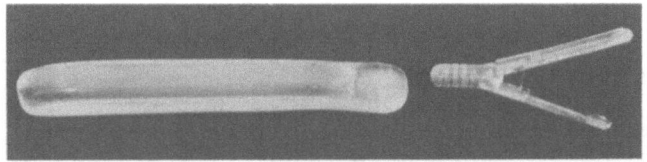

Figure 3. Loeffler prosthesis. (From Furlow.[13] By permission of the American Diabetes Association.)

rod was blunt at one end and had lateral convolutions designed specifically for deeper implantation to prevent migration and erosion (Figure 2).[13]

In an attempt to prevent distal migration and instability of the prosthesis, Loeffler and Iverson[14] added a proximal bifurcation of Pearman's centrally placed silicone rod. Tudoriu[15] modified the centrally placed silicone rod by adding a Teflon bifurcation distally, again designed to enhance stability (Figure 3). The latest attempt at a centrally placed prosthesis was the Gerow device (Figure 4).[16] This did improve on earlier devices by providing for sufficient bulk to fill both corpora, but implantation required incision of the intracorporeal septum and did not provide for proximal stabilization. Despite all the design alterations, use of the centrally placed prosthesis was fraught with complications of pain, migration, and instability.

In 1973 Morales and associates[17] reported on 15 cases in which paired double-limbed polyethylene rods were implanted. Each corpus was dilated and exact measurements were obtained. The distal end of the prosthesis was trimmed to a length that provided for a snug fit, thus preventing instability or migration. Although the prosthesis was functionally satisfactory, the diameter of the rods was inadequate to produce normal penile girth.

In 1975 Small and associates[18] introduced paired silicone semirigid rod implants. The device allows for adequate penile length, girth, and stability (Figure 5). This prosthesis, more than any other, has established the concept that prosthetic surgery is a practical, uncomplicated, and reliable means of

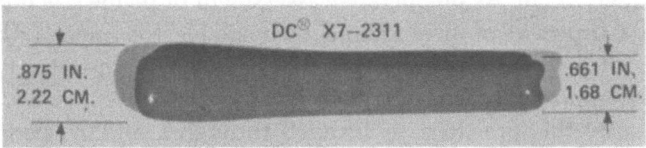

Figure 4. Gerow prosthesis. (From Furlow.[10] By permission of the J.B. Lippincott Company.)

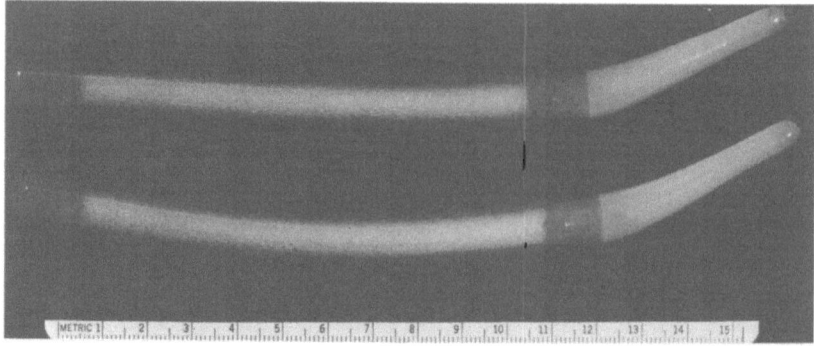

Figure 5. Small–Carrion prosthesis (manufactured by Heyer–Schulte Corp., Goleta, California). (From Furlow.[13] By permission of the American Diabetes Association.)

correcting erectile impotency, and it has become the standard by which newer developments in penile implant surgery are judged.

The great shortcoming of all rigid or semirigid rod prostheses proved to be concealment. To provide a more physiological implant, Scott and associates[19] introduced the concept of the inflatable penile prosthesis in 1973.

CURRENTLY USED PROSTHESES

SEMIRIGID RODS

Small–Carrion Prosthesis

Since its introduction in 1973,[20] this prosthesis has become accepted worldwide and has been implanted in more than 20,000 patients. Small–Carrion implants are cylindrical paired rods, each composed of an outer silicone shell filled with an inner silicone sponge. (Over the years, medical-grade silicone has proved to be highly compatible with the tissues.) Several sizes are available: diameters are 9, 11, and 13 mm; and length ranges from 12 cm through 21 cm. As preoperative assessment of penile size is difficult, the entire assortment of sizes should be available for implantation. The prosthesis kit includes a set of sizers that is used intraoperatively to determine the appropriate length and diameter.

Ordinarily this prosthesis is inserted through a midline perineal incision that allows for access to both corpora (Figure 6). Additional routes of access to the corpora include the infrapubic, dorsal, penoscrotal, and dorsal subcoronal. All currently used rod prostheses may be inserted

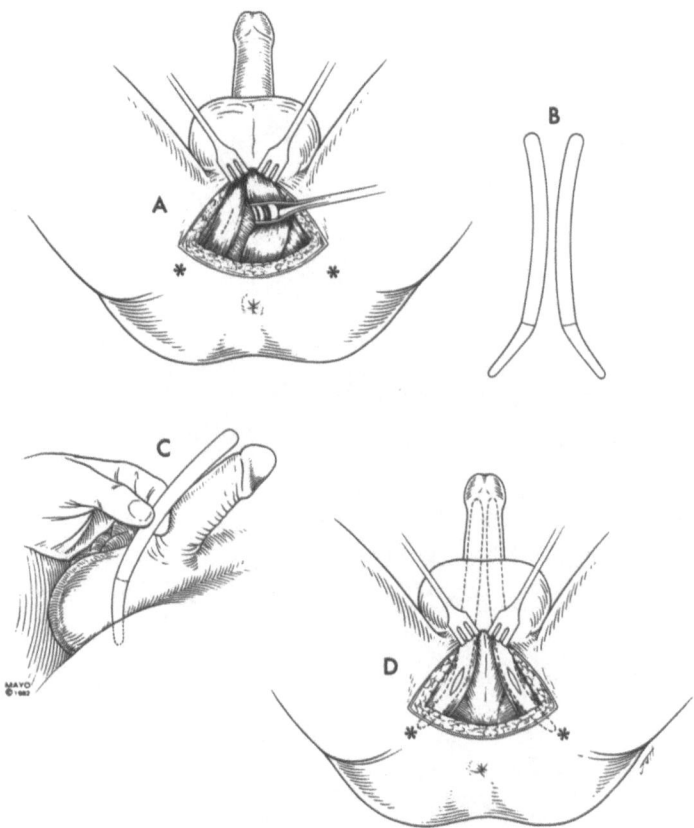

Figure 6. Surgical procedure for insertion of Small–Carrion prosthesis. (From Furlow.[10] By permission of Mayo Foundation.)

through these incisions. However, flexibility of the prosthesis generally makes the more proximal or distal access the easiest.

Appropriateness of length is important with all devices. There is a natural tendency for the surgeon to select the longest possible implant. Unfortunately, oversizing can lead to the so-called SST deformity, which results in a downward curvature of the glans penis or in development of pain or erosion of the rods due to pressure necrosis.

Finney Flexirod Prosthesis

Introduced by Finney[21] in 1977, this prosthesis was designed to be an improvement on the double-rod semirigid penile implant.[22] The proximal stability achieved by the Small–Carrion devices was to be preserved, but

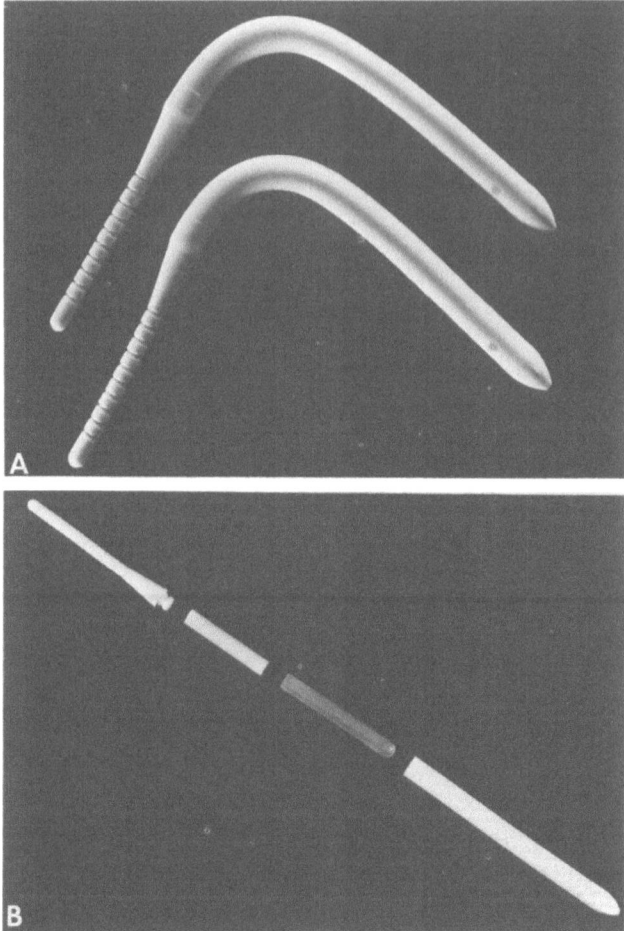

Figure 7. Finney prosthesis. A: Flexirod implant. B: Inserts giving hinged construction (manufactured by Medical Engineering Corporation Surgitek, Racine, Wisconsin). (From Furlow.[10] By permission of the J.B. Lippincott Company.)

the flexibility and ultimate concealability of the penile shaft was to be enhanced (Figure 7). A simple hinge was provided by placing a portion of soft silicone rubber at the base of the penis, but the remainder of the penile shaft was of more rigid silicone material. Since the proximal–distal penile measurement varies considerably, the implant was designed for adjustment of length to place its hinge portion at the base of the penis. In addition, the proximal end was designed to be trimmed to the appropriate length. Distal diameters available are 9, 10.5, 12, and 14 mm.

In the majority of cases, implantation of the Flexirod prosthesis has been accomplished via the dorsal penile approach—a longitudinal incision through the tunica albuginea into each corpus, done with care to avoid the midline and the neurovascular bundle (Figure 8). Since the Finney prosthesis is soft and flexible, it can be inserted easily into the corpus with a twisting motion.

Jonas Silicone–Silver Prosthesis

In an attempt to provide adequate penile rigidity for intercourse, maintain simplicity, and enhance concealment, Jonas[23,24] introduced the silicone–silver malleable paired-rod prosthesis (Figure 9). These rods are formed principally of silicone rubber surrounding a woven silver-wire insert, but the tip and midportion are of softer silicone, which reduces the risk of rod

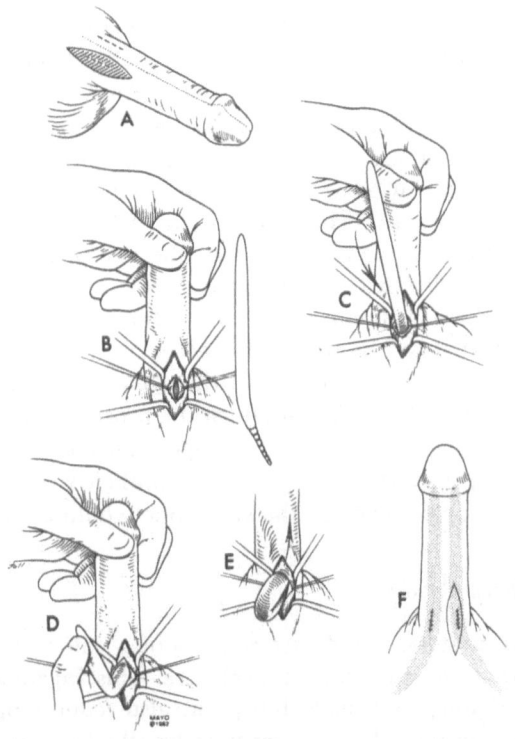

Figure 8. Surgical insertion of the Flexirod prosthesis. (From Furlow.[10] By permission of Mayo Foundation.)

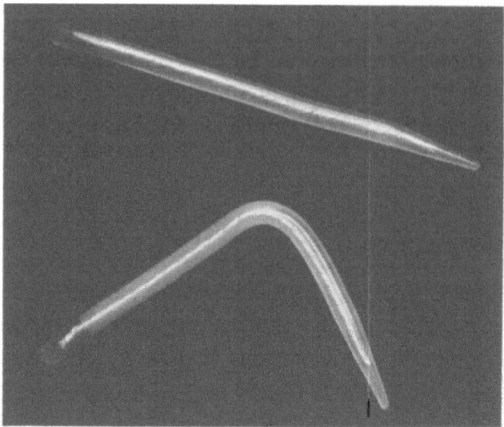

Figure 9. Jonas prosthesis. (From Furlow.[10] By permission of the J.B. Lippincott Company.)

perforation through the glans and enhances flexibility of the rod at its midportion. The prosthesis is manufactured in three diameters (9.5, 11, and 13 mm) and in ten lengths from 16 to 25 cm.

Having a full set of prostheses at surgery is recommended, for the exact determination of size is made at that time. Ordinarily a dorsal sub-coronal skin incision is used, with care to avoid the neurovascular bundle in the midline (Figure 10). The tunica is incised, allowing dilatation of both corpora, and girth is estimated from the size of dilator that can be passed proximally with ease. A calibrated sizer is available for estimation of length. Since there is abundant material at the conical-shaped proximal end of each rod, that can be trimmed if necessary for a better fit.

Concern has been expressed about the eventual fatigue and fracture of the silver-wire insert. Testing in which the prosthesis was twice flexed 90° at 90 bends/min showed some breakage after 6000 cycles. With additional testing up to 30,000,000 cycles, no broken wires perforated the silicone. This testing far exceeds the stress one would anticipate in use.

AMS 600 Malleable Prosthesis

Introduced in 1983, this device consists of a pair of tapered silicone rods containing a woven stainless steel core. This ingenious device not only provides rigidity and malleability but also reduces operating room inventory by requiring only three separate lengths to be in stock (12 cm, 16 cm, and 20 cm). The exact length to be implanted is achieved by adding rear tip extenders in 1-cm increments. Each rod is 13 mm in width. How-

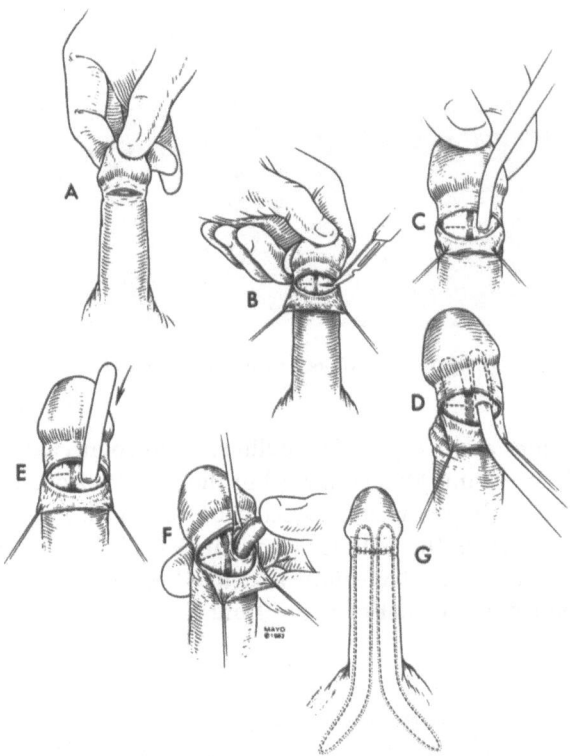

Figure 10. Surgical procedure for insertion of Jonas silicone–silver prosthesis. (From Furlow.[10] By permission of Mayo Foundation.)

ever, an outer skin may be removed to reduce the diameter to 11 mm. Thus, three different pairs of rods will be sufficient to fit 30 different penile sizes (Figure 11).

The device may be implanted in a manner similar to that used for the other semirigid prostheses.

INFLATABLE PENILE PROSTHESIS

Unique and truly creative was the Scott inflatable penile prosthesis introduced in 1973.[19] This was designed to satisfy the requirements of suitable penile rigidity for intromission and penile flaccidity for concealment and comfort. Over its 10-year history, several subtle changes in the device have greatly improved its function and reliability (Figure 12). This hydraulic system utilizes two inflatable cylinders made of silicone—one

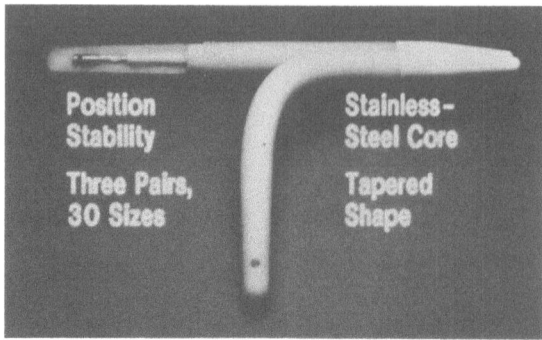

Figure 11. AMS 600 malleable prosthesis.

to be placed into each corpus. The cylinders are connected by tubing to an inflate–deflate pump that rests within the subcutaneous tissues of the scrotum. In turn, the pump is connected by tubing to a reservoir placed beneath the fascia of the anterior abdominal wall. The entire device is filled with a radiocontrast medium that has been diluted to an osmotic concentration similar to that of tissue fluid.

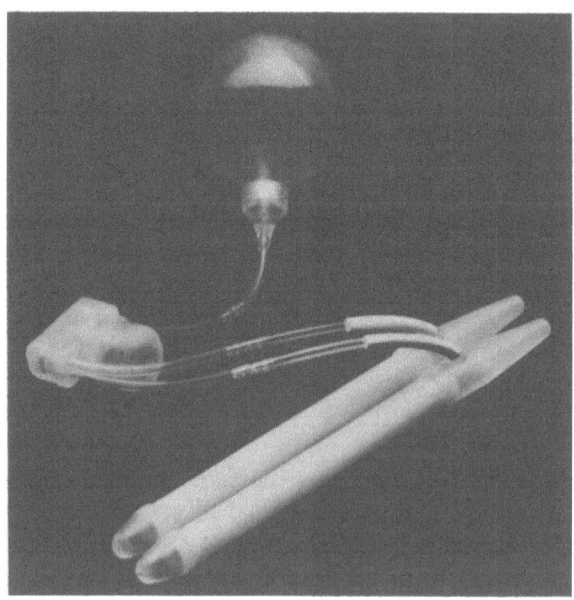

Figure 12. AMS 700 inflatable penile prosthesis (manufactured by American Medical Systems, Inc., Minnetonka, Minnesota).

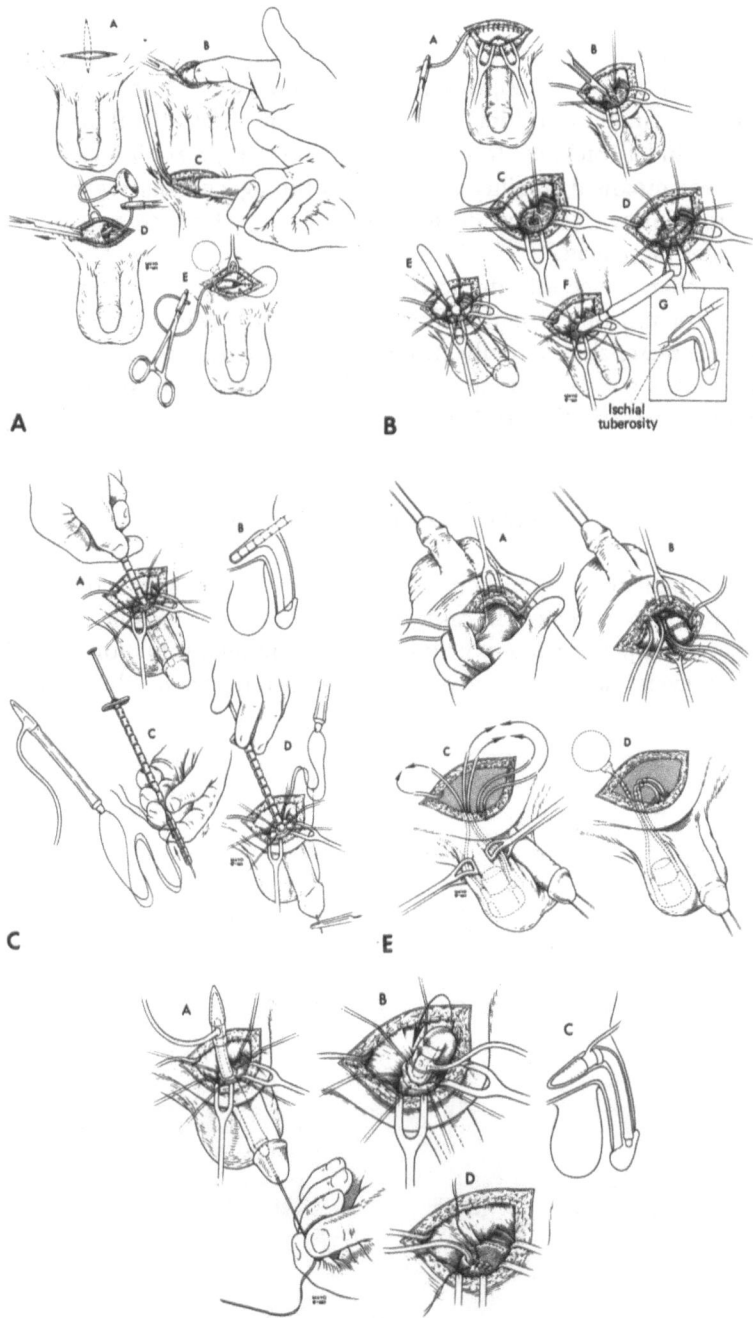

Figure 13. A–E: Implantation of AMS 700 inflatable penile prosthesis: suprapubic approach. (From Furlow.[10] By permission of Mayo Foundation.)

The entire device may be inserted by either the infrapubic (Figure 13) or the scrotal (Figure 14) approach. Significant design additions have been, including (1) nonkink tubing, (2) dip coating to prevent leaking, (3) increased cylinder thickness to prevent ballooning, (4) rear-tip extenders to provide for proximal stability and reduced tubing–cylinder wear, and (5) use of the Furlow insertion device, which has greatly increased the ease of cylinder placement.[25]

A similar device introduced in 1983 uses polyurethane (Bioflex) for cylinder construction (Mentor Corporation, North Minneapolis, Minnesota). This material, reportedly strong and durable, was chosen to prevent cylinder leaks and ballooning, which occurred with early models of the inflatable prosthesis (Figure 15).

SELECTION OF PATIENTS

Most patients seeking help for impotence are strongly motivated to get the problem corrected. In cases without an obvious organic etiology—such as radical pelvic surgery or trauma—a thorough evaluation including hormone levels, blood sugar, psychological screening, penile blood pressure

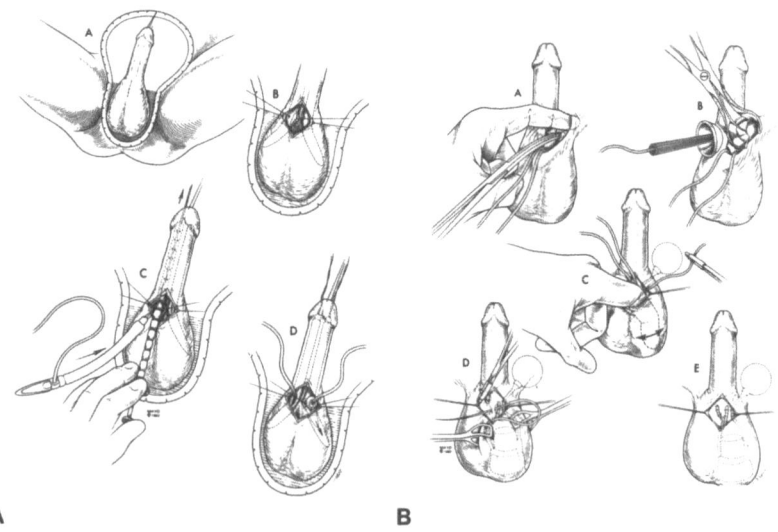

A   B

Figure 14. A and B: Implantation of AMS 700 inflatable penile prosthesis: scrotal approach. (From Furlow.[10] By permission of Mayo Foundation.)

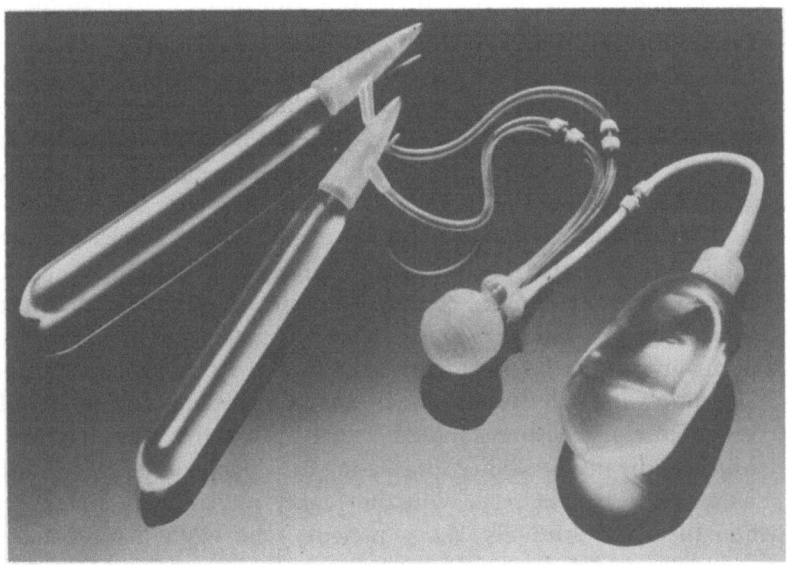

Figure 15. Mentor inflatable penile prosthesis (manufactured by Mentor Corp., Minneapolis, Minnesota).

evaluation, and nocturnal penile tumescence should lead ultimately to the correct categorization. But although possible causes for erectile impotence are numerous, only a few can be managed easily with conservative measures. An obvious example is antihypertensive medication that causes difficulty in sustaining a full erection: the patient may well respond to reduction or adjustment of the dosage. Patients with psychogenic erectile dysfunction are best managed initially with proper counseling; yet some of them are refractory to conventional therapy, and there may not be a simple solution to the erectile difficulty.

Proper screening and workup identify those patients who will respond to conservative nonsurgical management. There will be a residue of patients—depending on the clinical setting—who are strongly motivated to overcome their erectile dysfunction, and in these cases there is no alternative to consider except surgery.

Surgery implies either a penile prosthesis or revascularization. At present, only the occasional patient who has a limited segmental vascular lesion can be considered an ideal candidate for revascularization. Furthermore, the long-term results of correction by revascularization techniques have varied. To regain erectile function by virtue of ones own tissues is certainly appealing, but until revascularization techniques can reliably correct vasculogenous erectile dysfunction, the only reasonable approach in the majority of cases is a penile prosthesis.

Most patients who have filtered their way through the diagnostic maze have received information about penile prostheses. Much of this information has been gained from the lay press through numerous articles dealing with sexual dysfunction. The information generally has been accurate, and it has done much to broaden awareness of the problem of erectile dysfunction and of the corrective methods available. However, since it is desirable that the patient be informed about impotence and penile prostheses well before consultation with the implanting surgeon, one should not presume that the problem has taken care of itself. Many of the manufacturers of prostheses have such material in suitable form and will supply it to physicians who deal with impotence. It can be mailed to the patient along with a standard sexual-dysfunction questionnaire.

Much of the responsibility for steering the impotent patient to further evaluation or treatment rests with the family physician or sexual-dysfunction therapist. Formerly, many patients who might have benefited from a prosthesis did not consider it because the primary physician failed to make the suggestion or because of preconceived negative biases about such devices. Currently, however, most practitioners have been educated as to the therapeutic options for erectile dysfunction, and suitable cases are much less often missed.

For the implanting surgeon, the key to patient selection is the patient's understanding and motivation. Although patients are strongly encouraged to include their sex partners in making a decision as to a penile prosthesis, this is not absolutely necessary. Nonetheless, one should avoid situations where the patient plans to surprise his partner with the prosthesis. Experience has shown that such withholding of information may lead to poor satisfaction of the partner, and it may indicate additional underlying behavioral difficulties best managed with other techniques. It is best that the patient's regular sex partner be at least informed as to the patient's plans.

The implantation of a penile prosthesis will not assure sexual gratification, and potential patients and partners must accept this possibility. Although the experienced implanting surgeon can estimate the potential for success from his assessment of the patient's outward psychological makeup, in select situations it is best to have the likelihood of success confirmed by a psychologist or psychiatrist. This is especially true in cases of refractory psychogenic sexual dysfunction and those of individuals seeking modification of a previously inserted prosthesis that has not been satisfactory.

The definition of a successful implant is difficult, but the patient must recognize that a functional prosthesis will be only one facet of a satisfactory sexual relationship and that the prosthesis alone will not guarantee success. Patients must accept the knowledge that a rigid penis will only ensure intromission. Orgasm and ejaculation may or may not follow. However, the patient should be assured that if these functions are possible with a flaccid penis, they will probably occur after implantation.

SELECTION OF DEVICE

If there is no physical impairment of the penis (i.e., Peyronie's disease, previous priapism, previous radiation therapy), those patients who have expectations not disproportionate to the potential for success and are willing to accept the risks inherent in prosthetic surgery will be candidates for a penile prosthesis.

The modern implanting surgeon should have the facility to offer the patient either a semirigid rod prosthesis or an inflatable device. Obviously, each type has its distinct advantages and disadvantages. Advantages of the rods are (1) ease of implantation, (2) relatively low cost, (3) infrequency of mechanical failure, (4) enablement of intromission, (5) convenience for wearing of external collecting devices, and (6) high percentage of patient–partner satisfaction. Disadvantages are (1) inadequacy of concealment capability, (2) unphysiological function, and (3) increased difficulty of transurethral surgery.

The inflatable device, being more complex mechanically, has the disadvantages of (1) requiring some dexterity of the patient to manipulate the pump, (2) more frequent mechanical malfunction, (3) increased cost, and (4) more involved surgery for implantation. Beyond enablement of intromission, its distinct advantages are (1) enhanced concealment and (2) more physiological function.

Most patients, when presented with the advantages and disadvantages of each kind of device, make their own choice—which is influenced also by socioeconomic status, life-style, age, and medical history. Yet in special situations, the surgeon may be compelled to offer advice. If the patient has a disabling curvature from Peyronie's disease and is to receive an inflatable prosthesis, it may be necessary to combine a penile-straightening procedure with the implantation. A rod device, however, may override the inherent bend in the penis and thus make straightening unnecessary. Similarly, if the patient formerly has had priapism or already has undergone insertion and removal of a penile prosthesis, the matrix within the corpus will be scarred and fixed. In this circumstance, dilatation is difficult, and it may be possible only to insert a rod device.

From my experience with many cases of erectile dysfunction due to various causes in patients of all adult ages, it appears that the inflatable and rod prostheses are chosen with nearly equal frequency. One factor that has worked against the patient's selection of the inflatable device has been its potential for malfunction and the need for a reparative surgical procedure in the event of failure. The exact rate of malfunction is difficult to determine because the inflatable device has been continuously modified and improved. What is direly needed is assessment of several hundred patients who have received the same inflatable device and have been followed up for a 5-year period. We would then have a 5-year rate as a basis for appropriate advice to patients during the device-selection process. It is best to advise all patients considering implantation of an inflatable penile prosthesis that the device, like all mechanical equipment, may fail— but that if it does, it may be repaired with surgery.

RESULTS OF IMPLANTATION

Evaluation of the results of penile prosthetic surgery should include several considerations. (1) Did the prosthesis effect sufficient penile rigidity for intromission? (2) Was the patient satisfied with the intromission? (3) Was the patient's partner satisfied with the intromission? (4) Was the prosthesis acceptable between episodes of intercourse? (5) Were there any surgical complications? (6) Or medical complications? Unfortunately, most reports dealing with results of implantation do not take all facets of the problem into account.

Small reported excellent surgical results in 589 (97%) of 610 patients who had received the Small–Carrion prosthesis[20] (Table 1).

Finney reported satisfactory surgical results of 98% of 521 implantations, only seven having been followed by a complication (infection or extrusion) that required removal of the prosthesis.[21] He emphasized that no adequate studies have been devoted to patient or partner satisfaction with the Flexirod, but it was his impression that "new partners are more enthusiastic than some spouses who have lived with their impotent mate, often for years, and as a result are less interested in sex."

Jonas,[26] the developer of the silicone-silver penile prosthesis, reported surgical success in 94% of his cases, again demonstrating that rod-type prostheses are an excellent means of establishing penile rigidity with a minimum of surgical complications. In a more thorough study, Krane et al.[27] reviewed 29 cases in which the Jonas prosthesis had been implanted. There were two surgical failures due to erosion. Answers to a questionnaire disclosed that 17 (89%) of 19 patients had experienced satisfactory intercourse and 16 (89%) of 18 partners had expressed satisfaction with coitus. Some difficulty with concealment was reported by 20% of the patients.

In a similar review of 100 cases with the Jonas prosthesis, Benson et al.[28] found that surgical success had been achieved in 93, and 90 patients were satisfied with their surgical result, each stating that it was his opinion and the opinion of his sexual partner that the prosthesis was satisfactory for intercourse. However, 20 of these 90 patients reported difficulty with penile concealment. Of the ten who were dissatisfied with the prosthesis, three had erosion and seven said the penis was not long or rigid enough. Ultimately, the rod prostheses in three of them were replaced with an inflatable device. Among the 100 implantations of the Jonas prosthesis, 56 were done under local anesthesia, with hospitalization averaging only 2.8 days.

Thus it appears that rod prostheses may be implanted with surgical success rates exceeding 95% and patient–partner satisfaction rates approximately 85%. But the problem of concealment, although not well documented in the literature, is inherent in all rod prostheses. The malleability of the Jonas device is a response to this problem. When queried, however, approximately 20% of patients expressed concern about their appearance with the prosthesis.

Surgical success of implantation of the inflatable penile prosthesis is best determined several months afterward. Barry et al.[29] compared Flexirod and inflatable devices with respect to continuing function of first implants (Fig. 16). Their data confirm the fact that the inflatable device, being mechanical, may malfunction: continued satisfactory service at 42 months was projected for 68% of the inflatable implants and for 96% of the nonmechanical Flexirod prostheses.

Montague[30] reviewed his data on 169 patients with penile prostheses, which included 121 inflatable implants. Of the latter, 70 had been implanted through a lower abdominal incision, and ultimately 34 of those required revision for leaks or kinks. The remaining 51 inflatable devices were implanted through a scrotal incision, and only four of these have required revision. Montague pointed out that his conversion to the scrotal approach for implantation coincided with the introduction of rear-tip extenders and other technical improvements that have greatly enhanced the reliability of the inflatable prosthesis.

After a review of 175 cases, Furlow[31] conceded that mechanical complications do occur and that revision may be required at some time, sooner or later. However, up to 95% of the patients should have a satisfactory functional result.

Gerstenberger et al.,[32] studying patient–partner satisfaction in 175 cases, found that the rate, initially 79%, increased to 89% after modifi-

Table 1. Diagnosis and Surgical Results in 610 Patients [a]

Diagnosis	No. of patients	Results		Comments
Postprostatectomy, cystectomy, abdominal–perineal resection	87	Excellent:	85	Bilateral perforation at glans; 1 patient had
		Poor:	2	radiation therapy
Aortobifemoral bypass	15	Excellent		—
Postpriapism	13	Excellent:	11	Unable to implant intracorporeal prosthesis
		Poor:	2	
Psychogenic	84	Excellent:	83	One patient had prolonged discomfort in glans, gradually cleared; 1 patient never satisfied with size and underwent insertion of inflatable implant; 2 patients originally had inflatable penile implant
		Poor:	1	
Arteriosclerotic or hypertensive vascular disease (and medications)	157	Excellent:	154	One implant too small and replaced 6 wk postoperative; erosion through glans with loss of 1 implant: 2 patients; bilateral perforation at glanular–meatal junction with initial urinary retention; 1 patient originally had inflatable penile implant
		Good:	2	
		Poor:	1	
Spinal cord injury	32	Excellent		Eighteen implanted solely for sexual dysfunction
Post-electrical burn	1	Excellent		Required urethroplasty

Condition	No.	Rating		Comments
Peyronie's disease	44	Excellent: Good: Poor:	40 3 1	Plaque incised, 12; penis not straight, 3; erosion of 1 implant in patient where plaque not incised
Pelvic fracture	26	Excellent: Good:	25 1	Lost 1 prosthesis secondary to infection; an occasional patient required a different-length prosthesis on each side
Post-groin explosion	1	Poor		Had 1 prosthesis but subsequently removed because of poor tissue healing
Diabetes mellitus	124	Excellent: Good: Poor:	120 1 3	Urinary retention, 1; septicemia and loss of both implants, 2; perforation of 1 implant; urethroplasty and subsequent erosion of other implant, 1
Epispadias, exstrophy	1	Good		Small phallus
Hypogonadism	3	Excellent		One patient had replacement of testicular implants
Scleroderma	1	Good		Lost 1 implant secondary to surgical perforation at glans
Neurological disease (i.e., multiple sclerosis)	8	Excellent		—
Chronic renal disease	13	Excellent: Poor:	12 1	Because of persistent pain of unknown cause, both implants were removed from 1 patient

ᵃ Total patients: 610; excellent: 589; good: 9; poor: 12; surgical success: 96% (excellent only). Modified from Small.[20]

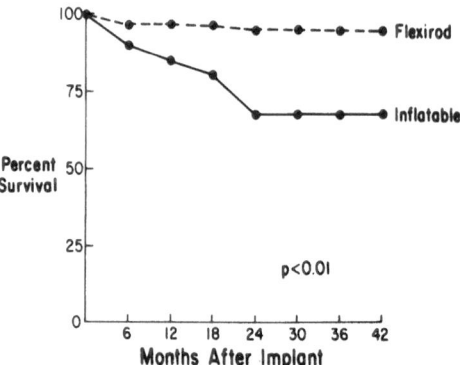

Figure 16. Survival curve comparison of first penile prosthesis implants. (From Barry et al.[29] By permission of the Professional Medical Services Company.)

cation of unrecognized complications. This supports the findings of Malloy and Voneschenbach, who reported a 90% satisfaction rate (35 of 39).[33]

COMMENT

The overriding benefit of an inflatable penile prosthesis is its greater physiological normality. Theoretically, this should be studied in a group of patients who undergo sequential implantation of both the inflatable and semirigid-rod penile prostheses. Since this protocol is not practicable, we must infer from personal experience and published data the relative superiority of these two categories of prostheses. To date, considering all aspects of both rod and inflatable prostheses, the patient has an excellent opportunity to regain penile rigidity and ultimately engage in satisfactory sexual relations, regardless of which device is implanted. As mentioned before, the best approach is to offer the well-informed patient an alternative of either a semirigid rod or an inflatable prosthesis.

PHILOSOPHICAL CONSIDERATIONS

It is clear that great strides have been made in the management of erectile dysfunction through the development of penile prostheses, and numerous patients have benefited from this creative concept. One may question the wisdom of using a technique that destroys the erection-producing tissue in the corpus when ongoing research in the areas of electrical stimulation, pharmacology, and microvascular surgery show promise. But as in all medical problems, we must do what is best for the patient in the current state of the art.

It is likely that significant technological advances in the development of penile prostheses will continue, but not until reliable, time-tested alternatives are developed will there be a true therapeutic option for erectile dysfunction.

REFERENCES

1. Bogoras N: Über die volle plastische Wiederher stellung eines zum Koitus fähigen Penis (Peniplastica totalis). *Zentralbl Chir* 63:1271–1276, 1936
2. Frumkin AP: Reconstruction of the male genitalia. *Am Rev Soviet Med* 2:14–21, 1944
3. Bergman RT, Howard AH, Barnes RW: Plastic reconstruction of the penis. *J Urol* 59:1174–1182, 1948
4. Scardino PL: Cited by Goodwin WE, Scott WW: Phalloplasty. *J Urol* 68:903–908, 1952
5. Goodwin WE, Scott WW: Phalloplasty. *J Urol* 68:903–908, 1952
6. Beheri GE: Surgical treatment of impotence. *Plast Reconstr Surg* 38:92–97, 1966
7. Loeffler RA, Sayegh ES: Perforated acrylic implants in management of organic impotence. *J Urol* 84:559–561, 1960
8. Lash H, Zimmerman DC, Loeffler RA: Silicone implantation: Inlay method. *Plast Reconstr Surg* 34:75–80, 1964
9. Pearman RO: Treatment of organic impotency by implantation of a penile prosthesis. *J Urol* 97:716–719, 1967
10. Furlow WL: Surgery for male impotence, in Glenn JF (ed): *Urologic Surgery*, ed 3. Philadelphia, JB Lippincott, 1983, pp 837–851
11. Pearman RO: Insertion of a silastic penile prosthesis for the treatment of organic sexual impotence. *J Urol* 107:802–806, 1972
12. Lash H: Silicone implant for impotence. *J Urol* 100:709–710, 1968
13. Furlow WL: Diagnosis and treatment of male erectile failure. *Diabetes Care* 2:18–25, 1979
14. Loeffler RA, Iverson RE: Surgical treatment of impotence in the male: An 18-year experience with 250 penile implants. *Plast Reconstr Surg* 58:292–297, 1976
15. Tudoriu TH: Penile implants (parts I and II). *Br J Sexual Med* 4:27, 1977
16. Annexton M: Treatment of impotence by penile implants. *JAMA* 241:13–17, 1979
17. Morales PA, Suarex JB, Delgado J, et al: Penile implant for erectile impotence. *J Urol* 109:641–645, 1973
18. Small MP, Carrion HM, Gordon JA: Small–Carrion penile prosthesis: New implant for management of impotence. *Urology* 5:479–486, 1975
19. Scott FB, Bradley WE, Timm GW: Management of erectile impotence: Use of implantable inflatable prosthesis. *Urology* 2:80–82, 1973
20. Small M: Prosthetic surgery for impotence: Small–Carrion penile prosthesis, in Barrett DM, Wein AJ (eds): *Controversies in Neuro-Urology*. New York, Churchill Livingstone, 1984, pp 491–508
21. Finney RP: Prosthetic surgery for impotence: Finney–Flexirod prosthesis, in Barrett DM, Wein AJ (eds): *Controversies in Neuro-Urology*. New York, Churchill Livingstone, 1984, pp 509–520
22. Finney RP: New hinged silicone penile implant. *J Urol* 118:585–587, 1977
23. Jonas U: Silikon–silber penisprosthese. *Aktuel Urol* 9:179–182, 1978
24. Jonas U, Jacobi GH: Silicone–silver penile prosthesis: Description, operative approach and results. *J Urol* 123:865–867, 1980
25. Furlow WL: Inflatable penile prosthesis: New device for cylinder insertion. *Urology* 12:447–449, 1978

26. Jonas U: Prosthetic surgery for impotence: Silicone–silver penile prosthesis, in Barrett DM, Wein AJ (eds): *Controversies in Neuro-Urology*. New York, Churchill Livingstone, 1984, pp 521–530

27. Krane RJ, Freedberg PS, Siroky MB: Jonas silicone–silver penile prosthesis: Initial experience in America. *J Urol* 126:475–476, 1981

28. Benson RC Jr, Barrett DM, Patterson DE: The Jonas prosthesis—Technical considerations and results. *J Urol* 130:920–922, 1983

29. Barry JM, Giesy JD, McDuffie R: Actuarial survivals of inflatable and flexible, hinged penile prostheses. *Urology* 20:605–607, 1982

30. Montague DK: Experience with semirigid rod and inflatable penile prosthesis. *J Urol* 129:967–968, 1983

31. Furlow WL: Inflatable penile prosthesis: Mayo Clinic experience with 175 patients. *Urology* 13:166–171, 1979

32. Gerstenberger DL, Osborne D, Furlow WL: Inflatable penile prosthesis: Follow-up study of patient–partner satisfaction. *Urology* 14:583–587, 1979

33. Malloy TR, Voneschenbach AC: Surgical treatment of erectile impotence with inflatable penile prosthesis. *J Urol* 118:49–51, 1977

11

Erectile Impotence: Training and Research Needs

R. TAYLOR SEGRAVES, HARRY W. SCHOENBERG, and
KATHLEEN A. B. SEGRAVES

Erectile problems are quite common. As reviewed in previous chapters, approximately 10% of healthy young males have been reported to complain of erectile dysfunction.[1] In patients with chronic diseases, the prevalence of impotence probably exceeds 30%.[2-4] It is clear that these problems are a source of considerable personal distress to many of these men and that because of personal embarrassment many patients do not volunteer such information to their physicians. It appears that physicians as a group have been remiss in not directly inquiring about sexual function in our patients. This omission on our part is unfortunate as many of these men might be helped by recent advances in diagnosis and treatment and thus avoid considerable personal suffering. Failure to inquire about sexual function may contribute to poor health care in other areas as well. It is clear that many pharmacological agents are associated with sexual side effects, and these symptoms may explain noncompliance with certain medical treatment programs.[5] Even in cases where the pharmacological agents can-

R. TAYLOR SEGRAVES and KATHLEEN A. B. SEGRAVES • Department of Psychiatry, Tulane University Medical Center, New Orleans, Louisiana 70112.   HARRY W. SCHOENBERG • Department of Surgery, Section of Urology, University of Chicago, Chicago, Illinois 60637.

not be changed because of life-threatening disease, a frank discussion of this with the patient might engender greater cooperation.

Within the past 5–10 years, it has become respectable for academic physicians to be concerned with the diagnosis and treatment of sexual difficulties. Accordingly, there has been a tremendous growth of research and clinical interest in this area. It is clear that any physician regardless of his professional training must exert considerable effort to remain abreast of current information. For many physicians, this type of time commitment is unrealistic. In many cases, the only practical solution to appropriate treatment planning is the use of multidisciplinary teams. Clearly, each member of the team has to be comfortable with, knowledgeable about, and interested in human sexuality. Sexual function lies at the interface of various biological and psychological systems. Clearly, the multidisciplinary team should include psychiatric and nonpsychiatric physicians. The authors of this text have found such a collaborative effort personally rewarding as well as a service to our patients.

The need for multidisciplinary-team evaluation of patients became increasingly obvious to us when we realized that many cases cannot be neatly dichotomized into organogenic or psychogenic etiologies. All too often, one observes mixed etiologies where an interaction of both factors is involved. For example, it is not uncommon to observe diabetics with similar degrees of autonomic neuropathy with quite dissimilar outcomes in sexual function. In such cases, the physicians need to collaborate to find the minimal intervention that will be effective for the given patient. Some diabetics can adapt to decreased erectile turgidity and postpone penile prosthesis surgery until the problem considerably worsens. Other diabetics may find such an adaptation impossible for characterological reasons and thus be immediate candidates for surgery.

TRAINING

Most physicians in current practice did not receive formalized training in the diagnosis and treatment of sexual problems in medical school or residency training. This is true of psychiatrists and urologists as well as other subspecialists. It is only comparatively recently that medical schools have included human sexuality as part of the required curriculum.[6] Frequently, such courses are taught by nonphysicians. When physicians are involved in such courses, nonpsychiatric physicians are frequently conspicuously absent. Many of these courses have concentrated on making future physicians more comfortable with the topic of sexuality. It is still unclear how effective such courses are in influencing actual physician-patient interaction. Although the authors agree that the goal of increasing physician comfort with sexuality in themselves and their patients is laudable, the authors strongly feel that future physicians also need clear instruction on recent developments in diagnosis and treatment. Nonpsychiatric physician involvement in such courses is critical so that the students are made aware of recent advances in the understanding of the biological basis of human sexuality. It is quite possible that lack of knowledge regarding effective interventions is a greater impediment to physicians inquiring about their patients' sexual problems than the element of personal discomfort about sexuality.

NEED FOR FUTURE RESEARCH

The potential for future advances in our understanding of human sexuality is almost limitless. Unfortunately, this limitless potential is a function of our abysmal lack of current information. The vascular mechanisms underlying the erectile process are unknown. The role of venous constriction, if any, in tumescence is unclear,[7] and the previously accepted concept of "polsters" within arteriovenous shunts, redistributing blood flow to cavernosus spaces and thus producing erections, has recently been questioned.[8] It was previously accepted as established fact that penile erection was mediated predominantly by the parasympathetic nervous system and that the responsible neurotransmitter was acetylcholine.[9] However, more recent evidence has suggested a significant role for adrenergic fibers.[10–16] Cerebral structures mediating sexual arousal and erection are virtually uninvestigated in the human, and some controversy even exists regarding sexual pathways in the spinal cord.[17] As previously reviewed, the role of androgens in erectile function per se is unclear.[18] There is a pressing need for basic science investigation to delineate the physiology of tumescence and detumescence.

Patients still present for treatment and must be responded to by clinicians even in the absence of basic information about the physiology of erection and ejaculation. Although pure research into basic mechanisms of sexual function is important, there is a pressing need for applied research. As previously reviewed, nocturnal penile tumescence testing has not proved as useful in differential diagnosis as original reports suggested.[19] Clearly, there is a need to identify men for whom false positive (organic patterns) will be found. Similarly, it is unclear whether major affective disease which interrupts many basic physiological patterns also suppresses sleep tumescence. Although pudendal nerve conduction tests represent a major diagnostic breathrough, basic data as to degree of abnormal conduction necessary to produce neurogenic impotence are lacking. Doppler study of penile blood flow is clearly useful in documenting major arterial occlusion. However, normal erection requires approximately a sevenfold increase in blood flow into the corpora cavernosa.[20] It is possible that significant vascular impairment may not be detected in the flaccid penis. Revascularization surgery for vasculogenic impotence is clearly in its infancy and hampered by a lack of knowledge of the pelvic hemodynamics of normal erection.[21] As previously mentioned, the authors encounter approximately 15% of their cases of supposedly organogenic impotence for which a probable etiology cannot be found.

Although Dr. Levine presented an excellent review of the state of the art in treating psychogenic impotence (Chapter 4), it is clear that minimal evidence is available concerning the natural history of untreated erectile problems. There is minimal evidence on spontaneous remission rates or on the differential effectiveness of varying psychiatric treatment approaches.[22] It is also clear that many of the high success rates in behavioral treatment of impotence have occurred in highly selected self-referred patients. Many patients seen in medical clinics refuse a psychiatric referral or do not comply with conventional psychological treatment approaches.[23,24] Clearly, alternative treatment approaches need to be found for such men. As experience with behavioral sex therapy has become more widespread, it is becoming obvious that many cases of psychogenic impotence do not respond to behavioral sex therapy or any of the current psychiatric treatment approaches.

In conclusion, the more we know about erectile function, the more we realize how much more we need to know. Fortunately, current knowledge allows the well-informed clinician to establish a probable etiology and a helpful intervention in most cases. Hopefully, the future will provide information that will allow us to extend the number of patients for whom a definitive diagnosis and optimal treatment regime can be implemented.

REFERENCES

1. Nettleblatt P, Uddenberg N: Sexual dysfunction and sexual satisfaction in 58 married Swedish men. *J Psychosom Res* 23:141–147, 1979
2. Ellenberg M: Impotence in diabetics: the neurologic factor. *Ann Intern Med* 75:213–219, 1971
3. Sherman FP: Impotence in patients with chronic renal failure or dialysis. *Fertil Steril* 26:221–223, 1975
4. Bulpitt CJ, Dollery CT: Side effects of hypotensive agents evaluated by a self-administered questionnaire. *Br Med J* 3:485–490, 1973
5. Slag MF, Morley, JE, Elson MK, et al: Impotence in medical clinic outpatients. *JAMA* 249:1736–1740, 1983

6. Lief HI: Sex education in medicine: retrospect and prospect, in Rosenweig N, Pearsall FP (eds): *Sex Education for the Health Professional: A Curriculum Guide.* New York, Grune & Stratton, 1978

7. Krane RJ, Siroky MB: Neurophysiology of erection. *Urol Clin North Am* 8:91–102, 1981

8. Benson GS, McConnell JA, Schmitt WA: Penile polsters: Functional structures or atherosclerotic changes? *J Urol* 125:800–803, 1981

10. Benson, GS, McConnell JA, Wood JG: Adrenergic innervation of the human bladder body. *J Urol* 122:189–191, 1979

11. Dail WG, Evan AP: Experimental evidence indicating that the penis of the rat is innervated by short adrenergic neurons. *Am J Anat* 141:203–217, 1974

12. Domer FR, Wessler G, Brown RL, et al: Involvement of the sympathetic nervous system in the urinary bladder internal sphincter and penile erection in the anesthetized cat. *Invest Urol* 15:404–407, 1978

13. Dorr LD, Brody MJ: Hemodynamic mechanism of erection in the canine penis. *Am J Physiol* 213:1526–1531, 1967

14. Benson GS, McConnell JA, Lipshultz LI, et al: Neuromorphology and neuropharmacology of the human penis. *J Clin Invest* 65:506–513, 1980

15. Holmquist B, Olin T: Angiography of the internal pudendal artery at electrical stimulation of the pelvic nerves and at injection of posterior pituitary hormones. *Scand J Urol Nephrol* 3:291–296, 1969

16. McConnell J, Benson GS, Wood J: Autonomic innervation of the mammalian penis: A histochemical and physiological study. *J Neural Transm* 45:227–238, 1979

17. Wagner G, Green R: *Impotence: Physiological, Psychological, Surgical Diagnosis and Treatment.* New York, Plenum Press, 1981

18. Schwartz MF, Kolodny RC, Masters WH: Plasma testosterone levels of sexually functional and dysfunctional men. *Arch Sex Behav* 9:355–366, 1980

19. Wasserman MD, Pollack CP, Speilman AJ, et al: Theoretical and technical problems in the measurement of nocturnal penile tumescence for the differential diagnosis of impotence. *Psychosom Med* 42:575–585, 1980

20. Newman HF, Northup JD, Devlin J: Mechanism of human penile erection. *Invest Urol* 1:350–353, 1963

21. Michal V, Kramar R, Bartak V: Femoro-pudendal by-pass in the treatment of sexual impotence. *J Cardiovasc Surg* 15:356–359, 1974

22. Segraves RT, Knoph J, Camic P: Spontaneous remission in erectile impotence. *Behav Res Ther* 20:89–91, 1982

23. Segraves RT, Schoenberg HW, Zarins CK, et al: Characteristics of erectile dysfunction as a function of medical care system entry point. *Psychosom Med* 43:227–234, 1981

24. Segraves RT, Schoenberg HW, Zarins CK, et al: Referral of impotent patients to a sexual dysfunction clinic. *Arch Sex Behav* 11:521–528, 1982

Index

Abdominoaorticoiliac artery surgery, 186
Abdominoperineal colon resection, 9, 186
α-Adrenergic blocking agents, 33, 160
Adrenoleukodystrophy, 8
Affective disorders, 11
Age factors
  in impotence, 4
  in penile prosthesis implantation, 204–
    205
  in premature ejaculation, 4
  in sexual drive, 173
  in testosterone levels, 142, 145, 146
Aggression, 136
  hormonal factors, 138–139, 143–144
Alcoholism, impotence in, 8, 26–27, 159
Alzheimer's disease, 72
Amitriptyline, 38
Amoxapine, 39
Amphetamines, 45
Amylnitrite, 46
Amyloidosis, 79
Androgen(s), *see also* Testosterone
  aggression and, 138–139, 143–144
  brain sexual differentiation and, 116–123
  copulatory behavior and, 122–144, 145–
    148, 151
  gonadotropin release and, 116–120
Androgen function screening, 179
Androgen replacement therapy, 25, 144–
  150, 151
Aneurysmectomy, abdominal, 9
Anticholinergic agents, 42–43
Antihypertensive agents, 10, 27–34, 159
Antiserotoninergic agents, 26
Aortobifemoral bypass, 111–112

Aortoiliac vascular reconstruction, 9
Aphrodisiacs, 24–27
Arousal, components, 101
Arterial obstruction, vasculogenic
  impotence and, 7, 76–77, 105–113
Atenolol, 32
Autonomic neuropathy, 8

Baclofen, 43
Barbiturates
  androgenization and, 117, 119
  impotence and, 160
Behavioral therapy, 13, 102–103, 166
Bendrofluazide, 29
Beta blockers, 32, 159
Bethanidine, 34
Blood flow, penile, 107
  Doppler studies, 13, 109, 180, 244
  measurement, 108–110, 178, 179, 190
Brachial systolic pressure, penile, 108, 109
Brain
  androgen effects, 116–144
    on sexual differentiation, 116–123
  castration effects, 123
Brain lesions
  libido decrease and, 70
  sexual dysfunction and, 8, 70–73
Bromocriptine, 26, 151
Butaperazine, 37
Buttock atrophy, 105, 108
Butyrophenones, 37

California Psychological Inventory, 172,
  180
Carbonic anhydrase inhibitors, 43

247

Cardiovascular disease, 6–7, 9
Castration
  behavioral, 137–138
  brain response, 123
  copulatory behavior and, 125, 127, 129
  erection and, 25
  sexual activity decrease and, 25
Cerebral hemisphere disease, 70–73
Character neurosis, 92
Chemotherapy, 185
Chloridazepoxide, 40
Chlorpromazine, 36, 49
Chlorprothixine, 36
Chlorthalidone, 29
Cimetidine, 11, 40–42
Circannual rhythms, 124–125, 126, 127
Clofibrate, 11, 42
Clomipramine, 39
Clonidine, 31–32
Clorazepate, 40
Cocaine, 46
Collagen vascular disease, 77, 80
Conjoint therapy, for psychogenic
    impotence, 95, 96, 97–98, 99
Copulatory behavior
  androgen effects, 122–144, 145–148, 151
    circannual rhythms, 124–125, 126, 127
    exteroceptive stimuli and, 125–138
    castration and, 125, 126, 127
    components, 120–123
    olfactory stimuli and, 129–135
    stereotypical, 120–123
Cystectomy, 9
Cystoprostatectomy, 161

Debrisoquine, 34
Derogatis Sexual Functioning Inventory,
    172–174
Desire inhibition, 70, 94–95, 169
Desmethylimipramine, 39
Developmental experiences, psychogenic
    impotence and, 96–97
Diabetes mellitus
  ejaculatory reflex in, 168, 169
  erections in, 168, 170
  impotence in, 5, 12, 242
    diagnosis, 168
    peripheral nervous system
      involvement, 78–79
    psychogenic, 186

Dialysis, renal, 5–6, 79–80
Diazepam, 40
Digoxin, 42
L-Dihydroxyphenylalanine, 26
Disulfiram, 43
Diuretic agents, 28–29
Dominance, 136, 139, 140
Dopamine, 25
Dopamine agonists, 25–26
Doppler ultrasound probe, of penile blood
    flow, 13, 109, 180, 244
Drugs
  fertility-inhibiting, 23
  impotence-related, 10–12, 23–63, 159–
    160, 187
    anticholinergic, 42–43
    antihypertensive, 10, 27–34, 159
    aphrodisiacs, 24–27
    carbonic anhydrase inhibitors, 43
    cardiovascular, 42
    mechanisms of, 47–50
    monoamine oxidase inhibitors, 37–38
    psychiatric, 34–39
    tricyclic antidepressants, 38–39
Dystrophy, adiposogenital, 73

Ejaculation, 168
  in diabetes, 168, 169
  drug effects on, 23, 30, 31, 34, 35–36, 37,
    39, 43, 45, 47
  innervation mechanisms, 67
  painful, 37, 38
  premature
    age factors, 4
    incidence, 4
    opiate-related, 47
    psychogenic impotence and, 184
    treatment, 39
  retrograde, 184
  stages, 48
Elderly patients, sexual activity by, 3, 4
Emphysema, 9
Endocrine evaluation, 150–151
Endocrinopathies, hormonal therapy for,
    151
Endorphins, 118
Enkephalins, 118
Epididymis, innervation, 67
Epilepsy, 70–71
Erectile dysfunction, see Impotence

Erection
  adequate, 176
  castration effects, 25
  in diabetes, 168, 170
  early-morning, 167, 168, 169
  hemodynamics, 13, 48, 107, 108–110,
    178, 179, 180, 190, 244
  masturbation and, 167, 168, 169
  penile circumference in, 175, 178
  physiology, 47–48, 107, 178, 243
  in psychogenic impotence, 167
Estradiol, 119
Estrogen(s)
  in brain sexual differentiation, 119
  copulatory behavior effects, 122
Estrogen therapy, 159
Excitement inhibition, 93–94
Exhibitionism, 70, 71

Fenfluramine, 44
Fertility
  drug effects on, 23
  marijuana effects on, 27
  in paraplegia, 74, 75
Fluphenazine, 36–37
Follicle-stimulating hormone, 116, 117, 150
Frölich's syndrome, 73

Ganglionic-blocking agents, 34, 159
Gender identity disorder, 91
Genitalia, innervation, 67
Gonadotropin release, 76
  androgen regulation of, 116–120
Gonadotropin-releasing hormone, 116, 150
Gonadotropin therapy, 151
Guanethidine, 31
Guanoclor, 34
Guanoxan, 33–34
Guilt, 11

Heart failure, sexual activity and, 9
Heroin, 11, 46, 47
Homosexuality, ego-dystonic, 92
Homosexuals, impotence therapy for, 99
Hormonal factors, 115–158, see also names of
    specific hormones
  in aggression, 138–139, 143–144
  in brain sexual differentiation, 116–123
  in copulatory behavior, 122–144, 145–
    148, 151

Hormonal factors (Cont.)
  endocrine evaluation of, 150–151
  in gonadotropin release, 116–120
  in impotence, 144–152
Hormonal therapy, 44, 151
Hydralazine, 32–33
Hydrochlorothiazide, 29
5-Hydroxytryptophan, 26
Hypertensive arterial disease, 5, 7
Hyperthyroidism, 12
Hyperprolactinemia, 12
  Leydig cell dysfunction and, 148, 149
  nocturnal penile tumescence and, 177–
    178, 179
  situational erectile failure and, 177–178,
    179, 184, 189
Hypersexuality, 71–72
Hypogonadism, 12, 149, 179
Hypotension, idiopathic orthostatic, 80
Hypotensive agents, see Antihypertensive
    agents
Hypothalamic–pituitary axis disease, 73–
    74
Hypothalamus
  in gonadotropin release, 116
  neuroanatomical function, 68, 69
  in sexual differentiation, 116, 117
Hypothyroidism, 12

Iliac artery occlusion, 8, 105, 106, 107, 109,
    110
  treatment, 112
Imipramine, 38
Impotence
  age factors, 4
  alcohol-related, 8, 26–27, 159
  diagnosis, 1–13, 162
  diseases associated with, see specific diseases
  estrogen therapy and, 159
  etiology evaluation
    endocrine evaluation, 150–151
    laboratory procedures, 180, 188–189
    medical history, 179–180, 184–187
    multidisciplinary, 180–181, 242
    nocturnal penile tumescence testing,
      175–178
    organic versus psychogenic, 166–179
    personality questionnaire, 170–175
    physical examination, 180, 186, 188
    psychiatric evaluation, 180

Impotence (*Cont.*)
  screening protocol, 179–190
  sexual history, 167–170, 180, 181–184
  familial factors, 4
  future research needs, 243–244
  hormonal factors, 144–152
  incidence, 2, 3–7, 12, 66, 166, 241
  occupational exposure and, 44
  organogenic
    diagnosis, 12–13, 166–179
    incidence, 66, 166
    psychogenic impotence differentiated
      from, 166–179
    of unknown origin, 244
  pharmacological, 23–63, 159–160, 187
    anticholinergic agents, 42–43
    antihypertensive agents, 10, 27–34,
      159
    aphrodisiacs, 24–27
    carbonic anhydrase inhibitors, 43
    cardiovascular drugs, 42
    incidence, 66
    monoamine oxidase inhibitors, 37–38
    psychiatric drugs, 34–37
    tricyclic antidepressants, 38–39
  pituitary–gonadal axis abnormalities, 8
  prolactin and, 148–150
  psychiatric conditions and, 11–12
  psychogenic
    categories, 93–94
    conjoint therapy for, 95, 96, 97–98, 99
    cure rates, 100
    developmental experience and, 96–97
    diagnosis, 97
    differential diagnosis, 11, 167–179
    erectile response in, 167
    etiology, 11–12, 88
    fear of women and, 91–93
    homosexual, 99
    incidence, 12
    penile prosthesis and, 205–206
    premature ejaculation in, 184
    primary, 91–93
    psychological evaluation, 87–97
    secondary, 89–91
    sensate focus therapy, 99–100, 102–103
    sex partner's role, 95–96
    sexual drive and, 93–95
    sexual relationships and, 11
    situational, 96

Impotence (*Cont.*)
  spontaneous improvement, 100
  therapeutic failure, 101
  treatment, 13–14, 97–102
    renal dialysis and, 5–6, 79–80
    stress and, 7
    surgery-related, 9, 80, 160, 161, 186
    testosterone and, 145–148, 150–151
    treatment, 13–14
      physician training and, 242–243
  vasculogenic, 105–113
    nocturnal penile tumescence and, 109
    patient's history, 107–108
    penile blood flow measurement, 108–
      110, 178, 179, 180, 190, 244
    treatment, 9, 13, 111–112, 231–232,
      244
Indoramin, 34
Innervation, of genitalia, 67

Ketamine, 43
Klüver–Bucy syndrome, 71–72

Laboratory procedures, in impotence
    evaluation, 180, 188–189
Laurence–Moon–Bardet–Biedl syndrome, 73
Lebetalol, 32
Leriche syndrome, 77
Levadopa, 73
Leydig cells
  dysfunction, 146, 148, 149, 150
  pheromonal stimulation, 142
Libido decrease, *see also* Sexual drive
  adrenoleukodystrophy and, 8
  brain lesions and, 8, 70
  diuretics and, 28, 29
  etiology, 94–95, 184
  hormones and, 44, 169
  pharmacological, 30, 31, 32, 35, 37, 39,
    43, 46, 47, 49
Lithium, 40
Lobectomy, 70–71
Luteinizing hormone, 116, 117, 150
Lymphadenectomy, 9, 161, 186

Marijuana, 27, 46
Masochistic perversion, 91–92
Masturbation, erectile behavior during, 167,
    168, 169

Masters and Johnson Research Institute, 99
Medical history, 179–180, 184–187
Menstrual cycle, pheromones and, 136
Mesoridazine, 36
Methadone, 11, 46–47
Methantheline, 11
Methyldopa, 29–30
Minnesota Multiphasic Personality
    Inventory, 171–172, 180, 181
"Monkey gland" preparations, 25
Monoamine oxidase inhibitors, 37–38
Multiple sclerosis, 5, 6, 75–76
Myocardial infarction, 6–7

Naproxen, 44
Neuroanatomy, 66–70
Neuroleptic drugs, 49
Neurological disease, impotence and, 65–85
    cerebral hemisphere lesions, 70–73
    hypothalamic–pituitary disease, 73–74
    neuroanatomical factors, 66–69
    peripheral nervous system in, 78–80
    spinal cord disease, 74–78
Neurological examination, 81–82
Neurological history, 81
Nocturnal enuresis, 36
Nocturnal penile tumescence testing, 1–2,
    189, 243
    limitations, 175–178
    organogenic impotence findings, 166
    in renal disease, 6
    vasculogenic impotence findings, 109

Occlusive vascular disease, 7, 76–77, 105–
    113
Occupational exposure, 44
Olfactory stimuli, copulatory behavior and,
    129–135
Opiates, 46–47
Orgasm
    prolongation, 46
    seizure-related, 70
Ovary, innervation, 67

Parachlorophenylalanine, 26
Parkinson's disease, 73
Pelvic steal syndrome, 108, 170, 178, 190
Pelvis
    radiation exposure, 9, 80, 162

Pelvis (Cont.)
    surgery, 9, 161
Penile prosthesis implantation, 219–240
    acrylic splints, 220
    concealment, 233, 235
    device selection, 233–234
    history, 13, 219–222
    implantation results, 203–212, 234–238
    inflatable, 227–230
        advantages, 233
        AMS 700, 228, 229, 230
        disadvantages, 205, 233, 234
        implantation results, 235, 238
        Mentor, 230, 231
        patient satisfaction, 205
    patient selection, 230–233
    prevalence of use, 197, 208–209
    psychiatric evaluation for, 197–218, 232
        alternative treatment, 201–202
        etiology detemination, 200
        outcome data and, 203–212
        patient satisfaction, 204–206
        psychological contraindications, 200–201
        psychological status, 210–211
        regular use, 208–209
        screening approaches, 213–215
        screening goals, 199–202
        sex partner satisfaction, 206–208
        sexual relationship effects, 211–212
        surgical goals, 202–203
    psychogenic impotence and, 205–206
    semirigid rods, 222–227
        advantages, 233
        AMS 600 malleable, 226–227, 228
        disadvantages, 233, 235
        Finney flexirod, 223–225, 234, 235
        Gerow, 221
        implantation results, 234–238
        Jonas silicone–silver, 225–226, 234–235
        Lash–Maser silicone, 220–221
        Loeffler, 221
        patient satisfaction, 205
        prevalence of use, 197
        Small–Carrion, 221–223, 234
    sex partner and, 206–208, 215, 232, 234
    surgical procedures, 222–223, 224, 226,
        227, 229, 230
Penis
    blood flow measurement, 13, 108–110,
        178, 179, 180, 190, 244

Penis (Cont.)
  vascular anatomy, 105–107
Performance anxiety, 88, 89, 91, 94, 101
Perhexiline, 44
Peripheral nervous system disease, 78–80
Peripheral vascular disease, 7–8, 105–113
Perphenazine, 37
Personality questionnaire, 170–175
Peyronie's disease, 9, 32, 233
Phenelzine, 37–38
Phenobarbital, 120
Phenothiazines, 11
Phenoxybenzamine, 33, 160
Phentolamine, 33
Pheromones, 131, 132–135, 136
Physical examination, 180, 186, 188
Physician–patient interaction, 181, 242–243
Pindolol, 32
Pituitary disease, 151
Pituitary–gonadal axis abnormalities, 8
Plethysmography, of penile blood flow,
  109
Potency, components, 101
Prader–Willi syndrome, 73
Prazosin, 34
Pregnancy, 75, 76
Priapism, 9
  drug-related, 32, 36
  etiology, 160
  penile prosthesis implantation and, 233
  treatment, 160–161
Proctectomy, 9
Proctocolectomy, 161
Progestrin, 44
Prolactin, 148–150, 168
Propranolol, 11, 32
Prostate gland, innervation, 67
Prostatectomy, 161, 162, 186
Protriptyline, 39
Psychedelic drugs, 46
Psychiatric conditions, 11–12, see also
    Psychiatric evaluation; specific
    psychiatric conditions
Psychiatric drugs, 34–37
Psychiatric evaluation
  of impotence, 180
  of etiology, 4, 11–12, 88–97, 166–170
  of penile prosthesis candidates, 197–218,
    232
    alternative treatment, 201–202

Psychiatric evaluation (Cont.)
  etiology determination, 200
  outcome data and, 203–212
  patient satisfaction, 204–206
  psychological contraindications, 200–
    201
  psychological status, 210–211
  regular use, 208–209
  screening approaches, 199–202
  sex partner satisfaction, 206–208
  sexual relationship effects, 211–212
  surgical goals, 202–203
  of psychogenic impotence, 87–97
Psychological testing, 2, see also names of
    specific tests and personality questionnaires
Psychotherapy, 13, 102–103, 166
Psychotropic drugs, 10, 11
Puberty, true isosexual precocious, 73–74
Pudendal arteries, in vasculogenic
    impotence, 105–107, 112
Pudendal nerve velocity studies, 178, 179,
    243–244

Radiation, pelvic exposure to, 9, 80, 162
Renal disease, 79–80
Renal failure, 5–6, 160
Renal transplantation, 6, 160
Reserpine, 30–31
Revascularization surgery, 111–112, 231–
    232, 244
Riley–Day syndrome, 80

Schizophrenia, 11
Seizures, 70
Seminal vesicles, innervation, 67
Sensate focus, 99–100, 102–103
Serotonin, 25–26
Serotonin antagonists, 25–26
Sex offenders, hormonal therapy, 44
Sex partners, see also Sexual relationships
  alternate, 170
  hormonal status, 146, 152
  penile prosthesis implantation and, 206–
    208, 215, 232, 234
Sex therapy, 201–202
Sexual activity, see also Copulatory behavior
  brain disease and, 70–73
  castration and, 25
  by elderly, 3, 4

Sexual activity (*Cont.*)
emphysema and, 9
heart failure and, 9
neuroanatomical basis, 66–70
postcoronary, 6–7
psychotropic drugs and, 45–47
Sexual differentiation, of brain, 116–123
Sexual drive
age factors and, 173
psychogenic impotence and, 93–95
Sexual dysfunction, *see also* Impotence
neurological disease-related, 70–78
Sexual history, 167–170, 180, 181–184
Sexual perversions, brain disease-related, 70
Sexual relationships
penile prosthesis implantation and, 211–212
psychogenic impotence and, 11, 90–91, 95–96
Sexuality training, 242–243
Social stress, 137–138, 140, 141
Sperm count decrease, drug-related, 38
Spermatogenesis, 116
Spinal cord
diseases, 74–78
innervation, 67–68
trauma, 74–75
Spinal-cord-injured patients, 8
Spironolactone, 29
Spondylosis, cervical, 78
"SST syndrome," 223
Stress, 7, *see also* Social stress
Substance abuse, 45–47
Surgical procedures, impotence related to, 9, 80, 160, 161, 186
Syphilis, 78
Systolic pressure, penile, 108–109

Testes, innervation, 67
Testicular hormones, as aphrodisiacs, 25
Testosterone
brain sexual differentiation and, 108–119

Testosterone (*Cont.*)
copulatory behavior and, 122, 123
circannual rhythms, 124–125, 126, 127
exteroceptive stimuli and, 125–138
hypothalamic implantation, 123–124
impotence and, 2, 145–148, 150–151
libido decrease and, 169
plasma levels
aging effects on, 142, 145, 146
circannual, 124–125, 126, 127
diurnal, 128
social stress and, 138
Testosterone therapy, 2, 151, 165
Thioridazine, 35–36, 37, 49–50
Thiothixine, 37
Thyroid function abnormalities, 8, 12, 189
Tranquilizers
androgenization and, 119
sexual side effects, 35–37
Trauma
spinal cord, 74–75
urethral, 161–162
Tricyclic antidepressants, 38–39
Trifluoperazine, 37
Tumescence, *see also* Nocturnal tumescence testing
adequate, 176

Urethra trauma, 161–162
Urological problems, 12
Uterus, innervation, 67

Vascular disease, 7, 76–77, 105–113
Vitamin B_{12} deficiency, 77–78

Widowers, psychogenic impotence, 11, 90
Wives, *see also* Sex partners
of psychogenic impotent men, 95–96, 97–98
Women, *see also* Sex partners
fear of, 91–93